Medical Ethics

Medical Ethics

Second Edition

Edited by Michael Boylan

WILEY Blackwell

This edition first published 2014
© 2014 John Wiley & Sons, Inc

Edition history: Prentice Hall (1e, 2001)

Wiley-Blackwell is an imprint of John Wiley & Sons, formed by the merger of Wiley's global Scientific, Technical and Medical business with Blackwell Publishing.

Registered Office
John Wiley & Sons, Ltd, The Atrium, Southern Gate, Chichester, West Sussex, PO19 8SQ, UK

Editorial Offices
350 Main Street, Malden, MA 02148-5020, USA
9600 Garsington Road, Oxford, OX4 2DQ, UK
The Atrium, Southern Gate, Chichester, West Sussex, PO19 8SQ, UK

For details of our global editorial offices, for customer services, and for information about how to apply for permission to reuse the copyright material in this book please see our website at www.wiley.com/wiley-blackwell.

Library of Congress Cataloging-in-Publication Data

Medical ethics / edited by Michael Boylan. – 2nd ed.
     p. ; cm.
   Rev. ed. of: Medical ethics / Michael Boylan. c2000.
   Includes bibliographical references.
   ISBN 978-1-118-49475-2 (pbk.: alk. paper)
   I. Boylan, Michael, 1952–   II. Boylan, Michael, 1952– Medical ethics.
   [DNLM: 1. Ethics, Medical. W 50]
   R724
   174′.2–dc23

                                        2013016777

A catalogue record for this book is available from the British Library.

Cover image: Llanrwst Bridge, Conwy River, Wales © Martin Stavars, martinstavars.com
Cover design by www.simonlevy.co.uk

Set in 10.5/12.5pt Dante by SPi Publisher Services, Pondicherry, India
Printed in Singapore by Ho Printing Singapore Pte Ltd

1   2014

For Arianne

Contents

Notes on Contributors

Felicia Niume Ackerman is professor of philosophy at Brown University.

Pieter V. Admiraal is an anesthesiologist at Delft, The Netherlands.

Ellen Agard was Greenwall Fellow in Bioethics at Johns Hopkins University and Georgetown University.

Margaret P. Battin is Distinguished Professor of Philosophy and Adjunct Professor of Internal Medicine in the Division of Medical Ethics and Humanities at the University of Utah.

Nick Bostrom is director of the Future of Humanity Institute at Oxford University.

Michael Boylan is professor and chair of the Department of Philosophy at Marymount University.

Daniel Callahan is senior research scholar and president emeritus at the Hastings Center.

Daniel Finkelstein is a professor of ophthalmology at the Wilmer Ophthalmological Institute and on the core faculty at the Bioethics Institute at Johns Hopkins University School of Medicine.

Leslie P. Francis is professor and chair of the department of philosophy and Alfred C. Emery Professor of Law at the University of Utah.

John-Stewart Gordon teaches at the University of Cologne, Germany.

Richard E. Grant, is an orthopedic surgeon at Einstein Medical Center in Philadelphia, Pennsylvania.

Jay A. Jacobson is professor of internal medicine and Chief, Division of Medical Ethics and Humanities, and member, Division of Infectious Diseases, University of Utah School of Medicine and Intermountain Medical Center.

Leon R. Kass is Addie Clark Harding Professor in the Committee for Social Thought at the University of Chicago.

Paul M. Kelly is Director of the Masters of Applied Epidemiology Programme at the National Centre for Epidemiology and Population Health, Australian National University, Canberra, Australia.

David Koepsell teaches at Delft University in The Netherlands.

John David Lewis (deceased) was associate professor in the philosophy, politics, and economics program at Duke University.

Mary B. Mahowald is professor emerita of philosophy at the University of Chicago.

Richard W. Momeyer is on the philosophy faculty at Miami University, Oxford, Ohio.

John T. Noonan Jr was professor of law at the University of California, Berkeley, from 1967 to 1986, and is now the senior judge on the U.S. Court of Appeals, 9th Circuit.

Rosamond Rhodes is associate program director and professor of bioethics at the Mt. Sinai School of Medicine.

Rebecca Roache is a James Martin Research Fellow at the Future of Humanity Institute at Oxford and a Senior Research Associate, Holywell Manor (Balliol College Graduate Centre).

Jan Russell is executive staff assistant in the school of nursing at the University of Missouri-Kansas City, Missouri.

Julian Savulescu is Uehiro Professor of Practical Ethics at Oxford University, UK.

Michael J. Selgelid is Senior Research Fellow in the Center for Applied Philosophy and Public Ethics (CAPPE) and the Menzies Centre for Health Policy at the Australian National University.

Anita Silvers is professor and chair of the Department of Philosophy at San Francisco State University.

Adrian Sleigh is Professor of Epidemiology at the National Centre for Epidemiology and Population Health, ANU College of Medicine and Health Sciences, The Australian National University.

Brian Smart is on the faculty at Keele University, UK.

Charles B. Smith is emeritus professor of medicine at the University of Utah School of Medicine.

Katharine V. Smith is program director in the school of nursing at the University of Missouri-Kansas City, Missouri.

Judith Jarvis Thomson is professor of philosophy at Massachusetts Institute of Technology.

Rosemarie Tong is Distinguished Professor in Health Care Ethics; Director Center for Professor and Applied Ethics, Department of Philosophy, The University of North Carolina at Charlotte, Charlotte, North Carolina.

Edward Wallach is J. Donald Woodruff Professor of Gynecology in the Department of Gynecology and Obstetrics at Johns Hopkins University School of Medicine.

Preface to the Second Edition

Medical Ethics is one of my three texts on applied ethics that is now being published by Wiley-Blackwell. The idea behind each of the books, in general, is to present some of the most pressing questions in applied ethics through a mixture of classic essays and some new essays commissioned precisely for these volumes. The result is a dialogue that I think readers will find enriching.

In addition to the essays, there is an ongoing pedagogical device on how to write an essay in applied ethics—using case response as the model. To this end, the major chapters of the book are followed by two sorts of cases: macro cases and micro cases. In macro cases the student takes the role of a supervisor and must solve a problem from that perspective. In the micro cases the student becomes a line worker and confronts dilemmas from that vantage point. Some felicity at both perspectives can enable the student better to understand the complication of applying ethical theories (set out in Chapter 1) to real-life problems.

Others using the book may choose instead to evaluate selected essays through a "pro" or "con" evaluation. This approach emphasizes close reading of an article and the application of ethical theory (set out in Chapter 1) to show why you believe the author is correct or incorrect in her/his assessment of the problem. In order to make this approach appealing to readers, some effort has been made to offer different approaches to contemporary questions in healthcare ethics.

What is new in this second edition?

- Half of the selections have been replaced (most with essays solicited especially for this volume).
- The book is introduced with a new discussion on Ethical Decision-Making by the editor.
- An original chapter on "health" provides a theoretical context for the succeeding essays.
- Two original essays discuss genetic enhancement (a new topic for discussion in this edition).
- A new section on gender, race, and culture has been added.
- A short story on organ allocation makes this section even more vivid to readers.
- A new subsection on international healthcare policy and ethics has been added.

It is my hope that this second edition will meet the needs of classroom instruction in a unique way while recognizing that the practice of medicine occurs within a diverse context that must be recognized in order to be effective. The world moves on and the healthcare field has to know when and how to adapt the principles of its historical practice to meet these demands.

As is always the case in projects like this there are many to thank. I would first like to thank all the scholars who have written original essays expressly for this edition. Their fine work has added a unique character to the book. To the anonymous reviewers of this book, a thank-you for your thoughtful comments. I would also like to thank Jeff Dean, my editor, for his support of the project, Robert Hine, my copy-editor, and the whole Wiley-Blackwell team.

I would also like to thank my research team at Marymount: Tanya Lanuzo and Lynn McLaughlin. Their expertise helped with my original essays that are in this volume. Finally, I would like to thank my family: Rebecca, Arianne, Seán, and Éamon. They continually help me grow as a person.

Source Credits

The editor and publisher gratefully acknowledge the permission granted to reproduce the copyright material in this book:

Chapter 3

"Rational Non-Interventional Paternalism: Why Doctors Ought to Make Judgments of What Is Best for Their Patients," by Julian Savulescu, originally published in the *Journal of Medical Ethics* 1995; 21: 327–31. Reprinted with permission of the BMJ Publishing Group.

"Ethical Issues Experienced by HIV-Infected African-American Women," by Katharine V. Smith and Jan Russell, originally published in *Nursing Ethics* 1997; 4: 394–402. Reprinted with permission of Edward Arnold Permissions.

"Should Informed Consent Be Based on Rational Beliefs?" by Julian Savulescu and Richard W. Momeyer, originally published in the *Journal of Medical Ethics*, 1997; 23: 282–8. Reprinted with permission of the BMJ Publishing Group.

"Cultural Diversity and Informed Consent," by Ellen Agard, D. Finkelstein, and E. Wallach, originally published in the *Journal of Clinical Ethics* 1998; 9, no. 2 (Summer): 173–6. © 1998 *The Journal of Clinical Ethics*, all rights reserved. Used with permission of *The Journal of Clinical Ethics*.

"On Treatment of Myopia: Feminist Standpoint Theory and Bioethics," by Mary B. Mahowald, is from *Feminism and Bioethics: Beyond Reproduction*, edited by Susan M. Wolf. Copyright © 1996 The Hastings Center. Used by permission of Oxford University Press, Inc.

"Culture and Medical Intervention," by Michael Boylan, was originally published in the *Journal of Clinical Ethics* 2004; 15(2, Summer): 187–99.

Chapter 4

"Killing and Allowing to Die," by Daniel Callahan, was originally published in the *Hastings Center Report* 1989; 19 (Special Suppl.): 5–6. Reprinted by permission. © The Hastings Center.

"Euthanasia in The Netherlands: Justifiable Euthanasia," by Pieter V. Admiraal, is reprinted by permission of the publisher, *Issues in Law and Medicine* 1988; 3(4, Spring). Copyright © 1988 by the National Legal Center for the Medically Dependent & Disabled, Inc. pp. 361–70.

Chapter 6

Ethical Reasoning

MICHAEL BOYLAN

What is the point of studying ethics? This is the critical question that will drive this chapter. Many people don't think about ethics as they make decisions in their day-to-day lives. They see problems and make decisions based upon practical criteria. Many see ethics as rather an affectation of personal taste. It is useful only when it can get you somewhere. Is this correct? Do we only act ethically when there is a *win-win* situation in which we can get what we want and also seem like an honorable, feeling, and caring person?

A Prudential Model of Decision-Making

In order to begin answering this question we must start by examining the way most of us make decisions. Everyone on earth initiates the decision making process with an established worldview. A worldview is a current personal consciousness that consists in one's understanding about the facts and values in the world. It is the most primitive term to describe our factual and normative conceptions. This worldview may be one that we have chosen or it may be one that we have passively accepted as we grow up in a particular culture. Sometimes the worldview is wildly inconsistent. Sometimes the worldview has gaping holes so that no answer can be generated. Sometimes it is only geared to perceived self-interest. And sometimes it is fanciful and can never be put into practice. Failures in one's personal worldview model will lead to failures in decision-making.

One common worldview model in the Western world is that of celebrity fantasy. Under this worldview, being a celebrity is everything. Andy Warhol famously claimed that what Americans sought after most was *15 minutes of fame*.[1] Under this worldview model we should strive to become a celebrity if only for a fleeting moment. What does it mean to be a celebrity? It is one who is seen and recognized by a large number of people. Note that this definition does not stipulate that once recognized the object is given positive assent. That would be to take an additional step. To be seen and recognized is enough. One can be a sinner or a saint—all the same. To be recognized

Medical Ethics, Second Edition. Edited by Michael Boylan.
© 2014 John Wiley & Sons, Inc. Published 2014 by John Wiley & Sons, Inc.

is to be recognized. If this is the end, then it is probably easier to take the sinner route. In this way, the passion for celebrity is at heart contrary to ethics.

Another popular worldview model is one of practical competence. Under this model the practitioner strives to consider what is in his or her best interest and uses a practical cost-benefit analysis of various situations in order to ascertain whether action X or action Y will maximize the greatest amount of pleasure for the agent (often described in terms of money). Thus, if you are Bernie Madoff (a well-known financial swindler) you might think about the risks and rewards of creating an illegal Ponzi scheme as opposed to creating a legitimate investment house that operates as other investment houses do. The risks of setting off on your own direction are that you might get caught and go to prison. The rewards are that you might make much more money than you would have under the conventional investment house model. Since you think you are smarter than everyone else and won't get caught, the prudential model would say—*go for it!* Madoff did get caught, but who knows how many others don't? We couldn't know because they *haven't been caught*. But even if you aren't caught, is that the best worldview approach? The prudential model says yes.

Possible Ethical Additions to the Prudential Model

Some people, including this author, think that the prudential model is lacking. Something else is necessary in order have a well-functioning worldview by which we can commit purposive action (here understood to be the primary requirement of fulfilled human nature). First, we have to accept that the construction of our worldview is within our control. What I suggest is a set of practical guidelines for the construction of our world-view: *All people must develop a single comprehensive and internally coherent worldview that is good and that we strive to act out in our daily lives*. I call this the personal worldview imperative. Now one's personal worldview is a very basic concept. One's personal worldview contains all that we hold good, true, and beautiful about existence in the world. There are four parts to the personal worldview imperative: completeness, coherence, connection to a theory of ethics, and practicality. Let's briefly say something about each.

First is *completeness*. Completeness is a formal term that refers to a theory being able to handle all cases put before it and to determine an answer based upon the system's recommendations. In this case, I think that the notion of the good will provides completeness to everyone who develops one. There are two senses of the good will. The first is the rational good will. The rational good will means that each agent will develop an understanding about what reason requires of one as we go about our business in the world. In the various domains in which we engage this may require developing different sorts of skills. In the case of ethics it would require engaging in a rationally based philosophical ethics and abiding by what reason demands.

Another sort of good will is the affective good will. We are more than just rational machines. We have an affective nature, too. Our feelings are important, but just as was the case with reason, some guidelines are in order. For ethics we begin with sympathy. Sympathy will be taken to be the emotional connection that one forms with other humans. This emotional connection must be one in which the parties are considered to be on a level basis. The sort of emotional connection I am talking about is open and between equals. It is not that of a superior "feeling sorry" for an inferior. It is my conjecture that those who engage in interactive human sympathy that is open and level will respond to another with care. Care is an action-guiding response that gives moral motivation to acting properly. Together sympathy, openness, and care constitute love.

When confronted with any novel situation one should utilize the two dimensions of the good will to generate a response. Because these two orientations act differently it is possible that they may contradict each other. When this is the case, I would allot the tiebreaker to reason. Others demur.[2] Each reader should take a moment to think about their own response to such an occurrence.

Second is *coherence*. People should have coherent worldviews. Coherence also has two varieties: deductive and inductive. Deductive coherence speaks to our not having overt contradictions in our worldview. An example of an overt contradiction in one's worldview would be for Sasha to tell her friend Sharad that she has no prejudice against Muslims and yet in another context she tells anti-Muslim jokes. The coherence provision of the personal worldview imperative says that you shouldn't change who you are and what you stand for depending upon the context in which you happen to be.

Inductive coherence is different. It is about making sure one's life strategies work together. When they don't work together we have inductive incoherence: in inductive logic this is called a sure loss contract. For example, if a person wanted to be a devoted husband and family man and yet also engaged in extramarital affairs he would involve himself in inductive incoherence. The very traits that make him a good family man—loyalty, keeping one's word, sincere interest in the well-being of others—would hurt one in being a philanderer, which requires selfish manipulation of others for one's own pleasure. The good family man will be a bad philanderer and vice versa. To try to do both well involves a sure loss contract. Such an individual will fail at both. This is what inductive incoherence means.

Third is *connection to a theory of being good*, that is, *ethics*. The personal worldview imperative enjoins that we consider and adopt an ethical theory. It does not give us direction, as such, to which theory to choose except that the chosen theory must not violate any of the other three conditions (completeness, coherence, and practicability). What is demanded is that one connects to a theory of ethics and uses its action-guiding force to control action.

The final criterion is *practicability*. In this case there are two senses to the command. The first sense refers to the fact that we actually carry out what we say we will do. If we did otherwise, we'd be hypocrites and also deductively incoherent. But secondly, it is important that the demands of ethics and social/political philosophy be doable. One cannot command another to do the impossible! The way that I have chosen to describe this is the distinction between the utopian and the aspirational. The utopian is a command that may have logically valid arguments behind it but is existentially unsound (meaning that some of the premises in the action-guiding argument are untrue by virtue of their being impractical). In a theory of global ethics if we required that everyone in a rich country gave up three-quarters of their income so that they might support the legitimate plight of the poor, this would be a utopian vision. Philosophers are very attracted to utopian visions. However, unless philosophers want to be marginalized, we must situate our prescriptions in terms that can actually be used by policy makers. Beautiful visions that can never be should be transferred to artists and poets.

How to Construct Your Own Model

The first step in creating your own model for which you are responsible is to go through personal introspection concerning the four steps in the personal worldview imperative. The first two are global sorts of analyses in which an individual thinks about who he or she is right now in terms of consistency and completeness. These criteria are amenable to the prudential model. They are instrumental to making whatever worldview one chooses to be the most *effective* possible. This is a prudential standard of excellence. What constitutes the moral turn is the connection to a theory of the good: ethics.

Thus the third step is to consider the principal moral theories and make a choice as to which theory best represents your own considered position. To assist readers in this task, I provide a brief gloss of the major theories of ethics.

Theories of ethics

There are various ways to parse theories of ethics. I will parse theories of ethics according to what they see as the ontological status of their objects. There are two principal categories: (i) the realist theories, which assert that theories of ethics speak to actual realities that exist,[3] and (ii) the anti-realists, who assert that theories of ethics are merely conventional and do not speak about ontological objects.

Realist theories

Utilitarianism is a theory that suggests that an action is morally right when that action produces more total utility for the group as a consequence than any other alternative. Sometimes this has been shortened to the slogan "The greatest good for the greatest number." This emphasis upon calculating quantitatively the general population's projected consequential utility among competing alternatives, appeals to many of the same principles that underlie democracy and capitalism (which is why this theory has always been very popular in the United States and other Western capitalistic democracies). Because the measurement device is natural (people's expected pleasures as outcomes of some decision or policy), it is a realist theory. The normative connection with aggregate happiness and the good is a factual claim. Utilitarianism's advocates point to the definite outcomes it can produce by an external and transparent mechanism. Critics cite the fact that the interests of minorities may be overridden.

Deontology is a moral theory that emphasizes one's duty to do a particular action just because the action itself is inherently right and not through any other sorts of calculations—such as the consequences of the action. Because of this non-consequentialist bent, deontology is often contrasted with utilitarianism, which defines the right action in term of its ability to bring about the greatest aggregate utility. In contradistinction to utilitarianism, deontology will recommend an action based upon principle. "Principle" is justified through an understanding of the structure of action, the nature of reason, and the operation of the will. Because its measures deal with the nature of human reason or the externalist measures of the possibility of human agency, the theory is realist. The result is a moral command to act that does not justify itself by calculating consequences. Advocates of deontology like the emphasis upon acting on principle or duty alone. One's duty is usually discovered via careful rational analysis of the nature of reason or human action. Critics cite the fact that there is too much emphasis upon reason and not enough on emotion and our social selves situated in the world.

Swing theories (may be realist or anti-realist)

Ethical intuitionism can be described as a theory of justification about the immediate grasping of self-evident ethical truths. Ethical intuitionism can operate on the level of general principles or on the level of daily decision-making. In this latter mode many of us have experienced a form of ethical intuitionism through the teaching of timeless adages such as "Look before you leap," and "Faint heart never won fair maiden." The truth of these sayings is justified through intuition. Many adages or maxims contradict each other (such as the two above), so that the ability properly to apply these maxims is also understood through intuition. When the source of the intuitions is either God or Truth itself as independently existing, then the theory is realist. The idea being that everyone who has a proper understanding of God or Truth will have the same revelation. When the source of the intuitions is the person himself or herself living as a biological being in a social environment, then the theory is anti-realist because many different people will have various intuitions and none can take precedence over another.

Virtue ethics is also sometimes called agent-based or character ethics. It takes the viewpoint that in living your life you should try to cultivate excellence in all that you do and all that others do. These excellences or virtues are both moral and non-moral. Through conscious training, for example, an athlete can achieve excellence in a sport (non-moral example). In the same way a person can achieve moral excellence, as well. The way these habits are developed and the sort of community that nurtures them are all under the umbrella of virtue ethics. When the source of these community values is Truth or God, then the theory is realist. When the source is the random creation of a culture based upon geography or other accidental features, then the theory is anti-realist. Proponents of the theory cite the real effect that cultures have in influencing our behavior. We are social animals and this theory often ties itself with communitarianism that affirms the positive interactive role that society plays in our lives. Detractors often point to the fact that virtue ethics does not give specific directives on particular actions. For example, a good action is said to be one that a person of character would make. To detractors this sounds like begging the question.

Anti-realist theories

Ethical non-cognitivism is a theory that suggests that the descriptive analysis of language and culture tells us all we need to know about developing an appropriate attitude in ethical situations. Ethical propositions are neither true nor false but can be analyzed via linguistic devices to tell us what action-guiding meanings are hidden there. We all live in particular and diverse societies. Discerning what each society commends and admonishes is the task for any person living in a society. We should all fit in and follow the social program as described via our language/society. Because these imperatives are relative to the values of the society or social group being queried, the maxims generated hold no natural truth-value and as such are anti-realist. Advocates of this theory point to its methodological similarity to deeply felt worldview inclinations of linguistics, sociology, and anthropology. If one is an admirer of these disciplines as seminal directions of thought, then ethical non-cognitivism looks pretty good. Detractors point to corrupt societies and that ethical non-cognitivism cannot criticize these from within (because the social milieu is accepted at face value).

Ethical contractarians assert that freely made personal assent gives credence to ethical and social philosophical principles. These advocates point to the advantage of the participants being happy / contented with a given outcome. The assumption is that within a context of competing personal interests in a free and fair interchange of values those principles that are intersubjectively agreed upon are sufficient for creating a moral "ought." The "ought" comes from the contract and extends from two people to a social group. Others universalize this, by thought experiments, to anyone entering such contracts. Because the theory does not assert that the basis of the contract is a proposition that has natural existence as such the theory is anti-realist. Proponents of the theory tout its connection to notions of personal autonomy that most people support. Detractors cite the fact that the theory rests upon the supposition that the keeping of contracts is a good thing, but why is this so? Doesn't the theory presuppose a meta-moral theory validating the primacy of contracts? If not, then the question remains, "what about making a contract with another creates normative value?"

For the purposes of this text, we will assume these six theories to be exhaustive of philosophically based theories of ethics or morality.[4] In subsequent chapters you should be prepared to apply these terms to situations and compare the sorts of outcomes that different theories would promote.

The fourth step, in modifying one's personal worldview (now including ethics) is to go through an examination of what is possible (aspirational) as opposed to what is impossible (utopian). This is another exercise in pragmatic reasoning that should be based on the agent's own abilities and situation in society given her or his place in the scheme of things. Once this is determined, the agent is enjoined to discipline herself or himself to actually bring about the desired change. If the challenge is great, then she or he should enlist the help of others: family, friends, community, and other support groups.

How Do Ethics Make a Difference in Decision-Making?

In order to get a handle on how the purely prudential worldview differs from the ethically enhanced worldview, let us consider two cases and evaluate the input of ethics. First, we will consider a general case in social / political ethics and then one from medical ethics. The reader should note how the decision-making process differs when we add the ethical mode. In most cases in life the decisions we make have no ethical content. It doesn't ethically matter whether we have the chocolate or vanilla ice cream cone. It doesn't ethically matter if we buy orchestra seats for the ballet or the nose bleed seats. It doesn't ethically matter if I wear a red or a blue tie today. The instances in which ethics is important comprise a small subset of all the decisions that we make. That is why many forego thought about ethical decision-making: it only is important in a minority of our total daily decisions. In fact, if we are insensitive to what *counts* as an ethical decision context, then we might believe that we are *never* confronted with a decision with ethical consequences.

To get at these relations let us consider a couple of cases in which the ethical features are highly enhanced. Readers are encouraged to participate in creating reactions to these from the worldviews they now possess.

Case 1: Social/Political Ethics
The Trolley Problem

You are the engineer of the Bell Street Trolley. You are approaching Lexington Avenue Station (one of the major hub switching stations). The switchman on duty there says there is a problem. A school bus filled with 39 children has broken down on the right track (the main track). Normally, this would mean that he would switch you to the siding track, but on that track is a car filled with four adults that has broken down. The switchman asks you to apply your brakes immediately. You try to do so, but you find that your brakes have failed too. There is no way that you can stop your trolley train. You will ram either the school bus or the car, killing either 39 children or four adults. You outrank the switchman. It's your call: what should you do?

Secondary nuance: what if the switchman were to tell you that from his vantage point on the overpass to the Lexington Avenue Station there is a rather obese homeless man who is staggering about. What if (says the switchman) he were to get out of his booth and push the homeless person over the bridge and onto the electric lines that are right below it? The result would be to stop all trains coming into and out of the Lexington Avenue Station. This would result in saving the lives of the occupants of the two vehicles. Of course it would mean the death of the obese homeless person. The switchman wants your OK to push the homeless man over the bridge— what do you say?

Analysis

This case has two sorts of interpretations: before and after the nuance addition. In the first instance, one is faced with a simple question: should you kill four people or thirty-nine? The major moral theories give different answers to this question. First, there is the point of view of utilitarianism. It would suggest that killing four causes less pain than killing thirty-nine. Thus one should tell the switchman to move you to the siding.

There is the fact that when the car was stuck on the siding, the driver probably viewed his risk as different from being stuck on the main line. Thus, by making that choice you are altering that expectation—versus the bus driver who has to know that he is in imminent danger of death. Rule utilitarians might think that moving away from normal procedures requires a positive alternative. Killing four people may not qualify as a positive alternative (because it involves breaking a rule about willful killing of innocents). Thus, the utilitarian option may be more complicated than first envisioned.

Rule utilitarianism would also find it problematic to throw the homeless person over the bridge for the same reason, though the act utilitarian (the variety outlined above) might view the situation as killing one versus four or thirty-nine. However, there is the reality that one is committing an act of murder to save others. This would be disallowed by the rule utilitarian. If the act utilitarian were to consider the long-term social consequences in sometimes allowing murder, he would agree with the rule utilitarian. However, without the long-term time frame, the act utilitarian would be committed to throwing the homeless person over the rail.

The deontologist would be constrained by a negative duty not to kill. It would be equally wrong from a moral situation to kill *anyone*. There is no *moral* reason to choose between the car and the bus. Both are impermissible. However, there is no avoidance alternative. You will kill some group of people unless the homeless person is thrown over the wall. But throwing the homeless person over the wall is murder. Murder is impermissible. Thus, the deontologist cannot allow the homeless person to be killed—even if it saved four or thirty-nine lives. Because of this, the deontologist would use other normative factors—such as aesthetics to—choose whether to kill four or thirty-nine (probably choosing to kill four on aesthetic grounds).

The virtue ethics person or the ethical intuitionist would equally reply that the engineer should act from the appropriate virtue—say justice—and do what a person with a just character would do. But this does not really answer the question. One could construct various scenarios about it being more just to run into the school bus rather than the car when the occupants of the car might be very important to society: generals, key political leaders, great physicists, etc. In the same way, the intuitionists will choose what moral maxim they wish to apply at that particular time and place. The end result will be a rather subjectivist decision-making process.

Finally, non-cognitivism and contractarianism are constrained to issues like "What does the legal manual for engineers tell them to do in situations like this?" If the manual is silent on this sort of situation, then the response is: what is the recommended action for situations *similar* to this in some relevant way? This is much like the decision-making process in the law where *stare decisis et non quieta movere* (support the decisions and do not disturb what is not changed). In other words, one must act based upon a cultural/legal framework that provides the only relevant context for critical decisions.

In any event, the reader can see that the way one reasons about the best outcome of a very difficult situation changes when one adds ethics to the decision-making machinery. I invite readers to go through several calculations on their own for class discussion. Pick one or more moral theories and set them out along with prudential calculations such that morality is the senior partner in the transaction. One may have to return to one's personal worldview (critically understood—as per above) and balance it with the practical considerations and their embeddedness to make this call.

Let us now consider a case from medical ethics.

Case 2: An Admission to the Emergency Room

You are an emergency room physician. A 35-year-old woman from Honduras is admitted with a severe upper respiratory infection. In the process of your examination of the woman, Gabriela (mother of four young children), you find a suspicious lump in her breast. You think that it should be subject to further tests (including imaging) that may indicate biopsy because it may be cancerous. The lump has nothing to do with the upper respiratory infection, but you are concerned. The woman says she does not want any tests done on her breast (she explains to a Spanish-speaking nurse who translates for you). Her husband wouldn't like someone cutting into her breasts. It would be very bad for her. She refuses to sign an informed consent form for the procedure. Instead, she signs a waiver of services recommended form.

You feel in a bind. You did a fellowship in oncology and have a pretty good suspicion that she may be in the early stages of breast cancer and action now will save her life. If you don't act, no one will know the difference. If you put her out and do the procedure anyway you might save her life but lose your job. Something tells you that there may be other options, but if you discuss these with a supervisor, you might place yourself at risk by going "on record." This could include a future lawsuit against you should the patient's husband sue the hospital. What should you do?

Analysis

From the prudential point of view the emergency room physician should take Gabriela's preference and let things go. It is probable that the patient will progress to breast cancer and die within a few years. However, you gave Gabriela every opportunity to proceed to further tests (at no expense to her). You also used a native speaker as interpreter so that there might be no miscommunication. She also signed a waiver of recommended services form. The staff lawyer says you won't be sued. The prudential option says, "Just sign the discharge papers."

If we expand the prudential point of view further, it is murkier. This is because the prudential point of view of the emergency room physician may be different from that of the patient, the patient's family, and others in the Hispanic community. The prudential viewpoint alone cannot answer this disparity.

When moral considerations are introduced into the decision-making process things work differently. First, let's consider non-cognitivism. There are two operational cultures working here: that of the United States and that of Honduras. This creates a problem.[5] Which should be considered to be primary? The domicile of the hospital is in the United States and thus under US laws. However, the personal worldview of the patient is strongly connected to Honduras. The popular culture of Honduras considers breast cancer to be the result of infidelity in marriage or drug abuse. This belief is contrary to world science, but nonetheless it represents attitudes within the group Gabriela lives in. Ethical non-cognitivism can highlight these difficulties but can give us no direction on which culture should be decisive.

Contractarianism can help here by highlighting the legal arena that represents the social contract codified within the United States. If contracts can be ranked by their enforcement power, then the laws governing informed consent and documenting refusal of treatment will trump other contracts (such as those within the local Honduras community within this American city). But contractarianism does not tell us *why*. It would permit the re-enforcement of the prudential position.

Utilitarianism will look at the community of people involved: Gabriela's family, Gabriela's community within the American city, and other cultural minorities that the hospital services. If cultural superstition is allowed to trump received medical practice, then lots of people will be at mortal risk. It would seem that some sort of intervention is necessary. This is risky because it can involve a lawsuit. The husband, family members, perhaps the family's priest, etc. should be briefed on the medical situation and why continued testing is necessary. They must confront superstitions and show them to be what they are: unfounded cultural beliefs that can result in the death of a loved one, Gabriela.

Deontology will support a similar outcome but will do so from the standpoint of the duties incumbent upon a physician according to the professional duties of medicine and from the duty to rescue all we can without incurring a similar risk upon ourselves.

Ethical intuitionism can go either way according to the moral maxim that is generated by one's considered reflections in equilibrium.

Thus, the realist moral theories will advocate a process that will support continued lobbying of Gabriela's family and support group for continued medical testing and the consequent actions that might be required should the tests be positive. The prudential and the anti-realist moral theories will tend toward either confusion or letting Gabriela go home without further testing.

Conclusion

This chapter began by asking the rhetorical question: "What is the point in studying ethics?" The examination of the question took us various places. First it took us to prudential decision-making and possible problems that many decision models face because of unreflective worldviews. Next, some suggestions were made to remedy this problem including the personal worldview imperative. Finally, the essay worked through two case studies in which difficult decisions were presented. In this context, the prudential models were supplemented with an overlay of some ethical theories that might offer more coherent direction in decision-making. My slant was toward the realist ethical theories and the swing theories interpreted realistically. However, each side was presented in order that readers might make up their own minds on how they intend to adopt the overlay of ethics into their worldview and into their decision-making model. This is an important, ongoing task. I exhort each reader to take this quest seriously. It may be just the best investment of time you've ever made!

Notes

1 Cited in *The Philosophy of Andy Warhol* (New York: Harcourt, Brace, Jovanovich, 1975). At an art exhibition in Stockholm he is reported to have said, "In the future everyone will be world-famous for fifteen minutes." Since that time, the quotation has morphed into several different formulations.

2 This is particularly true of some feminist ethicists. See Rosemarie Tong, "A feminist personal worldview imperative," in John-Stewart Gordon (ed.), *Morality and Justice: Reading Boylan's A Just Society.* Lanham, MD, and Oxford: Lexington/Rowman and Littlefield, 2009; pp. 29–38.

3 Another popular distinction is *natural* vs *non-natural*. This is a subcategory of realism. For example, the philosopher G.E. Moore was a realist about the existence of "good" but he felt that "good" was a non-natural property. Thus realists can be naturalists and non-naturalists. Anti-realists are neither natural nor unnatural—they don't think that the good (for example) actually exists at all: in or out of nature.

4 For the purposes of this book the words "ethics" and "morality" will be taken to be exact synonyms.

5 I examine this exact case in much greater detail in Michael Boylan, "Culture and medical intervention," *Journal of Clinical Ethics* 2004; 15(2): 187–99.

Overview: It is fitting to address what health is in a book on medical ethics. This is because medicine's mission is to advance health. If we don't know what health is, then medicine is lost without a map. In all three of these essays there are a few common answers to the problem that are in some ways useful, but certainly not comprehensive. For example, is being healthy to be at the median within some reference class? Certainly this is the way medical test results are often presented to the patient. However, there are certainly instances when being far away from the median is thought to be a desirable condition—such as being smart, or being athletically gifted, or being artistically talented. Perhaps there is more to the story? The essays in this chapter seek to explore this question.

Rosemarie Tong's point of focus is upon infertility—especially female infertility. Healthcare delivery can be seen from at least two critical vantage points: *clinical medicine*, which focuses upon a particular patient seeing her or his particular doctor about a particular problem, and *public health medicine*, which focuses upon groups of people sharing a particular condition that either is itself unhealthy or is a stepping stone to a chronic or fatal disease. For example, smoking and obesity among the general population lead to more respiratory diseases and lung cancer (the former) and diabetes along with musculoskeletal disorders (the latter). Using this bifurcated approach Tong examines how infertility can be addressed. The clinical approach looks at how IVF (*in vitro* fertilization) treatment performs, along with freezing female eggs before the patient is aged 35 so that they are more viable. Under the public health approach, various diseases (such as chlamydia) need to be routinely screened for and, where present, treated to keep women's reproductive tracts in the best possible condition. Also, there are exposures to chemicals in the workplace, among other factors. Tong makes a strong case for treating infertility first as a public health problem and then as a clinical problem.

In Anita Silvers' essay, the issue of health among the elderly is examined. This is certainly an important segment of the population to look at because elderly people go

Medical Ethics, Second Edition. Edited by Michael Boylan.
© 2014 John Wiley & Sons, Inc. Published 2014 by John Wiley & Sons, Inc.

to the doctor more often and have higher medical expenses. Should old people be thought of as "greedy geezers?" This perception can arise in the United States because Medicare (the social service medical plan that covers most of the elderly in the country) is funded by young people through payroll taxes. But Silvers argues against this charge. People are living longer lives and must adjust what they expect to be able to do. This is important for the personal worldviews of those who may have specific impairments as they age. The healthcare community must also adjust their expectations about what is healthy among the elderly. Without this adjustment, it might very well be the case that care may be denied "because those relying on prosthetics and mobility devices to locomote are not considered to be healthy enough." Silvers highlights some key issues in clinical medicine and healthcare policy.

Finally, in the last essay of this chapter, I set out various ways of understanding health: functional approaches (objectivism, uncompromised lifespan, and functionalism/dysfunctionalism). All three are shown to provide several key insights to health but are not sufficient to ground a general theory. Next, I examine the public health approach. Like Tong, I am very interested in this topic especially because of its ability to be translated into coherent public policy. Finally, there are the subjectivist approaches to health. Many of the subjectivist theories concentrate upon well-being. However, there are some difficulties here. For this reason, I advocate a self-fulfillment approach that is measured by an independent measure (to avoid the problems of the well-being approach). The independent measure involves a particular understanding of personal worldview. It is my contention that though all the aforesaid approaches to understanding what health is have merit, the strongest overall is the self-fulfillment approach.

Ethics, Infertility, and Public Health
Balancing Public Good and Private Choice[1]

ROSEMARIE TONG

Healthcare ethicists navigate comfortably in the realm of clinical ethics where the judgment of the individual patient reigns nearly supreme, and the principles of autonomy, beneficence, non-maleficence and justice are weighed against each other more or less carefully.[2] But they are less sure-footed in the realm of public health, where not the individual person but the whole community is the object of concern, and the main tug-of-war is between the competing values of individual freedom and the public good.[3] Nevertheless, like it or not, healthcare ethicists are increasingly being pushed into the public-health sector to address issues such as smoking,[4] drinking,[5] and, most recently, eating (obesity).[6] Moreover, they are being asked to address, as public health concerns, issues that used to be viewed as very private. Among these issues are a host of sexual practices and reproductive choices, including the subject of this presentation: infertility.

Many causes have come together to put a spotlight on infertility in developing as well as developed countries; but media coverage probably accounts for a goodly portion of the public's interest in infertility in the United States. Who hasn't heard of Octomom, a cash-strapped, single mother of six children, who used fertility drugs to produce enough embryos for eight infants most of whom were born with one or more serious medical conditions;[7] or the 66-year-old Romanian woman in an IVF program who gave birth to a 3.9 pound daughter, the sole survivor of a triplet pregnancy.[8] Here, I argue that even if infertility is not, strictly speaking a disease, it is still a disability that contributes to unhealthiness and often unhappiness. I also argue that a public health focus on infertility makes visible some ethical issues that have been neglected or inadequately addressed at the clinical level. My goal in making these arguments is to convince public health officials to use healthcare ethicists more systematically in developing a national plan for the prevention, detection, and management of infertility that is both socially just and attentive to the value of individual freedom.

Health, Disease, and Infertility

Understanding the concepts of health and disease is no easy matter because both of these concepts are variously defined. To begin with, health is not necessarily the absence of disease, disability, or defect because many persons with one or more of these "negativities" are quite healthy. For example, although persons with the gene(s) for Alzheimer's disease will probably manifest the symptoms of this degenerative neurological condition somewhere down the line, they may be able to lead healthy lives until they are well into their 60s, 70s, or even 80s.[9] Similarly, people who cannot see or hear, or who have had a limb amputated are often hale and hearty. But if health is other than the mere absence of disease, disability, or defect, then precisely what is health and why should we care about its definition?

Perhaps the most important reason to care about the definition of health—and disease, defect, or disability—is that the definitions of terms affect us in many ways, some of them very significant. For example, if we accept the World Health Organization's (WHO) definition of health as "a state of complete physical, mental and social well-being and not merely the absence of disease or infirmity,"[10] then most people are somewhat unhealthy. For instance, many individuals experience down-in-the-dumps days that fall short of clinical depression but are nonetheless de-energizing and demoralizing. Should healthcare practitioners provide these "unhappy campers" with ample supplies of Prozac or some other antidepressant to boost their low spirits? If so, it would seem that the business of healthcare practitioners—be they clinicians or public health officials—is to make everyone not simply healthy but also happy. After all, it makes just as much sense to define *happiness* as "a state of complete physical, mental, and social well-being" as it does to define *health* with these same words. But, even if the case can be made that clinicians should try to make their individual patients happy as well as healthy, public health officials do not always have this luxury. They need to be concerned about the good of society as a whole, a good that may be in opposition to any one individual's happiness and, in some instances, even health as in a triage situation where not everyone's healthcare needs can be met.

The natural or biological view of disease and health

Careful reflection on definitions of health—such as the WHO definition of health—puts into focus two competing views of health: namely, the natural or biological view and the normative or socially constructed view.[11] Those who hold the natural or biological view of health assume that all biological organisms, including human beings, are the product of a purposeful and organized biological evolution. They claim that health is best understood as the functioning of a biological organism in conformity with its natural design. On this conception of health, disease is the malfunction of a biological organism. For example, if the lungs are supposed to help human beings breathe, and an individual has emphysema, he is unhealthy.

A variant of the view that disease is some sort of organic malfunction is the notion that disease is a deviation from species-typical functioning.[12] So, if most people have a certain blood pressure, cholesterol level, or white blood cell count, then statistically significant departures from the typical condition are probable candidates for the label "disease." Among healthcare practitioners, physicians seem particularly fond of a statistical view of health, and it is this view of health that probably accounts for much of the weighing, measuring, and testing that occurs in physicians' offices. Despite the common sense appeal of this view, there is at least one problem with it. Bioethicist Arthur Caplan points out that just because a person deviates from a mean in a statistically significant way does not necessarily indicate that he or she is diseased.[13] For example, Olympic athletes are not viewed as diseased because they can run faster or jump higher than most people. Likewise, people whose IQs (intelligence quotients) or EQs (emotionality quotients) are extraordinarily high are viewed as anything but diseased. Instead, they are viewed as uncommonly blessed individuals.

A final variant of the natural or biological view of health is offered by physician-bioethicist Leon Kass. For him "health is a natural standard or norm…a state of being that reveals itself in activity as a standard of bodily excellence or fitness, relative to each species and to some extent to individuals, recognizable if not definable, and to some extend attainable."[14] Confessing that he cannot describe in sufficient detail a healthy human being, Kass instead offers a description of a healthy squirrel (why a squirrel, I have no clue). Writes Kass:

> [The ideally functioning squirrel] is a bushy-tailed fellow who looks and acts like a squirrel; who leaps through the trees with great daring; who gathers, buries, covers but later uncovers and recovers his acorns; who perches out on a limb cracking nuts, sniffing the air for smells of danger, alert, cautious, with his tail beating rhythmically, who chatters and plays and courts and mates, and rears his [sic] young in large improbably-looking homes at the tops of trees; who fights with vigor and forages with cunning; who shows spiritedness, even anger, and more prudence than many human beings.[15]

To be sure, squirrels (even super squirrels like this one) are not human beings; and built into Kass's description of the healthy squirrel/human being are several sexist and heterosexist assumptions that detract from its force, to say nothing of the grand assumption upon which it is founded: namely, the belief that there is a natural order that determines the function of each and every thing. Still, Kass's description of a healthy squirrel, with the needed translations into human terms, is not unreasonable for all its flaws.

The socially constructed view of health or disease

Unlike proponents of the natural or biological view of health and disease, proponents of the socially constructed view insist that assertions about values shape the meanings of health and disease. Thus, no matter how many facts we know about the functioning of a particular organ or system of organs, a deviation upward or downward from species-typical or species-average functioning will count as a disease or disability only if people regard the deviation as a disvalue—something to be avoided. Consider the debate that has swirled around homosexuality. Is it a sexual preference, a lifestyle choice, a sin, or a disease to be treated on account of its statistical deviation from the mean of heterosexuality? Originally classified as a disease by the American Psychiatric Association (APA), homosexuality was declassified as a medical problem by that same group in 1980.[16] Was this change in classification due to some new biological facts that had been discovered about homosexuality—for example, that homosexuals are far more numerous than previously thought, or that most individuals are bisexual? Or, instead, was the APA's declassification of homosexuality as a medical problem the result of its growing conviction that society should be equally accepting of individuals, whether they have a same-sex sexual preference or an opposite-sex sexual preference? In the estimation of those who think that the meaning of homosexuality is socially constructed, the answer to such questions is clear: labeling or not labeling homosexuality a disease is a value-based decision not a fact-based decision.

Another point that bolsters the socially constructed view of health and disease is the fact that what counts as a disease varies from culture to culture. In the United States, epilepsy is a recognized, neurological medical condition that is managed with prescription drugs. In Laos, epilepsy is a sign of spirit possession, something to be left alone for the good of the community.[17] Still, there are limits on viewing health and disease as socially constructed. There are some states of mind and physical conditions that virtually everyone values or disvalues. For example, it is very unlikely that anyone anywhere thinks it is better to have Ebola than not to have it.

Infertility as a Disvalued Dysfunction (Disease)

Reflecting on how best to understand disease and health—as biological fact or socially constructed value—my own view of disease resonates with Caplan's. He says that disease is a "'disvalued dysfunction' defined in terms of both human goals and the design of the human body (and the human mind, to the extent to which this can be known)."[18] Thus, it is not automatically certain that infertility is a disease or disability. On the one hand, it is a dysfunction, a departure from species-typical functioning—most couples can get pregnant if they try consistently for a year. On the other hand, infertility may or may not be a *disvalued* dysfunction. Worldwide, the fertility rate has gone down from 5 to 2.7, and, in the world's developed nations, it has plummeted from 5 to 1.5, a number far lower than the replacement rate required for a stable population size.[19] Japan's total fertility rate (2012 estimate) of 1.39 is very low,[20] and other nations with particularly low fertility rates are Russia, Poland, Romania, Ukraine, South Korea, Taiwan, Hong Kong, and Singapore.[21]

To be sure, some of the fertility crisis is the *voluntary* product of people not wanting many children or any children. Specifically, in some European countries, it has been reported that from 12 to 16% of women aged 18–34 intend to remain childless, or are inclined in the direction of childlessness.[22] Still, most of the fertility crisis is *involuntary*. For example, 7.3 million US women aged 15–44 want to get pregnant but experience difficulties conceiving or bringing a pregnancy to term.[23] Moreover, upward of 10–15% of heterosexual couples in the United States are infertile (i.e., unable to conceive during the previous 12 months despite trying).[24] From the vantage point of our species, what is noteworthy about these statistics is that both the number of involuntarily infertile people and the number of voluntarily fertile people are increasing at the same time. Admittedly, it is not as if the world is underpopulated,[25] but a species that cannot or will not reproduce itself in sufficient quantities is an imperiled species.

In this connection, consider the global implications of increased infertility. The whole emphasis on US aid to developing countries with large populations has been on controlling the size of their populations. Women and men have been offered contraceptives, most of them safe and effective,[26] and one of them—the condom for men—with the additional advantage of protecting against HIV AIDS.[27] However, international birth control efforts have not been without controversy. Consider the concerns raised about offering women in rural outposts of Africa the long-lasting contraceptive Norplant. Pressured by their spouses, some of these women dug the Norplant out of their arms. Serious infections sometimes resulted from these home surgeries.[28] Also consider the furor in India when poor men were incentivized with transistor radios, clothing, and cash to sign up for their free sterilizations. Some of them had no or little understanding that a vasectomy would end their reproductive capacities.[29] Not surprisingly, the one birth control technology that the United States has not offered pregnant women in developing countries is abortion. Because of moral and legal controversies over the status of the unborn fetus in the United States, abortion services have not been provided to women in developing countries who need them. Arguably, much in the way of human health and happiness might have been gained by providing these women with safe abortions. A 2009 study found that approximately 70 000 women died as a result of botched abortions, with 38 000 of those deaths occurring in sub-Saharan Africa.[30]

Although US efforts to help people in developing countries control the size of their populations have not been problem free, as just noted, they have been successful enough.[31] But what happens when the population size of some developing countries is decreasing at unfavorable rates? Will the United States be as eager to provide reproduction-assisting services as it was to provide reproduction-controlling services to people in developing countries? After all, recent statistics suggest that infertility in developing countries is a growing problem. The Demographics and Health Survey Program estimates that 167 million ever-married women aged 15–49 years in developing countries (excluding China) were infertile in 2002.[32] In some developing countries, infertility is three times higher than in developed countries. Among the causes of such high rates of infertility are pelvic infections, botched abortions, and botched deliveries. When there is no one available to perform a cesarean section, obstetric fistula generally occurs. The United Nations Populations Fund (UNFPA) estimates that worldwide there may be two million women with this condition. Husbands often abandon wives with fistula, and community support for these women is virtually non-existent. They are treated as lepers.[33] Though some of these infertile women may not be involuntarily infertile, most of them are.

Not being able to get pregnant is a prescription for disaster in countries where women who cannot conceive are viewed as useless or defective;[34] and, in such countries, it does not matter if the male member of a heterosexual couple is the one with the infertility problem: the woman will be blamed. Consequently, many infertile women—some of them very poor—are desperate for expensive drugs like Clomid and Pergonal. Moreover, in some countries, including developing countries, the demand for certain infertility treatments, including *in vitro* fertilization (IVF) may not be confined to *infertile* couples. For example, wealthy Chinese couples have come to the United States to undergo both IVF and pre-implantation genetic diagnosis (PIGD) in order to secure a male embryo.[35] Admittedly, the couples could have used amniocentesis to avoid a female child, but not without subjecting the women to at least one abortion and maybe more. Similarly, where having (biological) children is necessary for maintaining the family line, couples travel far from home to get pregnant. One of the advantages of seeking infertility services abroad is that it is easier to treat male infertility there. The infertile man has less face to lose abroad than in his native country, where "manhood" may be tied to getting one's wife pregnant.[36]

To be sure, infertility today is not a public health problem of the same magnitude that overpopulation was in the 1970s, but it is a growing problem worldwide, and for the one in six heterosexual couples in the United States who cannot get pregnant, it may be a prescription for heartbreak. Ours is a remarkably pronatalist society. The fact that 54% of US women work full time and 11% of women work part time in the paid job force[37] has not eliminated the socio-cultural norm that motherhood—biological motherhood—is the index of real womanhood.[38] Thus, it is not surprising that more and more people, including infertile people of modest means, are turning to fertility clinics to get pregnant.[39]

Clinical approaches to infertility

Because the initial assumption is that infertility is a female problem, it is usually the woman in a couple who makes the initial appointment at a fertility clinic. There she will be told what she probably knows from a preliminary Internet search, namely, that it is just as likely that her male partner is the one with "the problem." Indeed, 30% of infertility cases are due to a male factor, 30% to a female factor, 30% to a combined male and female factor, and 10% to unexplained causes.[40] Because male infertility factors like low sperm count, poor quality sperm, and minimally mobile sperm are easier to identify and treat than female infertility factors, most clinicians focus on male factors before moving on to female factors, which are harder to treat than male factors. Among the female factors for infertility are a wide range of ovulatory disorders, tubal problems, cervical problems, and uterine disorders. Treating women's infertility is a trial-and-error process, with incrementally increasing levels of treatment. In 2001, 1.1 million women in the United States made appointments at infertility clinics. Seventy-four percent received counseling, 59% underwent some testing, 46% received egg-stimulating drugs, 13% underwent intrauterine insemination (IUI), 8% underwent surgery for blocked fallopian tubes, and 3% used assisted-reproduction technology (ART).[41] If these statistics are accurate, it would seem that reproduction-assisting practitioners show considerable restraint in moving from non-invasive to invasive procedures.

Among the major ethical issues to address about assisted-reproduction technologies is their risk-benefit ratio. Although staunch IVF proponents insist that infants produced through IVF are at no greater risk for genetic damage than infants produced naturally, some recent studies suggest otherwise. According to a 2002 report in the *New England Journal of Medicine*, infants produced through IVF have an 8.6% risk of major birth defects—including heart and kidney problems, cleft palate, and undescended testicles—whereas babies produced naturally have only a 4.2% risk of these conditions.[42] In addition, IVF babies are 2.6 times more likely than naturally conceived babies to be born with a very low birthweight, a significant risk factor for cardiac and cognitive problems.[43] Still, the preponderance of IVF babies are born healthy: 91% compared to 95% of naturally conceived babies. Comments Dr Zev Rosenwaks, Director of New York Presbyterian Hospital's fertility program, "If you ask a couple if they would rather not have a child at all or try to have a child that over 95% of the time will be normal, I think they will choose to have the child."[44]

Much higher than the risks posed to IVF infants are the risks posed to the adults who use IVF. Many people do not realize how emotionally taxing, physically demanding, and financially costly IVF can be. Work schedules and marital relationships may be negatively affected, as the couple increasingly focus on making a baby happen.

Women enrolled in IVF programs take powerful, egg-stimulating drugs such as Clomid, Pergonal, and Follistim. Ovarian overstimulation and ovarian hyperstimulation are among the risks of these drugs. In addition, surgery to retrieve the eggs is also risky: adverse reactions to anesthesia, bleeding, and infection may occur. The chances of ectopic pregnancy, spontaneous abortion, or stillbirth are further factors for women in IVF programs to consider. To have worked so hard to get pregnant, only to lose the developing infant is particularly sad.

Conscientious clinicians are often troubled by their patients' desire to continue IVF treatments no matter what the risks to them. For example, clinicians may think that yet another cycle of IVF is counterindicated because the woman is too compromised health wise or her chances of getting pregnant and carrying a fetus to term are very slim. But the woman may insist that she is the one who has the right to decide when to start and stop infertility treatments, including the most aggressive ones.[45] Indeed, there have been cases in which women in their mid-fifties or even sixties have asked IVF practitioners to help them get pregnant. In some instances, the clinicians have acceded to their requests.[46]

As might be expected in the United States, a culturally and politically diverse society, the public is divided about postmenopausal pregnancies. There are those who insist that if a postmenopausal woman wants to get pregnant and clinicians have the means to help her, they should help her, even if the health risks of extending such help are very high. She, not they, should decide whether the health risks of IVF treatment do or do not outweigh the overall benefits to her. In contrast, others do not support IVF for postmenopausal women. They argue that it is irresponsible for a woman in her 50s or 60s to undertake a high-risk pregnancy that may result in serious harm to herself. They also point out that if a woman in her 50s or 60s bears a child, she will be in her late 70s when her child graduates high school. Should that child, they ask, be expected to care for her elderly parent if she gets Alzheimer's disease, for example? As compelling as this point may be to some, proponents of postmenopausal IVF respond that nowadays many grandparents rear their young grandchildren successfully.[47] They also stress that if it is socially permissible for men to "father" children in their 50s, 60s, 70s, and even 80s, then it should be socially permissible for women to "mother" a child in her 60s. Comments Robert Edwards: "if a man of 60 fathers a baby, then we buy him a drink and toast his health at a pub. But it is totally different with a woman of the same age."[48] To refuse to help infertile older women get pregnant simply because they are older is probably a sexist response to a group of women's legitimate treatment needs.[49]

Clinicians and their patients may also clash with respect to the number of embryos to insert into the uterus to achieve a pregnancy. In the early days of IVF, clinicians inserted as many embryos as possible into a woman's uterus, hoping that one would take; but nowadays clinicians are more concerned about the opposite problem, namely, too many embryos implanting.[50] Multifetal pregnancies are problematic because it is more difficult for most women to gestate twins, triplets, or quadruplets than to gestate a singleton. The strain on the heart can be considerable and bed rest may be prescribed.[51] In addition, it is hard to care for multiples, who are at increased risk for low birthweight, premature delivery, and disability.[52] Many couples' marriages dissolve because of the wear and tear caused by continuously having to do diaper or feeding duty;[53] to say nothing of paying all the childcare and physician bills. Nevertheless, many people in IVF programs get nervous when their clinician suggests that they do one single embryo transfer (SET), followed by a second one if the first fails, instead of transferring two embryos simultaneously into the woman's womb. They do not really believe that their chances of getting pregnant are about the same using SET as they are using standard IVF; and it does not seem to matter to them that the SET method carries a lower risk of multiples.[54] They would prefer twins to no baby at all.

With couples who desperately want a baby, convincing them not to implant more than one embryo is not always easy. So too it is not always easy to persuade couples carrying multiples to consider selective reduction and abort one or more of the fetuses for the benefit of the mother as well as of the surviving fetus or fetuses. Having invested so much in achieving a pregnancy, a couple may be reluctant to choose which embryo(s) to abort for fear of imperiling the whole pregnancy.[55] In addition, some couples will have religious reasons for rejecting selective reduction, viewing the technique as baby-killing. Interestingly, ART practitioners are now debating amongst themselves whether selective reduction below twins is ethical. Those who think that it is morally permissible to abort a healthy twin so that the woman gestates only a singleton argue that all multiple pregnancies, including twins, are more likely to compromise the health of either or both the mother and the embryos. Opponents of reducing twin pregnancies to singleton pregnancies argue that they have ethical problems engaging in this variation of selective reduction because they are performing an abortion for purely "social reasons" such as not wanting to take care of twins because of one's age (40 years and over) or one's low coping abilities.[56] At present, parents who want to reduce twins to a singleton are relatively rare, but their number is increasing. Mount Sinai Medical Center in New York, a hospital willing to help women gestate only one fetus, reported that in 1997, 15% of the selective reductions they performed were to a singleton. In 2010, 61 of the Center's 101 reductions were to a singleton. Of the 61 reductions selective to a singleton, 38 started out as twins.[57]

Often overlooked in discussions of IVF's overall risk-benefit ratio are the risks posed to egg donors. When infertile women in IVF programs fail to produce eggs, or produce few or unhealthy eggs, as is the case with many women over the age of 40, clinicians may suggest using an egg donor, typically a young woman with a generous supply of healthy eggs. There are several ways to structure an egg donor program. One way is to ask women with extra eggs in an IVF program to give them to women without any eggs. Here the fear is that the egg donor's eggs may not be of high enough quality, depending on her age and health. In addition, since the egg donor gets a 50–60% reduction in the total costs of IVF, less wealthy women are more likely to be "donors" than more wealthy women.[58]

A second way to secure donor eggs involves outright payment. Young women are solicited to sell their eggs for several thousand dollars. Prices fluctuate throughout the United States, but the average compensation in the United States is $4217, although one center reported paying $15 000.[59] The American Society of Reproductive Medicine (ASRM) considers compensation of $5000 or higher as "requiring justification," and deems compensation of $10 000 and above as "beyond what is appropriate;"[60] and the American College of Obstetricians and Gynecologists (ACOG) supports the guidelines outlined by the ASRM.[61]

Critics of commercial egg donation worry that egg donors may be tempted to sell their gametes simply because they are in serious need of money and willing to expose their bodies to risks they would otherwise avoid. But the women who sell their eggs reply that many tasks in life are risky and that competent adults have the right to bodily self-determination. Still, most conscientious clinics avoid using "super donors" who try to make a living, so to speak, by repeatedly exposing themselves to bodily risks that may harm them in the long run. The ASRM advises its members to limit successful donations from a single donor to 25 families per population of 800 000.[62] In addition, conscientious clinics provide egg donors as well as egg recipients with psychological counseling. They seek to avoid both heartache on the donor's part about the "baby I might have had, if I had kept my eggs for myself" and regrets on the recipient's part about "the baby inside of me not really being mine." Finally, although conscientious clinics match their donors and recipients for general appearance, they do not serve as intermediaries to get a couple the "perfect egg donor." Supposedly, some couples have used the Internet to secure eggs from very attractive and intelligent women for an extraordinarily high fee—over $50 000.[63] The question then becomes whether clinicians should help them have their "perfect baby."

A third way to structure an egg donor program is to use altruistic known donors. Although this way of running an IVF program has fallen out of popularity, most clinics are still willing to make exceptions to a commercial, anonymous donor policy. There have been and still are cases of daughters providing their mothers with eggs.[64] In some rarer instances, mothers have accorded their daughters the same favor.[65] Familial preferences about egg donation can get even more complicated than this, however. In one case a woman in her early 40s had gone through several unsuccessful IVF cycles. She wanted to use IVF one more time with any eggs she might have and any eggs her sister might have. Between the two of them, 17 eggs were harvested and inseminated. Three embryos were implanted and a healthy baby was born. The sisters both claimed they did not care whose eggs resulted in the baby. The husband of the rearing mother chimed in that he felt the same way.[66] Whether such special requests should be honored is, of course, a debatable issue. Interestingly, men with low sperm counts sometimes ask to have their sperm mixed with a brother's sperm so as to carry on a family line.[67] The wisdom of such pairings is doubtful. Unless guarded properly, siblings' relationships may weaken if squabbling starts over who is closest to the child.

IVF puts into the spotlight clinicians' complex negotiations with patients. Most recently, these negotiations have included IVF patients' demands to use pre-implantation genetic diagnosis for sex selection for social reasons,[68] and embryo selection for the purposes of "normalizing" or "enhancing" the fetus.[69] At the extreme are those who believe that when it comes to important and personal issues such as procreation, people should have nearly total freedom to get pregnant and choose irrespective of the risks to themselves.[70] At the other extreme are those who think that clinicians should be the ones to decide which people get pregnant[71] and which embryos get implanted.[72] Somewhere in between these two extremes of absolute autonomy and strong paternalism rests intelligent judgment. Over 150 years ago, philosopher John Stuart Mill claimed that when it comes to determining whose risk-benefit assessment is most likely to result in the most happiness for the most people, we have little more to rely on than the cumulative experience of humankind.[73] Although professional organizations like ACOG and ASRM, public health agencies like the Centers for Disease Control (CDC), and regulatory agencies like the Food and Drug Administration (FDA) may not have the gravitas of humankind's cumulative experience, they are certainly weighty enough to provide clinicians with reasonable guidelines for their practice. Morally speaking, in a diverse democratic society, it just does not get much better than fair-minded, measured reflection.

Public health approaches to infertility

As I have suggested, if clinicians are loathe to say "no" to their patients for fear of thwarting the principle of autonomy and/or losing business, perhaps public health agencies like the CDC, regulatory agencies like the FDA, and professional organizations like ASRM and ACOG may help them better to balance the values of personal liberty and the common good. These same groups may also remind clinicians that it is better to prevent disease than to treat disease. Among the preventable causes of infertility are tubal infertility, which affects 18% of the infertile couples in IVF programs. This condition is often the result of chronic pelvic inflammatory disease (PID), which can be prevented by early detection of chlamydia.[74] About 1 000 000 cases of chlamydia are reported to the CDC each year. African-American women are about eight times as likely to get chlamydia than White women, and there is increasing evidence that infertility rates are particularly high among poor racial and economic minorities because they have less access to regular healthcare.[75]

Other causes of infertility are environmental and/or occupational. There are about 84 000 chemicals in the workplace, some of which contribute to infertility, but little research is being done on them.[76] In addition, obesity and smoking contribute to infertility.[77] Recently, there has been a focus on maintaining the fertility of patients with cancer and HIV. Cancer patients need to know that sperm and eggs can be banked, that embryos can be frozen, and that the ovary can be relocated from the surgical field. HIV patients need to know that some of the drugs that promise to save them from an early death may render them infertile, and that if they intend to reproduce they had best bank their gametes before beginning a drug regimen.[78] More controversially, men and women may want to know they can freeze their gametes for possible posthumous use.[79]

Another way for public health groups to limit the harms associated with infertility treatments is to make sure that the public understands that not all clinics are equally successful in delivering a baby to infertile persons. Although a 1992 federal law required ART clinics to report success and failure rates to the CDC, implementation was slow, and studies continue to indicate that patients are often unaware of how low success rates actually are.[80] In 2009, the CDC found that 441 reporting clinics performed 146 244 IVF cycles in order to produce 45 870 infants.[81] Clearly, many IVF users are undergoing taxing treatments and spending thousands of dollars only to be disappointed.

Adding to the complexity of the situation is that other infertility treatments that are less costly but reasonably effective have not been studied nearly enough. For example, the success rates of ovarian stimulation followed by natural conception or intrauterine insemination are not being systematically tracked.[82] In addition, relatively little is known about success rates of using cryopreserved embryos versus never-frozen embryos.[83]

One of the main contributions public health groups can make to the oversight of the IVF enterprise is continuing to monitor the occurrence of multiples and setting up guidelines to limit their occurrence. Insufficient oversight of the IVF enterprise is unfortunate because of the role physicians in particular play in the reproductive drama. Judy E. Stern et al. comment that:

> Risk to the patient is of particular concern when treatment is elective because in such cases the patient would be healthy but for the medical intervention. Risk to the offspring in treatment of infertility is particularly significant in light of the fact that the offspring would not exist and thus would not suffer but for the medical intervention. This unique aspect of the treatment of infertility may impose a higher standard on physicians considering potential risks to these offspring.[84]

Although many physicians do adhere to such higher standards, some do not. They may find it difficult to say "no" to patients. They also may fear their patients will just take their business to some other, more accommodating fertility clinic. As late as 1995, the Institute for Science, Law, and Technology (ISLAT) collected data from 281 reporting clinics, some of which were still implanting as many as seven embryos during one IVF cycle. At that time, 37% of ART births were multiples as compared with 2% in the general population.[85] More recently, the CDC has reported that 32% of ART births are multiples as compared with 3% in the general population.[86] Thus, the percentage of ART multiples remains too high. All multiple births, even those of twins, pose serious health risks for both the mother and the infants; the human uterus is not designed to carry multiples. Thus, it may be prudent for the CDC to exert even more leadership and press for single embryo transfer (SET) for women under the age of 35 as the gold standard for ART clinics. It would be the clinic's responsibility to explain why deviations from this standard were necessary.

Another issue, and a controversial one at that, is for the CDC to educate women in particular about their "biological clocks." In the early 2000s some scientific studies were published stating that the best time for women to have children was between the ages of 20 and 35,[87] and that women who waited too long to become mothers risked infertility and possibly the disappointment of not being able to be biological mothers, technology notwithstanding. A number of women's groups reacted angrily to these studies, viewing them as scare tactics that might lure women out of the marketplace and back into the household.[88] This controversy was not resolved, but simply set aside. Perhaps now is the time for an informed public health agency like the CDC to initiate conversations about why, other things being equal, it may be preferable for women to get pregnant in their late 20s rather than in their late 30s or 40s. Recently, my mid-twenties graduate student went to her obstetrician-gynecologist. When the doctor found out that my student was going to law school, she immediately asked her if she had considered freezing her eggs so as to be able to postpone pregnancy until her 30s or 40s.

Routinizing the egg-freezing option may or may not be the way to go for all women, however. For example, Extend Fertility flashes the following message on its web page:

> As women, we lead rich and demanding lives…We have an astounding number of opportunities, and as a result, many of us choose to start our families later than our mothers and grandmothers…But in waiting longer to have children, many women face the real challenge of having successful, healthy pregnancies later in life…Freezing eggs offers women planning to have children after the age of 35 the opportunity to effectively slow down their biological clocks.[89]

To be sure, egg freezing seems like a good option for those women who are sure they do not want to get pregnant until they are well into their 30s. They have the security of knowing their banked eggs are probably of high quality and suited for use in the IVF process. Moreover, egg freezing or ovarian tissue freezing may be the only way a woman can maximize her chances of being a biological mother. For example, both of these techniques permit women with cancer or HIV to be treated without jeopardizing their reproductive future.[90] Still, it is not clear that actively encouraging fertile women to put motherhood on hold until their 40s when they may have to rely on IVF is in women's best interests. After all, the total costs of egg freezing and IVF are considerable,[91] and the older a woman is, the harder the pregnancy experience may be.[92]

Moreover, the chances of a live birth from IVF using frozen eggs is 1–10% compared to 17% with IVF using fresh eggs.[93] Moreover, it is worrisome that IVF practices like Extend Fertility market their egg-freezing services to women between 35 and 39 when it is known that it is far better to freeze eggs in one's late 20s or early 30s.[94] Clearly, there are many opportunities for public health agencies like the CDC to engage the public in informed discussions about "the biological clock."

Yet another issue for the CDC to address more aggressively is the lack of insurance coverage for costly treatments such as IVF. In 2004, only the following US states mandated infertility insurance coverage: Arkansas, California, Connecticut, Hawaii, Illinois, Maryland, Massachusetts, Montana, New York, New Jersey, Ohio, Rhode Island, Texas, and West Virginia; and most of these states' coverage for IVF was very limited.[95] And although Medicaid covers treatment for sexually transmitted diseases, it does not cover infertility treatments like IVF.[96] In fact, were it to cover IVF, the public would probably express outrage, as it did in the 1970s when someone interpreted Medicaid rules to provide women on welfare with coverage for insemination with donor sperm.[97]

But possible public outrage should not distract anyone interested in narrowing healthcare disparities and health status disparities. If infertility is a disease or disability, as I think it is, treatment for it should be provided. Left untreated, infertility can contribute to much psychological anguish, especially for those people who refuse to consider adoption or a childless life as a good option for themselves. The fact that only some states mandate infertility insurance coverage, and in limited ways at that, means that most people, including people without healthcare insurance, pay out-of-pocket for infertility services. Thus, only wealthy infertile people can absorb the costs of IVF—about $12 000 per cycle—without significantly affecting their financial well-being. To be sure, infertile people of more modest means can and do use a full array of infertility treatments, but they often go deep into debt in the process of trying to have a baby;[98] and poor infertile people know that no fertility clinic will treat them for free. Comments Maura R. Ryan:

> There is a marked disparity between the epidemiological profile of infertile women in the United States (who are likely to be under 30, African American, with a high school education and a low income) and the profile of those receiving infertility services (who are typically over 30, white, middle class, with an average of two and one-half years of college).[99]

Clearly, narrowing the healthcare gap between wealthy women and infertility insurance-covered women on the one hand, and poor women and women without any kind of insurance on the other hand is important for anyone who advocates social justice and agrees that infertility is a disease.

Conclusion

Bioethicist Leon Kass has made many distinctions between health and happiness, not all of them popular. Still there is wisdom in many of his views. He claims, for example, that acts like removing a normal breast because it interferes with a woman's golf swing or performing amniocentesis and then aborting the fetus if it is the "wrong" sex are:

...acts not of medicine but of indulgence or gratification in that they aim at pleasure or convenience or at the satisfaction of some other desire, and not at health. Now, some indulgences may be necessary in the service of healing, as a useful means to the proper end: I see nothing wrong in sweetening bad tasting medicine. But to serve the desires of patients as consumers should be the tasks of agents rather than doctors, if it should be the task of anyone.[100]

Interestingly, some fertility specialists admit that they are more in the happiness business than the health business. When critics questioned Dr Silber for transplanting an ovary from a sister into her sibling, some of his defenders supported the surgery as being just like any other organ donation. However, one of his defenders candidly admitted that the primary goal of an ovary transplant is making a woman happy and not necessarily healthy. Commented Dr Richard Gimpelson: "These other organs are donated to save someone's life. The ovaries are to make someone's life complete. It's a little bit different."[101] Actually, ovary transplant may be a lot different. Little is known about its health risks and benefits and yet this surgery is already being promoted to women as an option they should consider.

Clearly, when infertility practitioners push the envelope of infertility treatments, there is a role for the CDC and the FDA as well as ASRM, ACOG, and the American Association of Urologists (AAU). When medical treatment turns into unmonitored medical research, the public's health is at risk. Rather than encouraging women to view egg freezing and IVF as their treatments of choice, infertility practitioners should devote some of their time to fighting the causes of infertility, even if doing so means a downtick in their lucrative practice. The CDC is correct to emphasize how untreated sexually transmitted diseases may make women infertile. Treatment for such diseases should be very inexpensive, if not free, so as to decrease the health status gap between women who have good healthcare insurance and women who have no or inadequate healthcare insurance. In addition, the CDC should play a stronger role than it already does in researching the cost-effectiveness of IVF versus other, less high-tech options for treating infertility, and reporting the availability of insurance coverage for infertility treatments. Factors such as these latter two also contribute to the healthcare and health-status disparities that exist in the United States. Finally, the CDC, FDA, ASRM, ACOG, and AAU all need to demand greater accountability from fertility clinics with respect to multifetal pregnancies. Twins, triplets, quadruplets, and higher-numbered multiples seem very cute on popular magazine covers, but for every one of these adorable photos, there are thousands of multiples in intensive care units who may always suffer from one or another health condition because they were born too early or at an extremely low weight.

Infertility is indeed a public health concern that we all must address. Healthcare ethicists need to be included in the discussion loop more routinely so as to help strike a better balance between the values of individual freedom and the common good. However, the continuing leadership of the CDC, FDA, ASRM, ACOG, and AAU is also part of the cure for the infertility problem. For most people, creating a life remains one of life's most personally significant goals. Therefore, the more we can do to preserve the fertility of people, the better our collective as well as individual health and happiness.

Notes and References

1 This essay was presented in a much shorter version at the American Philosophical Association Eastern Division Meeting, 2011, and appeared in the *Newsletter on Philosophy and Medicine* 2012; 11(2): 12–17.

2 Tom L. Beauchamp and James E. Childress, *Principles of Biomedical Ethics*, 4th edn. New York: Oxford University Press, 1994.

3 Tom L. Beauchamp, Dan E. Steinbock, and Bonnie Steinbock (eds), *New Ethics for the Public Health*. New York: Oxford University Press, 1999.

4 Centers for Disease Control and Prevention, "Best Practices for Comprehensive Tobacco Control Programs." Page last updated November 15, 2012. http://www.cdc.gov/tobacco/stateandcommunity/best_practices/pdfs/2007/BestPractices_Complete.pdf [accessed February 25, 2013].

5 James F. Mosher and David H. Jernigan, "New directions in alcohol policy," in Tom E. Beauchamp and Bonnie Steinbock (eds), *New Ethics for the Public's Health*, New York: Oxford University Press, 1999; pp. 135–49.

6 "Experts address obesity and related health consequences," *Obesity, Fitness & Wellness Week* (25 August–1 September 2001: 17–18.

7 Anne Donchin, "In whose interest? Policy and politics in assisted reproduction," *Bioethics* 2011; 25(2): 97.

8 "No magic for older moms," *Wired*, last modified 17 January 2005; available at: http://www.wired.com/news/medtech/0,1286,66322,00.html?tw=wn_tophead_2 [accessed February 12, 2013].

9 Geoffrey Cowley, "Alzheimer's: unlocking the mystery," *Newsweek*, 2000; January 31, p. 48.

10 World Health Organization, *Preamble to the Constitution of the World Health Organization*, New York, June 19–22, 1956 (New York: adopted by the International Health Conference and signed on July 22, 1946).

11 Arthur L. Caplan, "The concepts of health, illness, and disease," in Robert M. Veatch (ed.), *Medical Ethics*. Sudbury, MA: Jones & Bartlett Publishers, 1977; pp. 57–73.

12 Susanne Brauer, "Age rationing and prudential life-span account in Norman Daniels' *Just Health*," *Journal of Medical Ethics* 2009; 35(1): 27–31.

13 Caplan (1977), p. 67.

14 Leon R. Kass, *Toward a More Natural Science: Biology and Human Affairs*. New York: The Free Press, 1985.

15 Kass (1985).

16 American Psychological Association, *Diagnostic and Statistical Manual of Mental Disorders III*. Washington, DC: APA, 1980.

17 Anne Fadiman, *The Spirit Catches You and You Fall Down*. New York: Farrar, Straus & Giroux, 1977; p. 21.

18 Caplan (1977), p. 71.

19 Richard Jackson, "The Global Retirement Crisis." Washington, DC: Center for Strategic and International Studies, and Citigroup; available at: http://csis.org/files/media/csis/pubs/global_retirement.pdf.

20 Central Intelligence Agency, "Country comparison: total fertility rate," https://www.cia.gov/library/publications/the-world-factbook/rankorder/2127rank.html [accessed February 25, 2013]

21 Central Intelligence Agency, "Country comparison: total fertility rate," https://www.cia.gov/library/publications/the-world-factbook/rankorder/2127rank.html [last accessed February 25, 2013].

22 Russell Shorto, "¿No hay bebés? Keine kinder? Nessun bambino? No babies?," *New York Times Magazine* 2008; June 29, pp. 34–41, 60–71.

23 Maurizio Macaluso, Tracie J. Wright-Schnapp, Anjani Chandra, Robert Johnson, Catherine L. Satterwhite, Amy Pulver, Stuart M. Berman, Richard Y. Wang, Sherry L. Farr, and Lori A. Pollack, "A public health focus on infertility prevention, detection, and management," *Fertility and Sterility* 2008; 93(1): 5.c2.

24 Mayo Clinic Staff, "Infertility," http://www.mayoclinic.com/health/infertility/DS00310 [accessed February 25, 2013].

25 The UN estimates the world's population has reached around 7 billion. United Nations Population Division, *World Population Prospects: The 2010 Revision*. New York: UN, 2011.

26 "Overview of Contraceptive and Condom Shipments FY 2011," https://dec.usaid.gov/dec/content/Detail.aspx?ctID=ODVhZjk4NWQtM2YyMi00YjRmLTkxNjktZTcxMjM2NDBmY2Uy&rID=MzIyODAz&utm_source=globalhealth&utm_medium=site&utm_campaign=fp [last accessed February 25, 2013].

27 Susan Weller and Karen Davis, "Condom effectiveness in reducing heterosexual HIV transmission," *Cochrane Review*, Issue 2 (2004): CD003255.

28 Gina Kolata, "U.S. experts applaud growth in options for contraception," *The New York Times* 1989; January 12, B17.

29 Donald P. Warwick, "Ethics and population control in developing countries," *Hastings Center Report* 1974; 4(3): 1–4.

30 Editorial, "Unsafe abortions: eight maternal deaths every hour," *The Lancet* 2009; 374: 1301.

31 United States Agency for International Development (USAID), "Family Planning." Last modified February 22, 2013. http://www.usaid.gov/what-we-do/global-health/family-planning.

32 Shea O. Rutstein and Iqbal H. Shah, "Infecundity, infertility, and childlessness in developing countries," *DHS Comparative Reports*. Calverton, Maryland and Geneva: ORC Macro and World Health Organization, 2004.

33 Centers for Disease Control and Prevention (CDC), "Infertility and public health." Last modified December 3, 2012. http://www.cdc.gov/reproductive health/infertility/publichealth.htm [accessed February 12, 2013].

34 Friday E. Okonofua, Diana Harris, Adetanwa Odebiyi, Thomas Kane, and Rachel C. Snowp, "The social meaning of infertility in southwest Nigeria," *Health Transition Review* 1997; 7: 206.

35 Carla K. Johnson, "Wealthy foreign couples travel to U.S. to choose baby's sex" *The Seattle Times* 2006, June 15; available at: http://seattletimes.nwsource.com/html/nationworld/2003062459_gender15.html [accessed February 12, 2013].

36 Daryn Eller, "Pros and cons of international fertility treatments." 23 January 2009; available at: http://www.conceiveonline.com/articles/pros-and-cons-international-fertility-treatments [accessed February 12, 2013].

37 *Women Employed*. Accessed February 12, 2013. http://www.womenemployed.org/index.php?id=20.

38 Susan J. Douglas and Meredith W. Michaels, *The Mommy Myth: The Idealization of Motherhood and How It Has Undermined Women*. New York: Free Press, 2004.

39 J. Farley Ordovensky Staniec and Natalie J. Webb, "Utilization of infertility services: how much does money matter?" *Health Services Research* 2007; 42(3): 973–4.

40 David A. Grainger and Bruce L. Tjaden, "Assisted reproductive technologies," in Marlene B. Goldman and Maureen C. Hatch (eds), *Women and Health*. San Diego: Academic Press, 2007; pp. 215–25.

41 Anjel Vahratian, "Utilization of fertility-related services in the United States," *Fertility and Sterility* 2008; 90(4): 1317–19.

42 Michael D. Lemonick, Janice M. Horowitz, Alice Park, and Sora Song, "Risky business?" *Time* 2002, March 18; available at: http://www.time.com/time/magazine/article/0,9171,1002016,00.html [accessed February 12, 2013].

43 Lemonick *et al.* (2002).

44 Quoted in Lemonick *et al.* (2002).

45 Christine Overall, *Reproduction: Principles, Practices, Policies*. Toronto: Oxford University Press, 1993; 181 pp.

46 "No magic for older moms," *Wired*, last modified January 17, 2005; available at: http://www.wired.com/news/medtech/0,1286,66322,00.html?tw=wn_tophead_2 [accessed February 12, 2013].

47 Kenneth R. Tremblay, Clifton E. Barber, and Laurel L. Kubin, "Grandparents as parents," Colorado State University Extension, last modified May 12, 2010; available at: http://www.ext.colostate.edu/pubs/consumer/10241.html [accessed February 12, 2013].

48 Bill Hewitt, "Turning back the clock," *People*, 1994, January 24; available at: http://www.people.com/people/archive/article/0,,20107350,00.html [accessed February 12, 2013].

49 Jacob M. Appel, "Motherhood: is it ever too late?," Huffington Post, last modified July 15, 2009, http://www.huffingtonpost.com/jacob-m-appel/motherhood-is-it-ever-too_b_233916.html [accessed February 12, 2013].

50 "Success rate climbs for in-vitro fertilization," *The Globe and Mail* (Toronto), 2008, December 15; available at: http:www.thegobeandmail.com/servlet/story/RTGAM.20081215.wivf1215/BNStory/national?Page=rssdid=RTGAM.20081215.wivf1215.

51 American College of Obstetricians and Gynecologists (ACOG), *Multiple Gestation: Complicated Twin, Triplet, and High-order Multifetal Pregnancy*, Practice Bulletin, no. 56. Washington, DC: ACOG, October 15, 2004.

52 Melinda A. Roberts, "Supernumerary pregnancy, collective harm, and two forms of the nonidentity problem," *Journal of Law, Medicine, and Ethics* 2006; Winter: 776–92.

53 Adriana Barton, "Disagreements over childrearing are growing cause of divorce," *The Globe and Mail* (Vancouver), 2010, September 13; available at: http://

www.theglobeandmail.com/life/family-and-relationships/disagreements-over-childrearing-are-growing-cause-of-divorce/article1705528/ [accessed February 12, 2013].

54 Macaluso et al. (2008), 5.c2.

55 Rush Padawer, "Unnatural selection" *The New York Times Magazine*, 2011, August 14, pp. 22–7.

56 Padawer (2011).

57 Padawer (2011).

58 Mark V. Sauer, "Should egg donors be paid? Exploitation or a woman's right?" *British Medical Journal* 1997; 314: 1403.

59 Roni Caryn Rabin, "As demand for donor eggs soars, high prices stir ethical concerns," *The New York Times*, 2007, May 15; available at: http://www.nytimes.com/2007/05/15/health/15cons.html [accessed February 12, 2013].

60 Rabin (2007).

61 ACOG Committee on Ethics, "Committee opinion: using preimplantation embryos for research," *Obstetrics and Gynecology* 2006; 108(5): 1305–17.

62 Committee Opinion, "Repetitive oocyte donation," *Fertility and Sterility* 2008; 90(Suppl. 3): S194.

63 Gina Kolata, "$50,000 offered to tall, smart egg donor," *The New York Times*, 1999, March 3; available at: http://www.nytimes.com/1999/03/03/us/50000-offered-to-tall-smart-egg-donor.html [accessed February 12, 2013].

64 The Ethics Committee, ASRM, "Family members as gamete donors and surrogate," *Fertility and Sterility* 2003; 80(5): 1124–30.

65 The Ethics Committee, ASRM (2003).

66 Sherman J. Silber, *How to Get Pregnant*. New York: Little, Brown & Co., 2007.

67 George Annas, "Beyond the best interests of the sperm donor," *Child Welfare* 1981; 15(13): 1969.

68 Kristen Philipkoski, "Sex selection just got easier: will girls be the chosen ones?" *Gizmodo*, last modified August 10, 2011; available at: http://gizmodo.com/5829757/sex-selection-just-got-easier-will-girls-be-the-chosen-ones [accessed February 12, 2013].

69 John A. Robertson, "Procreative liberty, embryos, and collaborative reproduction: a legal perspective" in Elaine Baruch, Amadeo F. D'Adamo, and Joni Seager (eds), *Embryos, Ethics, and Women's Rights: Exploring the New Reproductive Technologies*. New York: The Haworth Press, 1988; pp. 179–94.

70 Robertson (1988).

71 John A. Robertson, *Children of Choice: Freedom and the New Reproductive Technologies*. Princeton: Princeton University Press, 1994; pp. 223–7.

72 Robertson (1994).

73 Fred Wilson, "John Stuart Mill," Stanford Encyclopedia of Philosophy, last modified July 10, 2007; available at: http://plato.stanford.edu/entries/mill/ [accessed February 12, 2013].

74 Centers for Disease Control and Prevention (CDC), "Pelvic Inflammatory Disease (PID)—CDC Fact Sheet," last modified March 25, 2011; available at: http://www.cdc.gov/std/pid/stdfact-pid.htm [accessed February 12, 2013].

75 Centers for Disease Control and Prevention (CDC), "A Public Health Focus on Infertility Prevention, Detection, and Management," last modified December 28, 2009; available at: http://www.cdc.gov/reproductivehealth/Infertility/Whitepaper-PG2.htm [accessed February 12, 2013].

76 Centers for Disease Control and Prevention (CDC), "A Public Health Focus on Infertility Prevention, Detection, and Management," p. 3.

77 Centers for Disease Control and Prevention (CDC), "A Public Health Focus on Infertility Prevention, Detection, and Management," pp. 3–4.

78 Centers for Disease Control and Prevention (CDC), "A Public Health Focus on Infertility Prevention, Detection, and Management," p. 4.

79 UNC Press Blog, posted by Ellen, "Guest post: Karey Harwood on posthumous reproduction," last modified May 19, 2011; available at: http://uncpressblog.com/2011/05/19/guest-post-karey-harwood-on-posthumous-reproduction/ [accessed February 12, 2013].

80 Omo Franca, "Dealing with IVF failure," last modified December 28, 2007; available at: http://invitrofertilisation.blogspot.com/2007/12/dealing-with-ivf-failure.html [accessed February 12, 2013].

81 Macaluso et al. (2008), 5.e3.

82 Vahratian (2008), pp. 1317–19.

83 Georgia Reproductive Specialists, "Human embryo cryopreservation," 2007; available at: http://www.ivf.com/cryo.html [accessed February 12, 2013].

84 Judy E. Stern, Catherine P. Cramer, Andrew Garrod, and Ronald M. Green, "Attitudes on access to services at assisted reproductive technology clinics: comparisons with clinic policy," *Fertility and Sterility* 2002; 77(3): 537–41.

85 The Institute for Science, Law and Technology (ISLAT), "ART into sciences: regulation of fertility techniques," in Tom L. Beauchamp and LeRoy Walters (eds), *Contemporary Issues in Bioethics*, 5th edn. Belmont: Wadsworth Publishing Company, 1998; pp. 688–91.

86 Centers for Disease Control and Prevention (CDC), "Assisted reproductive technology (ART): Section 2: ART cycles using fresh, nondonor eggs or embryos (Part A)," last modified February 18, 2011; available at: http://www.cdc.gov/art/ART2008/section2a.htm [accessed February 12, 2013].

87 Editorial, "Which career first: the most secure age for childbearing remains 20–35," *British Medical Journal* 2005; 331: 588–9.

88 Rebecca Leung, "The biological clock," 60 minutes, last modified February 11, 2009; available at: http://www.cbsnews.com/stories/2003/08/14/60minutes/main568259.shtml?tag=untagged [accessed February 12, 2013].

89 Karey Harwood, "Egg freezing: a breakthrough for reproductive autonomy?" *Bioethics* 2009; 23(1): 40.

90 Centers for Disease Control and Prevention (CDC), "A Public Health Focus on Infertility Prevention, Detection, and Management," 2009.

91 International Council on Infertility Information Dissemination, Inc. (INCIID), "States mandating infertility insurance coverage," last modified November 9, 2004; available at: http://www.inciid.org/article.php?cat=statemandates&id=275 [accessed February 12, 2013].

92 Sharon Steinberg, "Ethics of postmenopausal pregnancy examined," Harvard Pilgrim Health-care, last modified August 2008; available at: https://www.harvardpilgrim.org/portal/page?_pageid=253,257749&_dad=portal&_schema=PORTAL [accessed February 12, 2013].

93 Harwood (2009), p. 56.

94 Harwood (2009), p. 56.

95 Editorial, "Which career first: the most secure age for childbearing remains 20–35," *British Medical Journal* 2005; 331: 588–9.

96 Staniec and Webb (2007), pp. 971–89.

97 Maura A. Ryan, *Ethics and Economics of Assisted Reproduction: The Cost of Longing*. Washington, DC: Georgetown University Press, 2001; 203 pp.

98 Kass (1985), pp. 159–60.

99 Tina Hesman Saey, "Local doctor pioneers ovary transplants," *St Louis Post-Dispatch*, 2007, February 12; available at: http://www.infertile.com/inthenew/lay/ov_trans_PD_02_12_07.htm [accessed February 12, 2013].

100 Kass (1985), pp. 159–60.

101 Hesman Saey (2007).

Too Old for the Good of Health?[1]

Anita Silvers

The greatest wealth is health.
Virgil (70–19 BC)[2]

Gold that buys health can never be ill spent.
John Webster (1580–1634)

The first wealth is health.

Ralph Waldo Emerson (1803–82)

It is health that is real wealth and not pieces of gold and silver.
Mahatma Gandhi (1869–1948)

Introduction: Goodness and Health

When asked whether they are hoping for a baby girl or baby boy, prospective parents often say, "We don't care, as long as it's healthy…" When asked how long they hope to live, older people often reply "As long as I have my health…" These expressions reflect a commonplace about the intrinsic value of health: health is an important good of the highest priority. But is health an absolute or relative state? And is there clear agreement on what health is?

The centrality of health's goodness is magnified by another commonplace idea, namely, that realizing the value of other basic goods depends on whoever seeks access to them being healthy first of all. And if health has such primacy both in itself and because of its effects, maintaining or improving people's health should take priority over other worthwhile aims. As a prudential personal policy, therefore, individuals should guard their health because health leads to other good things and because without health nothing else will seem good. Further, the public policy prompted by this view about the importance of health is that, above almost all other obligations, government must guard citizens' health. Further, healthcare justice seems to decree that unless health is distributed equitably among members of the population, there will be unfair disparities in people's capacity to take advantage of the opportunities that living in a democratic society provides. This latter contention about the connection of fair opportunity to health usually is interpreted as mandating a policy of equitable distribution of medical services. Thus a society's overall justness is said to depend importantly on its citizens all enjoying effective healthcare.

One version of the foundational role for other goods that health is thought to play makes being healthy a sufficient condition for enjoying other beneficial states. To illustrate, here is a Middle Eastern proverb that attributes such a power to health: "He who has health has hope; and he who has hope has everything."[3] And a similar idea prompted the eighteenth century essayist Joseph Addison to observe, "Health and cheerfulness naturally beget each other."[4] Health therefore is valuable not only in itself for the sense of well-being it provides to those who have it, but also instrumentally because valuable attitudes such as optimism, and admirable dispositions such as geniality, appear to be sparked by the combination of healthy body and healthy mind that constitutes the healthy human individual.

In a different version of the foundational claim, health is proposed to be necessary, even if not sufficient, for other important goods. Having one's health has been claimed to be necessary for taking advantage of or enjoying other basic goods, whether these be material (such as food and drink, or money) or intangible (such as beauty), personal (such as learning or liberty), or social (such as employment or association with other people). To the nineteenth century essayist Leigh Hunt, "The groundwork of all happiness is health."[5] To illustrate further, John Locke, whose political writing has influenced US political thinkers for more than three centuries, issued the following warning: "If by gaining knowledge we destroy our health, we labour for a thing that will be useless in our hands."[6]

Philosopher Lawrence Becker sums up this latter version of the primacy of health as follows: "Some level of good health is a necessary condition for almost everything we care about, both with respect to individual well-being and a sustainably productive, well ordered society." Notice that Becker talks about health as if its quantity can be discerned, or at least the level of its presence measured, in individuals and in societies as well.

Becker's judgment reflects a familiar kind of evaluation about people's health. Individuals are compared as to their success in caring for their health. Those most effective in maintaining personal health are more likely to be sought after as family partners, as work colleagues, and as associates for collaborative civic engagement and play. Also, nations are assessed as to their populations' health status, and comparisons both between different nations' populations, and of groups within a single national population, are made to identify disparities in levels of health among different groups of citizens.

Societies that achieve the greatest collective level of health for their populations may be emulated or envied as the most desirable locations in which to conduct business or to reside. Societies with high population health that is distributed fairly among different segments of the population often also are commended. Of course, such commendation is deserved only if individual citizens' levels of health are traceable not only to good genes or good luck, but to the just allocation of medical and other societal services.

Health thus is presumed to be a kind of thing attributable to individual persons, but also to collections of people like different economic or ethnic groups, or to entire nations. Health also is attributed to cohorts of different ages such as children and old people. But whether what counts as health remains constant throughout these different contexts is not clear. How can conceptualizations of health in infants and 90-year-olds be reconciled, for example, when neither the biological states of the elderly and the very young, nor their prognoses, have much in common? Yet to be healthy seems equally a desideratum for both very old and very young people.

Philosophers thinking about medicine often append another seemingly commonplace idea to the conventional celebration of health as a central good. They take health (or more precisely, engendering, improving, and preserving health) to be the medical profession's aim. Public policy, the ensuing argument goes, should value healthcare services because health is a basic good. From the reputedly indubitable goodness of health, plus the dubitable hypothesis that more healthcare will cause more health, it thus has seemed to follow that respectable theories of distributive justice should give access to healthcare priority over other kinds of resources that people (at least, some people) more readily could do without or would turn down. But we should not be lulled into thinking that the apparent lack of controversy about the goodness of health signifies consensus as to what health is, let alone about the distributions of health and health services people are owed.

Health—Neutral or Normative?

Health is both a neutral and a normative notion. In its neutral aspect, health refers to an individual's overall organic state. The processes that are conceptualized as creating the components of health may be narrowly construed as being strictly biological, or broadly construed as including social arrangements as well. In its normative aspect, conceptualizing health specifies or explains good health by delineating what constitutes the soundness of that state. Due to their normativeness, such ideas of health influence or have repercussions for healthcare policy and practice, including the political, economic, and cultural arrangements that position a healthcare system within society.

In regard to normativeness, there are several different ways of understanding how the idea of and facts about health can be a source of moral prescriptions, policy mandates, standards, and regulation. Some theorists take the normative dimension of health to emerge from the neutral one, hypothesizing that the vitality of the human organism is constituted by natural processes that maintain it at a close to optimal state as long as they work well. Here neutral claims about human biology are presumed to be preeminent, with normative claims supposedly reducing to factual claims about biological optimality or at least not extending much beyond these. Other theorists believe that the normative dimension of the idea of health will pervade any attempt at a neutral one, in that social values inevitably are among the drivers for distinguishing biologically desirable from detrimental processes.

Accordingly, for thinkers of the latter persuasion, the normative component of conceptualizing health is enlarged while the neutral aspect shrinks. Here the divisions between the organic conditions deemed optimal or pathological are held to be a function, at least in part, of diverse personal and social interests and policies rather than of organic processes distinctive or destructive of a natural human kind. On this view, the apparently bright line dividing who is considered healthy from who is not comes from the placement of societal spotlights rather than from a natural inner glow.

Of course, only some of us appreciate health thoughtfully, while others do so as an afterthought. And there also are individuals who seem so uncaring or reckless about health that they voluntarily engage in behaviors that impose injury or illness on themselves or others. In some cultural contexts a collective tendency to condemn such individuals for not taking care of themselves prevails, even to the extent of customarily speculating that individuals who become injured or ill bear responsibility themselves for suffering such outcomes. In other cultures bad luck or fate is blamed.

Our current cultural context leads us to expect that health deficits can and should be fixed. Some of us rely on the medical profession to take the lead in improving the sophistication of public judgment about (un)healthiness, especially in regard to silent symptoms such as elevation of blood pressure or prostate-specific antigens. Others, however, object to the medical profession's inflating ordinary people's worries about being healthy, especially as such anxieties can be exacerbated by medical practice that designates comparatively low-risk biological conditions as pathological and thereby demanding of prevention or cure. This kind of issue arises because of changing expectations about being healthy.

Definitions of Health

Various ideas of health have achieved prominence in the bioethics literature and influence in healthcare policy and practice as well. These represent different formats or structures for understanding this highly generalized concept that applies to diverse kinds of people whose situations vary enormously. In healthcare practice, certain tests or other evidence-based procedures may be designated as definitively determining whether persons and populations possess health and thereby are considered to fully capture what health is. But formulating a theory that advances a concept of health in the course of explaining biological or other phenomena might better support prediction, and thereby be a more generally informative format for comprehending what health is for people than any set of tests can be. And even more informative might be the addition of a viewpoint on the nature of health that is drawn from a theory of the place of health in our social as well as biological lives.

Adopting an understanding of health that is structured by one or a combination of these formats may require ignoring or ruling out some instances where ordinary usage would have it that references to health apply, but that are not compliant with a more narrowly refined definition. Concomitantly, a definition of health may be broadened beyond current usage, so that a larger proportion of an individual's propensities are medicalized—for example, tendencies to be inattentive or sad are medicalized as attention deficit disorder and depression. Although an enlightening definition of health need not comport with ordinary usage to be suitable, acceptability will be affected by the concept's normative commitments, which may be discerned by considering the impact of its adoption on health policy and healthcare practice. Of crucial importance in considering a particular idea of health is its prospective impact on healthcare justice, and specifically whether policies and practices built on the proposed understanding of health will promote or impede equitable access to, and treatment by, medical services.

One prominent idea of health construes it as normal biological functioning. This account equates health with the natural functioning of the human biological system. Natural human functioning is delineated in terms of what is typical of the human species.

On this idea, what is statistically typical of the species, or of a subgroup of the species, is presumed to be optimal or at least effective for maintaining the species or the prominence of the subgroup within the species. Further, reports about individuals' biological condition being typical, which are statistical descriptions, are elided with judgments that they are normal, which are evaluations that their biological components are properly formed and their physiological processes are working well. Within such a conceptual frame centering on normality, people with unusual biological properties or traits are readily thought of as malfunctioning, in part because a popularized (mis)understanding of evolutionary development throws suspicion on atypical biological conditions as being maladaptive. So what is advanced as being a detached scientifically descriptive approach to defining health turns out to be a covertly partisan criterion that imposes the functional modes standard for the most populous or otherwise dominant kind of human on everyone else. Historically, such seemingly scientific definitions have been applied to condemn females and racial minorities, among others, for being biologically defective.

A second prominent approach to defining health is openly, rather than stealthily, normative. An example of such an account is embedded in the aspirational policy that guides the mandate of the World Health Organization, a United Nations agency charged with pursuing "the attainment by all people of the highest possible level of health." The WHO constitution defines health as "a state of complete physical, mental and social well-being and not merely the absence of disease or infirmity" (WHO 1948). According to views like this, we should not think of health as merely the organism's natural biological state undisrupted by disease. Instead "health is a positive concept emphasizing social and personal resources, as well as physical capacities" (WHO 1986).

Notice that the WHO definition attributes both biological and social components to health. Initial attempts to explain the role of social factors conceived of these mainly as causes that directly depress or support individuals' biological condition. For example, the social factor of poverty leads to personal lack of food and the resulting starvation of people does direct biological damage to their bodies' cells. As thinking about the idea of health grew more perspicacious and nuanced during the last part of the twentieth century, acknowledgement of the influences of social organization became a presupposition of the concept.

To illustrate, as the journalist David Bornstein has observed, "Many health care professionals are aware that social conditions affect health more than medical care does."[7] Another reason for recognizing the social dimension of health was the observation that in social contexts favoring one-size-fits-all arrangements, biologically atypical individuals are much more likely to suffer constricted capacity to function and to have their biological condition labeled pathological than in one that responds to people's biological differences with flexibility, inclusive access, and support. An example is the inherited condition adermatoglyphia, labeled the "immigration delay disease," caused by a so-called disease allele that is an unstable version of the SMARCAD1 gene.[8] This allele causes affected individuals not to have fingerprints, which makes them dysfunctional, but only for purposes of obtaining proof-of-identity documents such as those needed to cross national borders. No other loss of function is attributed to this genetic condition; nevertheless it has been diagnosed as a disease.

Over the decades the WHO has expanded the sophistication of the approach to creating definitions by constructing classificatory systems that recognize the interaction of biological and social factors. The International Statistical Classification of Diseases and Related Health Problems (ICD) codes for diagnoses of pathologies and abnormalities, as well as evidence of diseases and injuries and their social circumstances. The International Classification of Functioning, Disability and Health (ICF) categorizes components of functional and dysfunctional states. Within the ICF framework, personal capacities and incapacities are cast as resulting from complex relationships among individuals' health conditions, their personal agency, and the accommodating or exclusionary nature of their physical and social environments.

These classifications, as well as others developed by various nations and by international organizations, are used for, among other purposes, measuring health outcomes to assess the comparative effectiveness of healthcare programs. Computing the size of the health improvements that alternative health resource allocation projects are likely to achieve is proposed to resolve such policy questions as which kinds of disease prevention efforts to deploy, which segments of the population to try to cure, and which governments are performing the best in regard to their population's health. The details of, as well as any general thesis embedded in, each definition of health influence the amount and kind of medical or rehabilitation care provided to people whom that definition designates as currently or prospectively unhealthy but as able to benefit from treatment.

In sum, what a society thinks health is affects not only who receives services, but also which services are received. Given the impact of how health is conceptualized on decisions about whose health merits care, we should be concerned with the details of whatever idea of health drives the distribution of medical resources. Normative definitions are conventions that go beyond biological fact to serve the social and political purposes of organizations that adopt them. Defining health in such persuasive ways suggests that nature endorses certain policy directions and practical choices.

To illustrate, statistical definitions invite pathologizing all whose biological constitution does not accord with the common pattern. Adopting this sort of definition of health encourages dismissing individuals who are shorter, slower, or sadder than the standard for persons, or are otherwise biologically anomalous, as being too ill or impaired to participate productively in social activities, at least until they are medically or surgically altered to approximate normality or in some other way fixed. This way of thinking in terms of biological homogenization rationalizes standardization of workplaces, educational processes, and social components, as those whom biology has not made to fit the supposed template for healthy humanity are deemed defective and therefore not eligible for social opportunity.

Another problem plaguing many normative definitions arises from disagreements about the propriety of broad, or instead narrow, definitional scope. Proponents of conservative conceptualizing argue that confining what constitutes health to biological conditions alterable by pharmaceutical, surgical, electrical, or similar manipulations of body parts focuses healthcare policy on problems remediable through medical intervention. They object to broader definitions that, they complain, conflate being healthy with that feeling of overall well-being that can elude even the most species-typical individuals. Proponents of expansive conceptualizing, on the other hand, argue that successfully cultivating health in people calls, at the very least, for nourishing, sheltering, and educating them, and organizing them into satisfying community roles. These two points of view clash in practice about such choices as whether promoting health demands dispelling unhappiness with pills, and whether medical insurers or instead school districts should be the providers of the behavioral instruction that may be therapeutic for autism.

Disputes of these sorts are rooted in people's divergent values about responsibility for health; they therefore cannot be resolved simply by shifting around non-normative components of the definition of health. To use such a definition, decisions about relativizing the standard it sets to cohorts and contexts must be made. For example, what assumptions about the effect of economic conditions should be incorporated into the concept so as to constrain interpretations of observations that signify health? Should the standard be applied differently in dissimilar economic contexts, so that prosperous and impoverished populations may be judged equally healthy despite differences in the levels of energy and initiative their people show? Or may contexts diverge sharply in regard to people's access to material goods without affecting the application of the standard, so that the lower levels of energy and initiative of populations deprived of nutrition, shelter, and similar sustenance may be judged unhealthy when compared with the higher levels of more economically favored peoples?

Each choice about relativizing the concept has its own policy and practice impacts. On the first of these choices about selecting context, economically disadvantaged populations will be deemed healthy, even if their energy and initiative do not rise to the standard of people in privileged populations. In other words, if the standard for judging whether a particular impoverished population is healthy is based on the levels of energy and initiative typical only of poor people generally, a poor population is more likely to seem healthy than if its members' energy and initiative are compared to the levels achieved by much better nourished and rested people.

Why limit the comparison of signifiers of health to poor people this way? Characterizing a population as healthy may be favorable for economic development that needs a supply of reliably healthy workers to attract private investment. So in this scenario a conception of health that contextualizes the judgment of population health just to a comparison class of people with similar economic status is beneficial as a marketing tool to try to remedy impoverishment.

On an alternative scenario, however, comparison of the same impoverished population with the higher levels of energy and initiative manifested by a dissimilar, economically privileged people results in the former group, which has sharply lower levels due to having little to eat, being designated as unhealthy. Why structure the comparison this way instead? Characterizing a population as unhealthy may procure international assistance, including nutritional supplements, from wealthier nations and from international organizations like the WHO. Thus, in a scenario different from the first one, being designated as an unhealthy population may be beneficial because an alternative strategy for obtaining resources is to be played out.

Ideas of health, and the standards for wellness they contain, therefore can vary in virtue of the comparison classes they invoke. Such definitional differences will affect the aims for which each conceptualization of health is applied, as well as how different kinds of people are judged in regard to those aims. The next section, which explores how conceptualizing health influences elder policy and practice regarding the aged, will illustrate in more detail issues that arise in the course of applying an idea of health that has impact on policy and practice to a non-dominant segment of the population.

Oldness

As the US demographic swells with a growing proportion of old people, what constitutes health for elders, and what healthcare should be provided for them, have become aggravated questions. The baby boomers (born 1946–64) were the largest cohort in US history at the time of their births. Seventy million boomers soon will double the number of Americans over age 65. Within two decades, boomers will join the "old old," people 85 and older. This fastest growing segment of the population is second only to children in needing care.

The unprecedented numerosity of the elderly has been attributed to increased use of medical technology to extend senescent lives. Boomers' lifespan (the longest length of time humans have been known to live) is not predicted to be greater than earlier generations. But successful campaigns to reduce early death have increased their life expectancy (the average number of years to be lived by a group of people born in the same year). Life expectancy for a generational cohort grows when fewer members of it die young. Preventative medicine such as vaccinations against infections like measles, smallpox, influenza, and polio reduced the number of deaths in the boomer cohort, as did campaigns for early detection of disease and against contamination of air and food by noxious substances. For example, in just the quarter century from 1985 to 2010, campaigns against smoking are calculated to have saved more than 50 000 lives in California alone.[9] Laws requiring buckling into seat belts also have increased life expectancy, one of several factors that have diminished accidental mortality in the generation born just after World War II as well as younger ones. Many such commendable efforts have combined to maintain the extraordinary size of the boomer cohort from childhood till now, when its members are entering the late stages of life. The boomer generation's numbers overwhelmed public education systems when its members started school in the mid-twentieth century. Now that they are becoming old, these same boomers are poised to stretch the medical care delivery system beyond current limits and perhaps beyond its capacity.

As a population cohort, the old may be deprived of financial resources and lack group medical insurance coverage because they no longer are employed. Private insurance plans would raise premiums based on advancing age because the risk of needing healthcare services increases after old age arrives. In contrast, the approach taken by public social insurance is that young people pay into the system through taxation while they are working and then in return the system pays out to provide medical care for them when they become old. Were it not for public plans that permit workers to pay into a system in order to provide for healthcare later, after they have ceased to work, many elders would find themselves unable to continue to afford medical care at the time of life they may need it most. But some people worry that the size of a retired boomer population may put sustaining healthcare for all of them beyond what the public system can pay.

In the face of such an increase of people seeking medical services, is it reasonable to expect that late life should be a time of healthy living? Or are aged individuals who demand medical services merely "greedy geezers." That is, does provision of healthcare to old people who need it impose unfair burdens on the young by consuming healthcare resources that, even if enormously generous, cannot effectively enable elders to enjoy the good of health?

In contemplating this conflict and considering the ethics of resolving it, at least two troublesome matters about elder policy must be resolved. Both arise from lack of clarity about the interaction of biological and social components in conceptualizing health and assigning health status. Both are exacerbated by the resulting lack of consensus about defining what constitutes health for old people.

When Is Old Age?

The first problem is to identify the boundaries of the aged population. When does old age start? Perceptions of being old vary with people's point of view, as thinking that someone is old can be affected by chronological standpoint. In a survey of US adults, respondents as a whole said old age begins at 68 years. But the subset of survey respondents over 65 years said old age begins at 75 years old, while the subset of respondents under 30 said having lived 60 years marks the start of being old.

Should being old be defined instead in terms of individuals' biological condition rather than their total years of life? Biological changes associated with being old include wrinkles due to loss of elasticity of the skin; grey or white hair or loss of hair; reduced hearing, vision, mobility, flexibility, agility, reaction time, and balance; deficits in cognition including memory; and diminution of reproductive function. At the cellular level, there appears to be a correlation between shortened telomeres and aging.

Telomere length does not match up consistently with chronological age, however. Telomere extension may be possible, having been demonstrated in laboratory mice and nematode worms. In regard to other biological changes associated with old age, not every individual undergoes these changes at the same time in life. Nor is every biological decrement associated with aging equally debilitating for everyone. Some people, for example, are devastated by the appearance of silver hair while others glory in it. Similarly, some people regret reduced reproductive capability while for others the change is liberating. Further, progress in such research fields as regenerative medicine (to replace worn-out or injured body parts with new organic ones) and bioengineered prosthetics (to manufacture non-organic replacement body parts) promise to make more and more bioengineered corporeal renewal available. Thus, modern medicine may place retrieval of youthful functional capacity within the reach of the old, if the price for such restorative medical services can be paid.

Biological markers alone thus seem too inconstant to signify definitively the line beyond which old age lies. So how, if not purely biologically, to characterize the group of people who are old so as to define this population? There is great variation in how biological senescence affects human activity and achievement. But people generally acknowledge old age to have set in when, along with their advanced years, they experience curtailment of social functioning. In other words feeling old or being treated as old seems to happen when people age out of productive social roles.

To illustrate, in sub-Saharan Africa men often are counted as old when they are 50 years old and women at 45. As in industrialized nations, old age is here defined mainly in relation to work identity. Where work roles demand youthful capacity for great physical exertion and stamina, people are likely to be considered old at an earlier age. Also, and especially for women, being viewed as no longer executing a reproductive role often prompts being designated as old. In the early nineteenth century agrarian Western nations also tended to take 50 years as the onset of being old, while today in these same but now industrialized places, being counted among the old usually occurs no earlier than age 60 or 65 because this is when eligibility for the benefits of retirement pension schemes most often begins. We may expect, therefore, that policies to raise standard retirement from the work force to age 70 or beyond, now being proposed in order to shrink the number of individuals drawing retirement benefits and to enlarge the number for whom payroll taxes are collected, will result in a redefinition of the time when being old begins.

In sum, neither chronology nor biology is a stable signifier of the onset of old age. When old age arrives is a movable number that is far from a purely natural one but instead results in some part from cultural, economic, and political arrangements. The nature of each society's productive roles, and the availability of healthcare that can keep people executing these roles, are two social factors that affect the designation of membership in the elderly population.

Health in Old Age

In addition to the puzzle about the age when being old starts, a second problematic matter has to do with how unhealthy the old are. As a generalization, old people no longer in the workforce are more frequent consumers of healthcare than young workers. That is to say, a larger proportion of this old cohort uses medical services compared with younger cohorts, although not every old person does. For example, the over-65 cohort is over-represented, with three times the proportion of seniors among the top 5% of healthcare dollar users in the nation as in the total adult population.

This is understandable because high medical expenditure is somewhat less concentrated, but not ubiquitous, among those over 65 than among younger people. Almost half the medical expenditure for all patients under age 65 is spent on the most expensive 5% of that patient population. In contrast, only about one-third of the healthcare expenditures for patients over age 65 is accounted for by the top 5% of medical services users.

In view of these distribution statistics, the following claim by Norman Daniels appears to be an overstatement: "When we reach age 65, we consume health care resources at about 3.5 times the rate (in dollars) that we do prior to age 65."[10] The comparative data are for the collective healthcare costs of entire cohorts, not for the personal costs of each old individual. The healthcare costs of an individual who has reached age 65 need not be higher than the amount that individual expended earlier for healthcare. Further, while healthcare costs for the old as a group cost 3.5 times more than for the young in 1985, by 2004 they declined to 3.3 times and still are trending downward, with the largest decline for any age cohort being for the age 85 and older group.

A captivating idea urges old people to pursue a program of successful aging. To age successfully is to prevent disease, maintain full function, and contentedly execute the activities of an admired social role. But this prescription too easily can promote expectations of not aging at all. To illustrate, it is hard to escape advertising that invites elderly men to keep medication for erectile dysfunction on hand so they are instantly ready to perform sexually whenever the opportunity presents itself. Such portrayals suggest people need not change when they grow old and their health in old age should remain as it was in earlier phases of life. If elders remain in the same health states as younger people, they will not use healthcare with more frequency than they did in youth.

On reflection, however, this program proves deceptive. Like the components of any well-used mechanism, people's physical components wear out, buckle, or warp or otherwise deform. Medical services may delay such degeneration, or replace deteriorated parts, and possibly the patient's renewed productivity may offset the price of treatment. Eventually, however, the promise of effective renewal must fade away, which revives the challenge of understanding health in old age. Indeed, the Roman philosopher Cicero famously contended that there is a special character to health when one becomes old. Upon feeling discomfort, distress, dizziness, or pain, younger people ordinarily ask how long before they feel well and what steps will hasten healing. But not the aged, for whom, according to Cicero, such feelings characteristically induce fear that their last days are about to arrive.

For the aged, therefore, having one's health cannot be having the health of younger people, so what, for them, can having one's health be? For working age adults, health is understood in terms of species-typical biological functionality in the performance of staple social roles. For children, health can be related to the same standard, measured in terms of their potential to develop biological functionality rather than to current possession of it, as well as their potential to execute adults' social functions when they have matured sufficiently to do so. But biological functionality appears to decline rather than develop for the old. Being old is identified with ebbing strength, eclipsed optimism, depressed initiative, and doubts about personal worth. Conjoining this characterization of being old with the definition of health in terms of species-typical biological functioning designates being old as a time of losing one's hold on the good of health.

Elderly people also suffer deprivation of social functionality, as when aged individuals are retired from activities of social contribution and remanded to dependencies reminiscent of childhood. Further, for the old the resilience to maintain stability both in one's self and for one's environment also is assumed to slip away. In sum, none of the familiar conceptualizations of health provides space for allowing health to be a good available for the old as well as the young, as for all these versions the functionality of individuals in the former population is measured by a standard that compares them to young people's functioning and finds them wanting.

Goodness of Health for Old Age

That familiar ideas of health are biased in this way exacerbates the controversy about the strength of old people's claims to healthcare. If the characterization of health as inconsonant with old age prevails, elders cannot be owed their health as there can be no obligation to provide old people with what they cannot have. And if, just because they are old, health definitively eludes the elderly, healthcare services for them must be seen as ultimately ineffective, which inflames complaints that expending resources for their healthcare is wasteful.

Adopting a formulaic account of health that compares old age to youth disparagingly leads to a call to reduce medical services for the old. No doubt such reasoning will be found persuasive in some quarters, and especially to policy makers whose strategy for lowering healthcare costs is to label some groups of medical services users as undeserving. Thus has the "greedy geezer" grievance aimed at old people been fueled and the flames of resentment against this part of our population fanned.

Yet the reasoning deployed to motivate the "greedy geezer" complaint is suspect. Defining a minority population invidiously so as to make its members seem undeserving insults justice. Similar distortions infamously have been introduced by wrongly invoking misrepresentations of women and racial and other minorities to manipulate policy and practice. Standardizing health by reference to the biological functions and societal roles that typify humans in mid-life similarly misrepresents people whose lives have passed that point. Healthcare practices built on this wrong idea require reshaping around a conception of health that is fair to people when they are in mid-life but remains fair to them when they have grown old. What change(s) can be made in our understanding of health so as to conceptualize the health manifested in old age not as an evil but as a good?

Two emendations of our thinking about health suggest themselves here. Both link elder health to achieving new ways of functioning, one emphasizing biological process, the other focusing on social positioning. Perhaps unexpectedly, therefore, both equate the good of elder health with functioning anew. Both foreground as valuable adaptive shifts in modes of functioning, which are rare in young individuals but common when people reach old age.

How does biological functionality manifest in old age, a stage of life when individuals are at higher than species-typical risk of encountering impediments to their usual modes of functioning? For this population, there is greater motivation to adopt or adapt to alternative modes. Recognizing this characteristic of the elder cohort is crucial for constructing a portrayal of health in old age. Such a picture must distinguish dysfunctions attributable to physical or cognitive deterioration from the disabling disorientation that often is their consequence, for these are different states. Adaptation to the former by assuming a new functional mode is a key protection against falling prey to the latter. While decline from species-typical physical and cognitive mid-life functional levels may be an inescapable aspect of life for the old, displacement from the kind of healthy living appropriate for their time of life does not necessarily accompany such functional change. Considering different modes of functional mobility illustrates, and thereby helps to elucidate, this point.

Elderly individuals' ability to walk often becomes compromised; accelerating mobility limitation is characteristic of advancing into very old age. Moreover, being unable to mobilize in the usual way disturbs how the physical world seems, as the person is deprived of the usual spatial experience, such as coming closer physically to objects or distancing them, and approaching and even grasping desired things or escaping unpleasant ones.

When their capacity for their former mode of mobilizing declines (from muscle or joint deterioration, stroke, loss of balance or vital capacity, or similar problems of old age), elders too often are confined to wherever caregivers place them, in chairs or beds, thereby constricting their sense of personal freedom to that of a small child in a stroller or crib. And when one cannot mobilize at will, the aspect of well-being associated with personal autonomy may be extinguished. Immobility thus can debilitate an individual's capacity for spatial judgment and perception, causing serious symptoms of disorientation as well. To be disoriented is to lose one's sense of position in relation to one's physical, temporal, and social surroundings, and to be befuddled in regard to one's identity and direction. This avoidable outcome of biological changes that come with age, and not necessarily those changes themselves, can destabilize health.

So it is not old age itself, nor even the characteristic advent of reduced function in old age, but instead a familiar yet escapable adjunct of such dysfunction that is inimical to health. For, to continue with the illustration, while mobility characteristically becomes compromised in the elderly, being old does not necessitate that disorientation ensues. A wide range of compensatory devices that provide alternative modes of mobilization exist. Users of these devices can approach and withdraw from destinations, thereby preserving their spatial orientation, and can retain their freedom to choose their own location in space. But often the existing health system plans do not make these available to old people, on the grounds that the elderly cannot be cured, for although these devices restore functionality, users still will not function in the species-typical way. Distressingly, such deprivations of a health resource, made on the ground that old people cannot retrieve normal health, often needlessly exacerbate the displacement experiences that corrode people's functional resilience, leading to further enfeeblement.

Whether such users are judged irremediably unhealthy and denied healthcare services because relying on prosthetics and mobility devices to locomote is not considered to be healthy enough, or instead are endorsed as beneficiaries able to achieve through these means the good of health as befits their age, will depend on whether the idea of health is relativized to humans generally or just to humans who have similar long spans of years. If the former, elders cannot help but seem unhealthy as a group, compared with groups of younger people. Moreover, vacillation about social contributions elders should make and concomitant social roles that they might flourish in adds to the shadows that darken discussions about health and healthcare for the old. For how can our healthcare allocation systems assess the prospects for elderly individuals' functionality, and more generally their well-being, if we are not in agreement about what it is appropriate for old people to do?

Conclusion

As previously discussed, what a society thinks health is affects not only who receives services, but also which services are received. Medicine (including bioengineering) can provide materials and devices, both organic and inorganic ones, that renew functionality by supplementing or substituting for debilitated or destroyed species-typical modes of biological functioning. But preventing our medical system from begrudging the dispensation of health care to old people calls for biologically sophisticated public discussion, together with a commitment to social justice, to forge more knowledgeable and more inclusive ideas about old age and elder health.

Notes and References

1 This essay was presented in a much shorter version at the American Philosophical Association Eastern Division Meeting, 2011, and appeared in the *Philosophy and Medicine Newsletter* 2012; **12**(4).

2 Ezine articles, "Top 40 Health Quotations." Available at: http://ezinearticles.com/?Top-40-Health-Quotations&id=5266 [accessed February 13, 2013].

3 Ezine articles, "Top 40 Health Quotations."

4 Ezine articles, "Top 40 Health Quotations."

5 Ezine articles, "Top 40 Health Quotations."

6 Ezine articles, "Top 40 Health Quotations."

7 David Bornstein, "Treating the cause, not the illness", *New York Times*, July 28, 2011; available at: http://opinionator.blogs.nytimes.com/2011/07/28/treating-the-cause-not-the-illness/ [accessed February 13, 2013].

8 Janet Fang, "Fingerprintless? Mutation causes 'immigration delay disease'." Smartplanet, August 10, 2011; available at: http://www.smartplanet.com/blog/rethinking-healthcare/fingerprintless-mutation-causes-8216immigration-delay-disease/6126 [accessed February 13, 2013].

9 Pacific Institute for Research and Evaluation (PIRE), "California anti-smoking laws save thousands of lives, new study finds." Available at: http://www.pire.org/detail2.asp?core=38853&cms=114 [accessed February 13, 2013]. PIRE is one of the nation's preeminent independent, non-profit organizations.

10 Norman Daniels, "Justice, health, and healthcare," in *Medicine and Social Justice*, 2nd edn, edited by Rosamond Rhodes, Margaret Battin, and Anita Silvers. New York: Oxford University Press, 2012; pp. 17–34.

Health as Self-Fulfillment[1]

Michael Boylan

Nothing is better than a diligent life.
Ancient Roman adage

Let me begin with a little story. There was once a king named Agamemnon who was a general in a foreign war (on behalf of his brother). The war lasted a long time. When he finally returned (with a princess from the losing side who was now his concubine) he was killed by his wife (who had a consort of her own). The principal reason that Clytemnestra gave for killing Agamemnon was that he killed their daughter Iphigenia out of "deer" necessity dating back to a dispute with Artemis. In the middle of this tragedy Zeus comments:

> It is true that man's high health (*hygeia*) is not content with limitation. Sickness (*nosos*) chambered beats against a common dividing wall. It is human destiny to set a true course in life, yet this course may be dashed against the sudden reefs of disaster.
> Aeschylus, *Agamemnon* ll, 1001–7 [Aeschylus, 1972; my trans.]

So what are we to make of our little tale? From the beginnings of the Western tradition in ancient Greece *health*, represented by the goddess Hygeia, stood within a context.[2] She was the daughter of Asclepius (god of medicine—who himself was the offspring of Apollo). Her siblings were Eros (god of love and directed desire), Peitho (goddess of eloquent persuasion), Panakeia, (goddess for all curing), Iaso (goddess of remedy and recuperation), Akeso (goddess of recovery), and Aglaea (goddess of natural beauty). Hygeia attended her father Asclepius (god of medicine) and pal'd around with Aphrodite (goddess of love, beauty, and sex). One day they had a feast to honor Hygeia's birthday. What began as panegyric for Hygeia quickly devolved into a dispute. Each sibling wanted *their* natures to be honored the most. This escalated into a fight concerning whom their father (Asclepius) loved best and who was grandfather Apollo's favorite. Each sibling made his or her case (based upon their natures), but there was no agreement and in the end the party degenerated into a disaster as everyone departed—everyone except poor Hygeia, whose feast it was!

What a sad story. But dry your eyes, the tale has a message: Hygeia (health) is not best understood by *any* single sibling. Instead we must understand health via a multilayered presentation. Certainly, medicine is about assisting us all toward good health. This means that the *aim* of medicine is promoting health. Thus, "health" is the foundational concern in medicine and medical ethics. But "health" means different things in different contexts. There have been several popular paradigms that have been advanced in recent years about health. These can be roughly grouped into three categories: (a) a functional approach that clinicians might take to be based upon some understanding of physiology; (b) a public health approach based upon some group allocation of goods that are primary to human agency; and (c) a more subjective approach based upon some understanding of well-being. Let's take a quick look at all three and then move toward one particular understanding of subjectivism.

Functional Approaches to Health

The first approach to be examined is the functional approach (also called "objectivism," biostatistical theory (BST), functionalism/dysfunctionalism, among others). The general approach of all these theories is to adhere to the methodological dream of the logical empiricists to create *value-free* science. BST has been advocated by Christopher Boorse (1975, 1976, 1977, 1997). BST takes a "body-state" to be diseased if it is operating below what is statistically normal for body-states of the same species, sex, and age (called the reference class). Health is thus defined as having all body-states operating at or above the normal efficiency level for the reference class (meaning there is an absence of disease). The intent is to make this a scientific measurement that is value free. One can measure body-states among humans (or among individuals in any other species) and create a normal range for functioning. The measurement device will thus produce data that are indicative of whether the individual in question is "normal" vis-à-vis her or his reference class. For example, there is the EQ_5D system that uses five basic dimensions: mobility, self-care, usual activity, pain/discomfort, and anxiety/depression. There are three levels in each dimension (Kind, 1998). With all permutations, the EQ_5D allows for 243 (3^5) health states—including death. However, the health states approach has come under criticism because it assumes that each disease presents with identifiable symptoms. But this is not always the case. The measuring system is also environmentally insensitive. For example, mobility might mean different things if one lives in a relatively flat, handicapped accessible city rather than a rural mountainous region.

However, it is true that a part of medicine is always in search of a reference class based either upon health states or upon some sort of measurable data on the functioning of biological organs and systems. When you get a blood test your platelet count, lipid count, and so on are all gauged in this way—likewise with other standard tests such as heart stress tests and the vaunted colonoscopy. So in this way Boorse and others of this ilk seem to have identified one sibling of Hygeia (health) that was properly invited to the party.

But there are some problems, too. These follow from the interpretation of what has been shown. It is not the case that we have a value-fee general account. This is because not all reference classes are considered to be equal (Kingma, 2007). For example, if we were to identify the reference class of heavy drinkers, then the normal range of liver function would be different from the range of liver function among the teetotal population. It would seem odd to say that the test results for liver function among the heavy drinkers would constitute health. In reply, Boorse might reply that the reference class of heavy drinkers is not the right kind of reference class. But to do this he would have to set forth a separate account of what makes a proper reference class. This would be grounded upon separate principles (another guest at the party). Also, other guests at the party, for example, evolutionary biologists or subjectivists, might have views of the grounding of health that are not physiologically grounded (DeVito, 2000).[3] Therefore, if Boorse wants to modify his claim to the vantage point of one single guest at the party, then there is no problem. However, if the claim is grander (being about health as such), then his argument fails in his design (Allmark, 2005; Hamilton, 2010).

A second approach in a similar vein is objectivism. According to this account, life is the value and health is associated with an "uncompromised" lifespan and disease with a compromised or shortened lifespan (Lennox, 1995). Everything is based upon the notion that the *summum bonum* is achieving and surpassing the normal lifespan. But this ignores the widespread phenomenon among many species of dying for the sake of the cohort in message warnings, and so forth—biological altruism (Sober and Wilson, 1998). Among humans, suicide and euthanasia are certainly sought by some suffering chronic, incurable pain. Also, there are those who willingly give up a kidney to save the life of another (usually a family member—DeVito, 2000). These organ donations statistically lessen the donor's lifespan. Thus, under the objectivist account such organ donations are instances of disease. Finally, there are those situations in which someone is in chronic pain to a high degree but the pain does not limit life expectancy. Can this person be said to be totally healthy? Thus, though there is an important insight about what mortality can tell us about general health and well-being, it is only one member of the party (Sen, 2009, ch. 7).

Finally, there is the functionalism/dysfunctionalism debate. This is generally carried on in the psychiatric community (Wakefield, 1992a, 1992b, 1993, 1997a, 1997b). Health in this context requires an understanding of healthy and unhealthy mental states. This is interpreted as having a functional mental state (controlled by a functional mental mechanism). What does it mean to have a dysfunctional mental mechanism? There seems to be no way around this being a socially constructed concept. For example, homosexuality is, on Wakefield's account (and Boorse's), judged to be a disorder or disease. This is totally based upon using *reproduction* and *mate selection* as the categories that define the reference group. Because homosexuals are a statistical minority of the population, they are "hurt" in these two areas because (a) they cannot naturally reproduce, and (b) they have fewer mates to choose from. Wakefield asserts that society would view these two conditions as a harm; therefore, homosexuals are "diseased" because of these two dysfunctions. However, this is very problematic because it imports social values in the assessment of normal function. Where do these come from? Some theories of evolutionary biology claim that homosexuality is adaptive because it creates more nurturers and thus increases group-level fitness (Sober and Wilson, 1998). Also, what about the possibility that the social group is prejudiced? For example, in the United States (for much of its history) there were fewer opportunities for Americans of African descent than for Americans of European descent? Does this mean that to be descended from Africa and living in America constitutes a disease? This author says *no*.

Definitions of mental health as seen within a functional arena can be useful. Autistic individuals are clearly not able to function in mainstream society in a manner that is in their own best interests. But what about other examples, such as deafness? Some deaf people value the deaf community as more viable than the mainstream community (Savulescu, 2002). This is certainly an issue that deserves further attention.

The addition of mental health to the picture of health is more complicated. There are certainly cases in which some references to normal functionality as supplemented by social adaptability are useful for determining mental health, but there are other cases in which we must pull aside another guest at the party in order to get an accurate depiction of health.

The above attempts all fail in their quest to become the universal definition of health because they base their approaches upon a value-free science. This was the dream of the logical empiricists (e.g., Bridgman, 1927; Hempel, 1950, 1951; Carnap, 1956). They saw raw objective observation sentences that were explained by theory statements that were, themselves, derived solely from induction that was probability based (thus purifying it from subjective value prejudices) as the holy grail of natural philosophy.

But the value-free dream of the logical empiricists has been largely rejected. This began with Quine in his "Two dogmas of empiricism" (Quine, 1953) and continued with Kuhn's *The Structure of Scientific Revolutions* (Kuhn, 1996), and ran its course via reformed-logical-empiricist Hilary Putnam in "The collapse of the fact/value distinction" (Putnam, 2002). This trend in the philosophy of science was partially driven by the philosophy of biology (because of biology's heavy clinical and laboratory observations), which exhibits its assumed values more clearly than the previous paradigm of the philosophy of physics (largely mathematically driven). Because science is not value free, those theories of health that depend upon a grand attachment to the outmoded logical empiricist worldview will not deliver on their claim.

The universal designs of this objective functionalism approach also fail because of the nature of biology. Whereas physics is largely driven by a universalist model that can be falsified by one instance (such as showing that E is unequal to mc^2 or that F is unequal to $m \times a$), biology is not. Aristotle, the inventor of biology, saw this in his depiction of the aims of biology, *epi to polu* (for the most part; see Boylan, 1984). What this means is that there are many exceptions in biology that do not exhibit themselves in physics. For example, if a baby human was born with only one hand, we would not say that the empirical generalization in biology that humans have two hands is false. This is because of the *for the most part* caveat. This variation between individuals within a species does not count against biological laws, but reinforces them via the theory of evolution, which requires variation within a species so that fitness is higher over a range of possible environments. This means that *diversity* and not *stasis* is the watchword. This variation extends to *health* as well (Hamilton, 2010). In the ancient Greek world of medicine acceptance of individual variation gave rise to various schools: *Empirics, Methodists,* and *Dogmatists* (Boylan, 2007). Each school placed a different emphasis upon how to acknowledge individual variation, ranging from the Empirics (the most) to the Dogmatists (the least). But even the Dogmatists (descending intellectually from the Hippocratic writers and Aristotle) asserted that *for the most part* was the way to understand the aspirational goal of biological laws.

Thus, this section has tried to show what is right and what is not right in understanding human health through the lens of the value-free functionalism.

Public Health Approach

A very popular guest at Hygeia's party in modern times is the group perspective. Some authors such as Amartya Sen have conjectured that public statistics on group longevity say something about how happy and capable people are within a society (Sen, 2009). Figures about infant mortality, morbidity due to certain types of disease, epidemiological data about who the sick are and any common forms of causation yield important information about community health. Individuals in the community can be protected by evidence-based medical responses, but the focus is upon the group.

There are at least two ways to understand the public health perspective on human health. Neither perspective is clinical, with its focus upon the individual and the physician. Instead, the focus is upon groups of people and maintaining environmental conditions that will minimize the spread of infectious disease via clean air, water, sanitation, vaccination, and access to basic medical care. This can be called the thin theory of public health. It is largely based upon prudential self-interest understood collectively. There is another vision of public health that extends this vision to basic human rights—such as those enunciated in the United Nations Universal Declaration of Human Rights. This can be called the thick theory of public health. I have been an advocate for the latter vision and believe that its broader mandate can only be supported by an appeal to normative ethics (Boylan, 2004b).

The difference between these two approaches is that the thin theory of public health views individuals as healthy if they aren't ill (defined as having known bacteria or viruses attacking the body causing a loss of function leading to diminished productivity in the workforce). This is often extended in the thin theory to include workplace injury, accident, and response to war and natural disaster. This viewpoint concentrates upon negative physical influences of various sorts upon the body and its physical systems—viewed collectively via an identifiable social/community group.

In contrast, the thick theory sets out that there is more about being healthy than merely being undiminished by one's physical systems—viewed via an identifiable social/community group. More is needed to demonstrate public health, namely various educational opportunities, human rights, and the ability to participate in one's community as an equal partner and to be able to strive towards one's vision of a life fulfilled (Boylan, 2004a).

What the public health perspective (in either of its two forms) has going for it is that it identifies groups of individuals within a context. There are natural and social environments in which we all live. While the thin theory focuses upon the natural environment, the thick theory combines the social and the natural contexts that permit individuals to act purposively according to their vision of the good. By focusing upon target groups, social changes can positively affect health within that target group. Darrick Tovar-Murray (2010) completed a small demonstration project to show the truth of this conjecture. Now it is correct that the context is not everything. One can live in an area that has a cholera outbreak and never get cholera. One can live under a repressive dictator and never get jailed for being an agent provocateur. Just because one lives in a bad natural or social environment does not insure that one will be a victim. What these deleterious environmental conditions do is to increase the probability that something bad will occur that will affect one's ability to execute purposive action. The public health perspective is thus important because it *can* affect the context of our action.

However, we must be clear that it does not guarantee it. One may have a relatively good natural and social environment and still fall prey to a fatal disease or be the victim of an unjust action. As was argued above, we are working in the land of statistical probabilities.

Given this structure of probabilities, one approach to public health is to view public preferences as a key determinant in creating the right sort of public health policy. Those who take this approach view public health much like economists view commercial choices in the marketplace. In the case of public health, the marketplace is perceived well-being. Thus certain health states are to be preferred to others on the basis of their contribution to well-being (Broome, 2002). At the individual level this leads to indifference curve choices in which the general public chooses to go after one health state, S, over another, S', because of its perceived link to health as understood through well-being (Hausman, 2006). This leads to a version of the social choice model for group evaluation of public health that is not unlike Sen's famous model (Sen, 1970). Social choice takes individual evaluations of preference rankings as its primary data. The bases of the preferences are subjective states and how we assess them. But unless we benchmark the bases of the assessment (say, upon some generally agreed group of core capabilities—so called "basic preferences"), then we risk people falsely judging how to rank various health states. This error can occur via *argumentum ad populum* (given our tendency as social creatures to jump on bandwagons).

Unfortunately, the average citizen is not an expert on health states or even on health-linked well-being as seen on the long range. Socrates used to ask whether the horse trainer would be a better person to ask about horses than the average person (ditto the shoe maker, flute player, and so on). Just as general consumer choices have often chosen the inferior over the superior—for example, the first IBM mainframe over the UNIVAC, VHS video tape over Betamax, the PC computer platform over Apple—so also have policy advisors made very bad collective preference choices, for example, the repeal of the Glass–Steagal Act in the United States or the non-regulation of derivatives and credit default swaps in the financial services industry.

There is something very appealing about seeing health via the public health guest to the party (thin, thick, or governed by social choice), but this perspective is general: often good for policy, but possibly inaccurate for individuals. It is one important perspective, but as we have seen before, there are many guests at this party.

Subjectivist Approaches

The last class of partygoers would be those who represent subjectivist approaches. These include the advocates of well-being broadly understood and well-being understood via the lens of self-fulfillment.

Well-being is a term that is used variously in different contexts. Derek Parfit (1984) suggests that there are three sorts of theories in this category: (a) *hedonistic theories*; (b) *desire-fulfillment theories*; and (c) *objective list theories*. The first path to well-being is merely to seek what one perceives will make one happier via some calculus that is made through a preference-hedonism model (cf. the public health preference model above). If X is thought to bring about more happiness than Y, X is preferred over Y. The very fact that the agent chooses X over Y indicates that the agent thinks that X will deliver the most happiness/pleasure. The criteria for this preference are calibrated via the personal worldview of the individual. Thus Freud near the end of his life might prefer to forego pain-killing drugs in order to maximize mental lucidity. This is a hedonistic calculation based upon Freud's personal theory of value (Griffin, 1977). Such an account is relative to the chosen personal theory of value. Unless one has created meta-ethical value criteria to steer the process, it is subject to very wide relativistic swings—some of which are in direct contradiction.[4]

In *desire-fulfillment theories* the model works this way: we should seek a course of life that will fulfill as many desires as possible. Parfit calls this approach the *success* orientation. The agent decides for him or herself what approach will yield success and thus fulfillment of as many desires as possible (thus ensuring well-being). In the context of health, one might choose to be an exercise enthusiast because undergoing that strategy can satisfy more physical desires than any other alternative. However, this could be turned on its head if I turn out to die from an inherited disease (despite my careful exercise routine). The very structure of the *desire-fulfillment theory* is such that it operates on a conditional "$p \rightarrow q$" structure (if p then q). However, if this model is faulty (as in the exercise example), then the conditional becomes contingent. This means that achieving the state "p" does not guarantee "q" (invalidating *modus ponens*), which also implies that one can fail to achieve q ($\sim q$), without assuming $\sim p$ (thus invalidating the logical rule of *modus tollens*). There may also be multiple ways of achieving q without invoking p. If "$p = 2$ hours daily of vigorous exercise" and "$q =$ not being sick from a bacterial/viral infection or subject to an organ failure," then it is easy to see that one might exercise and not stay well in the sense of q. Also, one might be well in the sense of q and not exercise. The reason for this harkens back to the objective functionalist theories of health discussed above.

Objective list theories seek a paternalist path toward well-being. Under this approach one acts according to a set of criteria that are generally agreed to lead to the fulfillment of as many desires as possible (thus ensuring well-being). This is very much like the success model of the previous paragraph except that the origin of the strategy is commonly accepted maxims. However, the problem raised with the exercise example would still hold here. The only real difference is the origin of the strategic approach. However, when thinking about health, we can think about the difference between these approaches as one in which first the agent chooses his or her path that they think will yield as much happiness as possible. The source of the strategy is a list of value priorities and factual understandings as found in the personal worldview.

In the second case the source of the strategies lies outside the agent—as well as the values and facts concerning the world (e.g., from the family physician). The agent then chooses to follow a regimen that is generally thought to improve one's chances of achieving "q."

There are many advocates of well-being as a way of understanding and achieving health. However, there are some detractors, too. One important attack on well-being as a master value comes from Thomas (Tim) Scanlon.[5] Scanlon distinguished three uses of "well-being": (a) the basis of individual decision-making (first person); (b) the basis of a concerned benefactor's action (third person); and (c) the answer to the "why should I be moral" question (first person). The first sense amounts to fulfilling desire. But rational choice (which should undergird theories of morality) cannot be based solely upon fulfilling desire—even rational desire expressed as a preference (see above). This is because of the connection with well-being that lacks the requisite boundaries.

These boundaries amount to the criteria of being choice worthy, which might lead some to theories such as Rawls (1971) or Sen (1970, 1992) (the second sense enunciated). But these also fail because the boundary line between agent and recipient is not clear. This is especially true when dealing in cases involving mental health. It is often the case that a person with diminished mental health might think that their well-being is just fine when most people (particularly their loved ones) might come to a different conclusion (e.g., those who cut themselves, or are suffering from anorexia, bulimia, bipolar syndrome, and so on). The subjective basis of well-being can be skewed when the agent's assessment capacity is impaired. Therefore, because of these reasons, the third sense of well-being is circular. Thus all three can fail and we must look further for a master underlying argument. Enter self-fulfillment.

Self-fulfillment

Self-fulfillment in the guise of functionalism has been raised before in the health debate (Allmark, 2005). This approach is generally tied to an understanding of Aristotle's *eudaimonia* as functionally "good souled" (where *soul* indicates a natural capacity of the human person, e.g., rationality). The idea of being "fulfilled" presupposes a standard that one works toward. The closer one gets to the terminus, the more fulfilled one is. The million dollar question is: "What is the standard for *Homo sapiens*?" Unless this question is answered, the self-fulfillment question devolves into the well-being question with all its various mazes of interpretation.

What makes this essay different is its connection of health to self-fulfillment as understood through an analysis of the personal worldview and my assumption that in life we all strive to achieve our vision of the good (Boylan, 2004a). I have written much on the personal worldview. The personal worldview is a compilation of all one's understandings of the world factually and normatively. I suggest a way to self-diagnose one's worldview via the personal worldview imperative: "All people must develop a single comprehensive and internally coherent worldview that is good and that we strive to act out in our daily lives" (Boylan, 2004a). There are four parts to this imperative: (a) a worldview must be comprehensive (leading to the development of the rational and affective goodwill); (b) a worldview must be internally coherent (deductively and inductively); (c) a worldview must connect to a normative theory of ethics; and (d) a worldview must be at least aspirational[6] and acted upon. I see this as a first-order meta-ethical theory that would give direction to how one would shape one's life. As I show elsewhere, I believe that this position dictates that everyone adopt cooperative theories of justice first in holistic ways of looking at the world (Boylan, 2004a, 2011). Let us examine these claims in relation to a common objector position.

The position I am thinking about centers around a personal worldview concept of life being like a daily hunt in the jungle for food. There are many snares in the jungle: wild animals might take *you* for food. You might be unsuccessful and eventually die in pursuing your quarry. Certainly those who have the hunting-in-nature metaphor view life as a continual struggle for survival. At any moment you may lose your hunting skills so that you will be forever lost. There is no one to help you. You are on your own to make it or fail. Success comes to those who deploy themselves most effectively.

Those who hold this worldview metaphor will be suspicious of those who are possible competitors. This is because they may take from them their daily kill. As this metaphor is translated into its modern referent, the animal carcasses become bank account balances. Everyone is after your money. The only way to protect yourself is to accumulate and hoard large amounts of reserve cash to protect you against a shortfall or an emergency (kind of like modern hunters putting meat into the deep freezer). The vision of being penniless on the street is constantly before the holder of this worldview as the worst case—*yet possible*—scenario.

Sometimes the hunting metaphor is combined with a war metaphor as in Thomas Hobbes' depiction of the state of nature:

> …there is no way for any man to secure himself, so reasonable, as Anticipation; that is, by force, or wiles, to master the persons of all men he can, so long, till he sees no other power great enough to endanger him (Hobbes, 1651/1997).

For Hobbes the metaphor is of a state of nature (forest, hill, and dale) in which all are equal—though not identical (e.g., you may be able to run faster than I, but I'm stronger than you: in the end the sums are equal). Because of this summative equality, and the fact of scarcity of resources, the result is that there is fierce competition that will inevitably lead to continual strife (war). This is the human condition according to Hobbes and is depicted via his state of nature metaphor.

Another fellow traveler is Friedrich Nietzsche, who seeks to describe the basic psychological nature of human kind in order to give a causal account from the agent's point of view:

> Suppose, finally, we succeeded in explaining our entire instinctive life as the development and ramification of *one* basic form of the will—namely, of the will to power, as *my* proposition has it…then one would have gained the right to determine *all* efficient force univocally as—*will to power*. The world viewed from inside…it would be "will to power" and nothing else (Nietzsche, 1886/1968).

For Nietzsche, the will to power is a psychological fact that finds metaphorical expression in *Beyond Good and Evil* and *On the Genealogy of Morals*. In some respects it is a deeper account than Hobbes' because it gives specification of *why* we are acquisitive. It is because, at base, we are psychological egoists whose quest in life is to exert whatever influence we can upon the world. There is a trust that those who can assert the most influence will also be driven by a love of nobility (beauty) that will keep them in check from being utter tyrants. Of course, skeptics of the regulative power of nobility (beauty) will see this depiction as one that devolves to mere *kraterism* ("to each according to his ability to snatch it"). Under this sparser interpretation, Nietzsche falls into the tradition of the hunting/war metaphor. (The more generous interpretation would put Nietzsche on the edges of the metaphor, given the tempering force of nobility [beauty].)

In either case "the will to power," as metaphorical expression, is seen in the context of other writers who assert the same thing. Like Hobbes, Nietzsche can be connected to a vision of life on earth as a competitive contest. We are all engaged in seeking to extend ourselves over our environment and over others.

One practical consequence of the hunting metaphor of life is *laissez faire* capitalism. We all strive to gain the goods, and the science of economics is created to describe (and not prescribe) the process. Since everything is all wrapped up tight in a theory of human nature, what could be more correct? This metaphorical expression measures our goodness in terms of the competitive acquisition of goods—money, status, and power. Thus, our primitive drive to be good is satisfied by the garnering of these goods in the highest amounts. The individual with the biggest heap at the end of the day is the winner!

If self-fulfillment is a legitimate way to understand health (one of the guests at Hygeia's party), then the competitive model sets the measure by which we can assess whether we are healthy: how much power have we achieved via competition within our frame of reference. The more power, the healthier we are. If one accepts that self-fulfillment is a legitimate way to understand health and if the best candidate for the scorecard is power, then QED.

In contrast to the highly competitive personal worldview paradigm, I would put forth an alternative model:

> Imagine that each of us is on a quest to be good. We are seeking a means to be good that will make our world (and us) better through intellectual excellence (theoretical and practical reason) and emotional excellence (love), that is, establishing the goodwill within ourselves. The quest may last a long time. The quest may end in failure. It is up to us to do our best to seek and obtain the object of the quest. In the process of our quest we may be required to undergo various ordeals and tests of our resolve and worthiness. It is the nature of human existence to sally forth on this quest and do our individual best at achieving the reward (though we may be humbled, scorned, and ridiculed in the process). This process thus represents a prescriptive view of a good human life. To be healthy is to be closer to the endpoint in the quest. The closer we are, the healthier we are.

THE COOPERATIVE GOODWILL THOUGHT EXPERIMENT

In the thought experiment an alternative is presented to the competitive worldview standpoint: the cooperative worldview standpoint as exhibited by the focus upon creating a good will. Though expressed differently both Aristotle and Kant, it holds that we ought to try to acquire various excellences in character that would create habits in us such that our decision-making apparatus (our will) would become increasingly good (as measured by our internal assessment via the personal worldview imperative).

There are several reasons why each of us should prefer the cooperative personal worldview over the competitive worldview—especially concerning health. First, there is some medical evidence that being hypercompetitive can lead to several serious medical conditions (Freidman and Rosenman, 1960; Al-Asadi, 2010; Haukkala *et al.*, 2010). Second, the nature of the competitive worldview is a zero-sum game while the cooperative worldview is not. The very nature of the competitive worldview is that there are limited goods sought after by many. It is much like the child's game of musical chairs. There are four chairs and six children. They walk politely around the chairs while the music is playing, but when the music stops, it is a mad dash for the chairs. Children are pushed away as the hyperaggressive ones win the day. Is this the community worldview we wish to promote? Will this lead to general public health? I think not. It will lead to a society of a few superwinners at the expense of the many. Such a worldview violates the personal worldview imperative because it violates the affective goodwill and the inductive understanding of consistency—as such it violates this first-order meta-ethical principle. In addition, I have argued elsewhere that such an outcome is inherently unjust (Boylan, 2004a).

So let's suppose that we proceed with a cooperative personal worldview that is in accord with the personal worldview imperative. What else is necessary to proceed along a path of health as self-fulfillment? To answer this, I would again foray to the ancient Western world and the biomedical writers—particularly the Hippocratic writers and Galen. What these writers found to be the case was that *balance* was the most critical factor to health. By balance they meant of course the balance between the four humors of the body: blood, phlegm, yellow bile (sometimes serum), and black bile (Hankinson, 2008; Gill, 2010). Of course, Aristotle advocated balance too, in his doctrine of the mean (and so did Confucius with his concept of *li*—balance presented via the metaphor of dance). What these ancient writers understood was that an essential key to health is balance because it encourages the development of *sophrosune*, or self-control (a master virtue when considering balance). Self-control is also crucial in achieving self-fulfillment. This is because deciding what one wants to do in life (constrained by the personal worldview imperative) is a process of reflection, self-control, and habits of excellence. These three menu items work together so that one can act autonomously toward a worthy goal in a balanced manner. The process looks like this:

1. One seeks balance to achieve self-control—basic fact of human nature.
2. Self-control allows one more successfully to carry out the personal worldview imperative (reflection that leads to the rational and affective good will)—Assertion [A].
3. A developed rational and affective good will allows one to develop habits of excellence that are directed toward one's chosen life plan—A.
4. A life plan chosen as per above will be the most choice-worthy path toward an agent's life goals (self-fulfillment) [1–3].
5. Because the process begins with balance, B, this property continues through all the steps as a property of the agent—Fact [F].
6. Balance supports personal health—5.
7. The choice-worthy path toward self-fulfillment supports personal health—4–6.

The self-fulfillment approach to health

What this approach to health offers is a subjectivist approach that has an objective structure (the personal worldview imperative) that can alleviate the common objections to well-being (the most prominent subjectivist theory discussed). Because of this, I think that it offers the best subjectivist understanding of health.

Conclusion

This essay began with Hygeia's party on Mount Olympus. There were many guests, each of which had a legitimate place to be there (no counterfeit invitations). I have tried to interpret this literary conceit to discuss the problem of health pluralistically—showing the proper roles of various perspectives, but also arguing that none of them gives a complete account.

From the point of view of most readers of this essay, the most personally relevant understanding of health is subjectivist. In order to avoid the common complaints against well-being not having an adequate external structure, this essay has set one in place within the context of self-fulfillment (within the context of the personal world-view imperative) and a personal measure of health as we lead our lives. In the end, we must judge ourselves after the lines of *The Eumenides* (the final work of the *Oresteia*):

> Home, home ever high aspiring,
> Daughters of Night, aged children, cavalier processional
> Bless these with silence…
> There shall be peace between Pallas Athena and the guests.
> Zeus, all knowing, met with Fate to confirm it
> Let us sing as we make our exit (lines 1033–47, my trans.).

Notes

1 This essay was presented in a much shorter version at the American Philosophical Association Eastern Division Meeting, 2011, and appeared in the *Philosophy and Medicine Newsletter* 2012; 12(4).

2 These relations are often parsed differently. This is because there are discrepancies among the primary sources. Since this is not an essay on philology, I will present these characters in the context of my initial story.

3 De Vito sets out additionally that if BST is correct, then any state that does not decrease lifespan or fecundity is not a disease, for example, flu, chronic pain, or bronchitis. Most would say that this is a major flaw with BST.

4 I have created such criteria in Boylan (2004a, chapter 2).

5 Scanlon's argument on well-being works this way:
  1. There are three uses of "well-being": (a) the basis of individual decision-making (first person); (b) the basis of a concerned benefactor's action (third person); (c) the answer to the "why should I be moral" question (first person)—Assertion [A] (Scanlon, 2000, p. 108).
  2. WB [well-being] 1a is experientially important to us all—Fact [F] (p. 108).
  3. WB 1a is sometimes understood as fulfilling desire—F (p. 113).
  4. Desire is not sufficient for rational choice—F (from Scanlon, 2000, chapter 1 / p. 114)
  5. Desire and its fulfillment cannot give an account of WB sufficient for morality—2–4.
  6. Rational desire understood as preference is often put forward as a ground for WB—F (p. 116).
  7. The good is not dependent upon preference (informed desire) but the reasons that make it worthwhile—A (p. 119).
  8. Rational desires understood as preferences cannot give an account of WB sufficient for morality—6–7.
  9. Some say that rational aims tied to WB create a motivation superior to desire—A (p. 121).
  10. [Motivation is important to morality]—F.
  11. Fulfillment of rational desire (broadly and specifically) must be tied to WB or the desire wasn't rational—A (pp. 121–3).
  12. Many rational desires have intrinsic aims (e.g., friendship and science) that are not connected to WB—A (p. 124).
  13. Though WB has some connections with rational aims, it is not the sole source of determination—9–12 (p. 124).

14. WB 1a does not have clear boundaries because it cannot account for why it is good—A (p. 127).
15. There is no limit to WB 1a—A (p. 129).
16. [What has no limits has no boundaries]—F.
17. WB 1a has a boundary problem—14–16 (p. 129).
18. In choosing the best life, the "most choice worthy" trumps "well-being"—A (p. 131).
19. WB is not primary and sufficient—17–18.
20. When one concentrates upon one's own WB, one becomes selfish—A (p. 137).
21. [Being selfish is bad]—A.
22. WB 1a can be counterproductive—20–21 (p. 133).
23. WB 1a is not a master value for morality—5, 8, 13, 17, 19, 22.
24. WB 1b is generally connected to morality via justice and benevolence, cf. Rawls and Sen—A (p. 139).
25. A benefactor may act to promote a choice-worthy life over one based upon WB (e.g., artist or labor organizer)—A (p. 135).
26. WB 1b implies a standard account of WB based upon promoting pleasure—A (p. 136).
27. The boundaries between the benefactor's and recipient's WB are unclear—A (p. 136).
28. The recipient does not have reason for merely promoting his pleasure—A (p. 136).
29. WB 1b is not a master value for morality—24–28.
30. WB 1c would require one to justify moral principles on grounds that presuppose what people are entitled to—A (pp. 137–8).
31. Premise #30 involves a circular claim—F (p. 138).
32. WB 1c is not a master value for morality—30–31.
33. Well-being is not a master value for morality—1, 23, 29, 32.

6 I interpret "aspirational" as being something that is attainable—though it may be very difficult to achieve. It is to be contrasted with "utopian," which is a goal that (though laudable) is practically impossible to achieve. For example, eliminating the common childhood diseases (that have known vaccines) in the world is aspirational while totally eliminating poverty is utopian.

References

Aeschylus (1972) *Aeschyli Septem Quae Supersunt Tragoedias* (D. Page, ed.) Oxford: Clarendon Press.

Al-Asadi, J.N. (2010) Type A behaviour pattern: is it a risk factor for hypertension? *Eastern Mediterranean Health Journal* 16(7): 740–5.

Allmark, P. (2005) Health, happiness and health promotion. *Journal of Applied Philosophy* 22(1): 1–15.

Boorse, C. (1975) On the distinction between disease and illness. *Philosophy of Public Affairs* 5: 49–68.

Boorse, C. (1976) Wright on functions. *The Philosophical Review* 85: 70–86.

Boorse, C. (1977) Health as a theoretical concept. *Philosophy of Science* 44: 70–86.

Boorse, C. (1997) A rebuttal on health. In J.M. Humber and R.F. Almeder (eds), *What is Disease?* Totowa, NJ: Humana Press, pp. 1–134.

Boylan, M. (1984) *Method and Practice in Aristotle's Biology*. Lanham, MD and Oxford: Rowman & Littlefield/UPA.

Boylan, M. (2004a) *A Just Society*. Lanham, MD and Oxford: Rowman & Littlefield.

Boylan, M. (2004b) The moral imperative to maintain public health. In: M. Boylan (ed.), *Public Health Ethics*. Dordrecht: Springer/Kluwer; pp. xvii–xxxiv.

Boylan, M. (2007) Galen on the blood, pulse, and arteries. *Journal of the History of Biology* 40(2): 207–30.

Boylan, M. (2008) *The Good, The True, and The Beautiful*. London: Continuum.

Boylan, M. (2011) *Morality and Global Justice: Justifications and Applications*. Boulder, CO: Westview.

Bridgman, P. (1927) *The Logic of Modern Physics*. New York: Macmillan.

Broome, J. (2002) Measuring the burden of disease by aggregating well-being. In: C. Murray, J. Salomon, C. Mathers, and A. Lopez (eds), *Summary Measures of Population Health*. Geneva: World Health Organization; pp. 91–113.

Carnap, R. (1950) *Logical Foundations of Probability*. Chicago: University of Chicago Press.

Carnap, R. (1956) *Meaning and Necessity*. Chicago: University of Chicago Press; pp. 205–21.

De Vito, S. (2000) On the value-neutrality of the concepts of health and disease: unto the breach again. *Journal of Medicine and Philosophy* 25(5): 539–67.

Friedman, M. and Rosenman, R.H. (1960) Overt behavior pattern in coronary disease. Detection of overt behavior pattern A in patients with coronary disease by a new psychophysiological procedure. *JAMA* 173: 1320–5.

Gill, C. (2010) *Naturalistic Psychology in Galen and Stoicism*. Oxford: Oxford University Press.

Griffin, J. (1977) Are there incommensurable values? *Philosophy and Public Affairs* 7(1) (Fall), 39–59.

Hamilton, R.P. (2010) The concept of health: beyond normativism and naturalism. *Journal of Evaluation in Clinical Practice* 16: 323–9.

Hankinson, R.J. (ed.) (2008) *The Cambridge Companion to Galen*. Cambridge: Cambridge University Press.

Haukkala, A., Konttinen, H., Laatikainen, T., *et al.* (2010) Hostility, anger control, and anger expression as predictors of cardiovascular disease. *Psychosomatic Medicine* 72: 556–62.

Hausman, D.M. (2006) Valuing health. *Philosophy and Public Affairs* 34(3): 246–74.

Hempel, C. (1950) Problems and changes in empiricist criterion of meaning. *Revue Internationale de Philosophie* 11: 41–63.

Hempel, C. (1951) The concept of cognitive significance: a reconsideration. *Proceedings of the American Academy of Arts and Sciences* 80(1): 61–77.

Hobbes, T. (1651/1997) *Leviathan* (R.E. Flathman and D. Johnson, eds). New York: W.W. Norton; Chapter 13, p. 60.

Kind, P. (1998) The EuroQuoL instrument: an index of health-related quality of life. In: B. Spiker (ed.), *Quality of Life and Pharmacoeconomics in Clinical Trials*, 2nd edn. Philadelphia, PA: Lippincott-Raven; pp. 191–201.

Kingma, E. (2007) What is it to be healthy? *Analysis* 67(2). 128–33.

Kuhn, T.S. (1996) *The Structure of Scientific Revolution*, 3rd edn. Chicago: University of Chicago Press.

Lennox, J. (1995) Health as an objective value. *Journal of Medicine and Philosophy* 20: 499–511.

Nietzsche, F. (1968/1886) Beyond good and evil. In: *Basic Writings of Nietzsche* (trans. W. Kaufmann). New York: Modern Library; pt II, sect. 36, p. 238.

Parfit, D. (1984) *Reasons and Persons*. Oxford: Oxford University Press; pp. 493–503.

Putnam, H. (2002) *The Collapse of the Fact/Value Dichotomy and Other Essays*. Cambridge, MA: Harvard University Press.

Quine, W. van O. (1953) *From a Logical Point of View*. Cambridge, MA: Harvard University Press.

Rawls, J. (1971) *A Theory of Justice*. Cambridge, MA: Harvard University Press.

Savulescu, J. (2002) Deaf lesbians, "designer disability" and the future of medicine. *Journal of Medical Ethics* 325: 771–3.

Scanlon, T.M. (2000) *What We Owe Each Other*. Cambridge, MA: Harvard University Press; pp. 108–38.

Sen, A., (1970) *Collective Choice and Social Welfare*. San Francisco: Holden-Day.

Sen, A. (1992) *Inequality Re-Examined*. Cambridge, MA: Harvard University Press.

Sen, A. (2009) *The Idea of Justice*. Cambridge, MA: Harvard University Press; pp. 164–7.

Sober, E. (1980) Evolution, population thinking and essentialism. *Philosophy of Science* 47: 350–83.

Sober, E. and Wilson, D.S. (1998) *Unto Others: The Evolution and Psychology of Unselfish Behavior*. Cambridge, MA: Harvard University Press.

Tovar-Murray, D. (2010) Social health and environmental quality of life: their relationship to positive physical health and subjective well-being in a population of urban African Americans. *The Western Journal of Black Studies* 34(3): 358–66.

Wakefield, J.C. (1978) Four basic concepts of medical science. In P.D. Asquith and I. Hacking (eds), *Proceedings of the Philosophy of Science Association* 1: 210–22.

Wakefield, J.C. (1992a) The concept of mental disorder: on the boundary between biological facts and social values. *American Psychologist* 47: 373–88.

Wakefield, J.C. (1992b) Disorder as harmful dysfunction: a conceptual critique of DSM III-R's definition of mental disorder. *Psychological Review* 99: 232–47.

Wakefield, J.C. (1993) The limits of operationalism: a critique of Spitzer and Endicott's proposed operational criteria for mental disorder. *Journal of Abnormal Psychology* 102: 160–72.

Wakefield, J.C. (1997a) Diagnosing DSM-IV—Part I: DSM-IV and the concept of disorder. *Behavior Research & Therapy* 35: 633–49.

Wakefield, J.C. (1997b) Diagnosing DSM-IV—Part II: Eysenck and the essentialist fallacy. *Behavior Research & Therapy* 35: 651–65.

Evaluating a Case Study
Developing a Practical Ethical Viewpoint

Your goal in this book is to respond critically to case studies on various aspects of Medical Ethics. To do this, you must be able to assess the ethical impact of some critical factor(s) in situations that pose ethical problems. One factor in assessing the case is the ethical impact of the project/policy/action. This chapter and Chapters 4 through 6 end with an "Evaluating a Case Study" section that focuses on a particular exercise. These sections include case studies to which you can apply the insight you gained from the readings and discussion in the chapter. Because the information presented in these "Evaluating a Case Study" sections is cumulative, you should be able to write a complete critical response to a case study by the end of Chapter 6.

Macro and Micro Cases

Beginning with this chapter, each chapter will end with cases for you to consider. The cases section is divided into two categories, macro and micro. Each type of case employs a different point of view.

Macro Case. The macro case takes the perspective of someone in an executive position of authority who supervises or directs an organizational unit. His or her decisions will affect many people and resonate in a larger sociological sphere.

Micro Case. The micro case examines the perspective of someone at the proximate level of professional practice, such as a nurse or doctor actually involved in the art of healing. Obviously, this case applies to more people than does the macro case.

Case Development. This book suggests one way to develop critical evaluations of ethical cases. In the "Evaluating a Case Study" sections, you will be asked to apply a specific skill to the cases presented. At the end of Chapter 6, you will be able to write an essay concerning the application of an ethical perspective to a specific problem.

Please note that although the cases presented here have fictional venues, they are based on composites of actual biomedical practice.

These end-of-chapter evaluations seek to bridge the gap between Normative Ethics and Applied Ethics. Skill in using Applied Ethics is very important, for this is where the practical decision making occurs. My approach in these essays is to allow you to employ techniques that you have been taught elsewhere in addition to those found in this text. Depending on your background in science or a health care field, you can write a critical response to a case study that demonstrates your professional acumen along with your sensitivity to the ethical dimensions found in the situation you are examining. Classes that have few students with scientific or biomedical backgrounds will deemphasize the fundamental details of science and health care and concentrate instead on a less technical response.

Biomedical personnel often become so enmeshed in the practice of medicine that they lose their ability to discern and react to possible ethical dilemmas, a difficulty experienced in all professions.[1] But this is wrong. The "Evaluating a Case Study" sections will help you analyze both ethical and practical situations. The approach will invoke a technique that rates a proposal as having three levels of complexity: surface, medium, and deep. The level of interaction allows you to see at a glance how the competing areas of interest and ethical value conflict.

The five "Evaluating a Case Study" sections are intended to sequentially lead you to develop the abilities to write a critical response to a case study: (a) Developing a Practical Ethical Viewpoint, (b) Finding the Conflicts (Chapter 3), (c) Assessing Embedded Levels (Chapter 4), (d) Applying Ethical Issues (Chapter 5), and (e) Structuring the Essay (Chapter 6).

At the end of Chapter 4 through 6, you will be presented case studies to which you can apply your newfound skills. By the end of the term, you should be able to create an ethical impact statement of some sophistication.

Let us begin first by choosing an ethical theory and then proceed to develop a practical viewpoint. Few people bother to choose an ethical theory; most pick-up a few moral maxims that they apply when the occasion seems appropriate. The manner of this acquisition is often environment dependent, that is, having to do with their upbringing, friends, and the community(ies) in which they live. As such, their maxims reflect those other viewpoints.

The Personal Worldview Imperative enjoins us to develop a single comprehensive and internally coherent worldview that is good and that we will strive to act out in our lives (see Chapter 1). One component of this worldview is an ethical theory. Thus, each of us must *develop* an ethical theory. This does not this mean that we must all start from scratch. Those before us have done much good work. But we must personally choose an ethical theory and assume ownership for it as being the most correct theory in existence. It is not enough merely to accept someone else's theory without any active work on our part. We must go through the process of personal introspection and evaluation to determine what we think is best and to be open to ways we can improve, the theory (in concept or in practice).

This process of making an ethical theory our own can take years. This course is only a few months. Does this pose a problem? Not really when you consider that part of the process of making an ethical theory our own involves provisional acceptance and testing of various moral maxims. Obviously, this testing has a limit. We should not test whether it is morally permissible to murder by going out and murdering various people. The testing I am advocating is a way to examine various moral commands and evaluate whether their application is consonant with other worldview values we hold. The process will perhaps go back and forth in a progressive dialectic until we have accepted or rejected the commands.

To begin this process of testing, we must identify the most prominent ethical theories and their tenets. Many books survey and evaluate the major ethical theories. In this series of textbooks *Basic Ethics in Action*, I have written one such survey entitled *Basic Ethics*. I would suggest that you refer either to that book or to another like it to obtain enough information to enable you to begin the process of choosing an ethical theory. A broad, brief account can be found in Chapter 1.

For the purposes of this book, I will highlight four major theories: Utilitarianism, Deontology, Intuitionism, and Virtue Ethics. To begin the process, I recommend that you choose a single theory from these four (or from others your instructor may offer) as your critical tool as you prepare for class. You might ask, How do I know which viewpoint to choose? This is a difficult question. It concerns the justification of the various ethical theories.

Many criteria can be used to justify an ethical theory. One criterion is Naturalism. Each theory presupposes a naturalistic or nonnaturalistic epistemological standpoint. Naturalism is complicated, for our purposes, let us describe it as a view that holds that no entities or events are in principle beyond the domain of scientific explanation. Cognitive claims are valid only if they are based on accepted scientific modes.

Ethical Naturalism states that moral judgments are also merely a subclass of facts about the natural world that can be studied scientifically. From this study, we can determine moral correctness as a corollary of certain facts that can be scientifically investigated (e.g., how much pleasure various alternatives will produce for the group). Thus, utilitarians believe that moral judgments *are* judgments about which alternative will be most beneficial to some group's survival.

A utilitarian might point to the scientific study of nature and say that the instinct to seek pleasure is evidenced in all species. Furthermore, an evolutionary advantage seems to exist for those species that act for the benefit of the group that does not exist for those that do not act in this way.

Many sociobiologists make this sort of claim. The main imperative of evolutionary theory is that a person's own genes be passed on to another generation. If passing on a person's own genes is impossible, the next best thing is to pass on the genes of the individual's relatives. Thus, seemingly altruistic behavior (such as a bird that stays behind in dangerous situations so that the group might survive) is really selfish because helping the group *is* helping the bird to pass on its genes (or those of its relatives).

Sociobiology, of course, is not universally accepted, nor is it necessary for a utilitarian to be a sociobiologist. However, this example does illustrate a type of justification that the utilitarian might make. He could move from the concept of group happiness in animals and extrapolate to humans. The supporting data are scientific; therefore, the theory is naturalistic.

Deontologists may or may not be naturalists. Since Deontology involves a duty-based ethics, the key question to be asked concerns how we know whether a binding duty exists to do such and such. Are all moral "oughts" derivable from factual, scientifically ascertainable "is" statements? If they are, then the deontologist is a naturalist. If they are not, then the deontologist is not a naturalist.

In his book *Reason and Morality*, Alan Gewirth claims to derive ought from is. There is no reference to knowledge claims that are not compatible with the scientific inquiry of natural objects. This would make Gewirth a naturalist. Kant and Donagan are somewhat different. Each refers to supernatural entities that are not scientifically supported. Kant spends considerable effort trying to define these boundaries in the "Transcendental Dialectic" section of his book *The Critique of Pure Reason*. This aside, neither Kant nor Donagan considered that a problem about integrating the factual and the normative existed.

If you are inclined to view reality as an extension of evolutionary biology or to believe that group advantage immediately entails a moral ought, then you are leaning toward Utilitarianism. If you think that people should act from pure duty alone without reference to anything except the rightness of the action, however, then Deontology is probably your preference.

The is-ought problem was sharpened by intuitionist G.E. Moore,[2] who rejected Ethical Naturalism because he believed it contained a fallacy (which he dubbed the *naturalistic fallacy*). This fallacy claims that it is false to define goodness in terms of any natural property. This is so because good is not definable and because good is not subject to scientific examination. This is true because the factual is realm is separate from the normative ought realm. The chasm between the two cannot be crossed.

Good for Moore is a unique, unanalyzable, non-natural property (as opposed, for example, to yellow, which is a natural property). Clearly scientific methods are of no use. Science can tell us things about yellow but can tell us nothing about the meaning of good. Other intuitionists also hold that we understand important moral terms and/ or moral maxims by cognitive means that are not scientific. Generally, these are immediate and cannot be justified in factual "is" language.

Intuitionism is therefore a non-naturalistic theory. Still, it has some remote connections to Naturalism. For example, one can point to the *plausibility* of accepting certain common moral maxims—such as a prohibition against murder—by reference to other societies. (In other words, since all societies prohibit murder, the prohibition against murder must be immediately apparent to all.) However, plausibility is not the same thing as exhaustive scientific demonstration. Justification in Intuitionism lies in its alleged unarguable truth that can be grasped in principle immediately by all.

If you are having trouble adopting any of the theories and believe that acceptance or rejection of an ethical theory comes to some sort of brute immediate acceptance, then you will probably want to accept Intuitionism as your ethical theory.

Finally, we turn to Virtue Ethics. This theory seems at first to be naturalistic. Aristotle lends credence to this when he talks about relying on the common opinions of people about what is considered to be a virtue. The common opinions could be gathered and reviewed much as a sociologist or anthropologist might do, and this "scientific" method would yield definitive results. Aristotle believed that some common agreement about a core set of virtues existed.

Justification, therefore, was not an issue for Aristotle. If we accept a worldview such as Aristotle presents, then we would all agree that everyone considers courage (for example) to be a virtue. The confirming data can be gathered and scientifically studied; ergo, it is naturalistic. The proof depends on the community that values these traits. This emphasis on community makes Virtue Ethics a favorite theory among those who call themselves *communitarians*. The communitarian begins with the group and its institutions and depends on individual members to submit to the authority of the group (or to change the group in ways it accepts).

How does Communitarianism affect today's pluralistic society? Some might argue that consensus about the virtues no longer exists nor does a single community to which we all belong. If there is no consensus as Aristotle envisioned, then what constitutes a virtue may collapse into a form of Intuitionism. For example, I think that X is a virtue. You think Y is a virtue. X and Y are mutually exclusive traits. You and I come from different communities/societies; therefore, we cannot come to an agreement. All each of us can say is I am right and you are wrong. Personal insight (Intuitionism) is all we have to justify our practices (to ourselves and to others).

If you believe that courage, wisdom, self-control, piety, and so forth are virtues in every society, then perhaps you will choose Virtue Ethics as your model.

To help you choose an ethical theory, try this exercise. Examine one or more of the following moral situations and (a) interpret what is right and wrong according to each of the four theories, (b) then give an argument that might be proposed according to each theory, and (c) state your own assessment of the strengths of each theory.

Situation One

You are the constable of a small, remote, rural town in Northern Ireland. The town is divided into the Catholics (20 percent minority) and the Protestants (80 percent majority). All Catholics live in one section of town on a peninsula jutting into the river just east of the main part of town.

One morning a young Protestant girl is found raped and murdered next to the town green. According to general consensus, a Catholic must have committed the crime. The Protestants form a citizens committee that demands the following of the constable: "We believe you to be a Catholic sympathizer, and we don't think you will press fast enough to bring this killer to justice. We know a Catholic committed the crime. We've sealed off the Catholic section of town; no one can go in or out. If you don't hand over the criminal by sundown, we will torch the entire Catholic section of town, killing all 1,000 people. Don't try to call for help. We've already disabled all communications."

You made every effort to find out who did it, but you made no progress. You could not find out. At one hour before sundown, you don't know what to do. Your deputy says, "Why don't we just pick a random Catholic and tell them he did it? At least we'd be saving 999 lives."

"But then I'd be responsible for killing an innocent man!" you reply.

Better one innocent die and 999 be saved. After all, there's no way the two of us can stop the mob. You have to give them a scapegoat," the deputy responds.

Describe how each ethical theory might approach this situation. Which one is most consonant to your own worldview, and why?

Situation Two

You are on the executive committee of the XYZ organization of health care professionals. Each year the committee gives an award to one of its members who displays high moral character in his or her work. This year you are among the four judges for the award. There is some disagreement among the judges, however, about what constitutes a good person. The judges, besides yourself, are Ms. Smith, Mrs. Taylor, and Mr. Jones. The candidates for the award are Mr. Big and Mrs. Little.

Ms. Smith said that the award should go to Mr. Big because he saved a man from drowning. However, Mr. Jones demurred, saying that Mr. Big's motives are suspect because the man he saved was in the midst of a very big financial deal with Mr. Big. If the man had been allowed to drown, Mr. Big would have lost a lot of money. Ms. Smith said motives are not important but that the goodness of the act counts and the man who was saved runs a big business in town. Many people besides Mr. Big would have been hurt if he had not saved the man.

Mr. Jones said the award should go to Mrs. Little because she performed a kind act of charity in chairing the town's United Way Campaign last year. Surely such an act could not be said to benefit Mrs. Little in any way (unlike Mr. Big).

Mrs. Taylor said that she is somewhat unsure about either Mr. Big or Mrs. Little because both of them have been recommended on the basis of a single good act. Mrs. Taylor believed that it would be better to choose a candidate who has shown over time to have performed many good actions and to be of good character. "After all," she said, "a single swallow does not make a spring." Mr. Jones and Ms. Smith scratched their heads at this remark and turned to you. Who is right?

Describe how each ethical theory might approach this situation. Which one is most consonant to your own worldview, and why?

Choosing an ethical theory is only the first step in developing a practical ethical viewpoint. A link between the normative theory and application of the theory is needed. In Chapter 1, I outlined my basic position concerning a personal worldview and how it might be utilized when applying an ethical theory. Precautionary reasoning is an example of one way to do this. According to this concept, a person must arrive at a level of potential agency ascription to fetuses, impaired humans, and nonhumans. Different people will arrive at different base levels at which they think it prudent to ascribe human agency (with all its ensuing rights) to some potential agent. A person may appeal to biological facts—such as the structure and development of the forebrain—for this. Another person may be more operational in evaluating seemingly purposive behavior. Still others may adopt other criteria.

The point is that one important aspect of developing a practical ethical viewpoint is to challenge ourselves to think about and provisionally accept certain tenets necessary to effectively apply ethical principles to practice. These concepts should allow professionals to connect normative theories to the real-life problems that confront them.

Before addressing ethical cases, try first to provisionally accept one moral theory. Then try to determine what connecting principles or concepts are necessary to translate theory to practice. Concentrate your efforts on these connections. They will be very useful to you as you address what you see as the important issues residing in each case.

Notes

1 For a fuller discussion of this see, *Basic Ethics*, chap. 7.
2 I cannot stress too much the impossibility of completely pigeonholing philosophers. In some important ways, Moore was an intuitionist because "good" had to be accepted as an unanalyzable, unnatural fact. Toward the end of *Principia Ethica*, however, he sounds much like an agathistic utilitarian, one who wishes to maximize the group's good. This mixture of labels among philosophers shows only that labels are limited in what they can do.

Ross and Rawls have deontological and intuitionistic aspects to their theories. Therefore, one label alone cannot adequately capture the spirit of their philosophy. In an introductory text, such as this one, labels are used to simplify—but hopefully not obfuscate—the dynamics present in these thinkers.

3

Physician, Nurse, and Patient
The Practice of Medicine

General Overview: This chapter explores some of the key practices that constitute the profession of medicine. To this end I have divided the chapter into four parts: Paternalism and Autonomy; Privacy and Confidentiality; Informed Consent; and Gender, Culture, and Race. These four make significant contributions in defining the practice of medicine and areas that are somewhat controversial. Many of the questions in one area overlap to another.

As an introduction to the traditional practice of medicine I first present the Hippocratic Oath, which has been a foundation for medical practice in the Western Tradition. I hope the reader will take a little time to look at it carefully as parts of it resonate throughout this book.

The Oath[1]

By Apollo (the physician), by Asclepius (god of healing), by Hygeia (god of health), by Panacea (god of remedy), and all the gods and goddesses, together as witnesses, I hereby swear that I will carry out, inasmuch as I am able and true to my considered judgment, this oath and the ensuing duties:

1. To hold my teacher in this art on a par with my parents. To make my teacher a partner in my livelihood. To look after my teacher and financially share with her/him when s/he is in need. To consider him/her as a brother/sister along with his/her family. To teach his/her family the art of medicine, if they want to learn it, without tuition or any other conditions of service. To impart all the lessons necessary to practice medicine to my own sons and daughters, the sons and daughters of my teacher, and to my own students, who have taken this oath—but to no one else.
2. I will help the sick according to my skill and judgment, but never with an intent to do harm or injury to another.

Medical Ethics, Second Edition. Edited by Michael Boylan.
© 2014 John Wiley & Sons, Inc. Published 2014 by John Wiley & Sons, Inc.

3. I will never administer poison to anyone—even when asked to do so. Nor will I ever suggest a way that others (even the patient) could do so. Similarly, I will never induce an abortion. Instead, I will keep holy my life and art.
4. I will not engage in surgery—not even upon suffers from stone, but will withdraw in favor of others who do this work.
5. Whoever I visit, rich or poor, I will concern myself with the well-being of the sick. I will commit no intentional misdeeds, nor any other harmful action such as engaging in sexual relations with my patients (regardless of their status).
6. Whatever I hear or see in the course of my professional duties (or even outside the course of treatment) regarding my patients is strictly confidential and I will not allow it to be spread about. But instead, will hold these as holy secrets.

Now if I carry out this oath and not break its injunctions, may I enjoy a good life and may my reputation be pure and honored for all generations. But if I fail and break this oath, then may the opposite befall me.

Within this oath are both a moral code for the profession of medicine and the outlines of a system of accreditation for new physicians via an apprenticeship. These two functions went a long way to establishing medicine as a profession that ordinary people could trust.

In the modern world there are many professional codes of conduct. One could look at the American Medical Association Code, the American Bar Association Code, among others. However, the Hippocratic Oath set the standard of what a professional code is. Certain key features will indicate why one should accept or reject such codes as solutions to the problems that have been outlined.

It is this author's opinion that among professional codes, the Hippocratic Oath is a good one. It balances between very specific prohibitions, such as not administering poison or not having sexual relations with one's patients, to more general principles such as "I will concern myself with the well-being of the sick" and "do no harm." These general principles are very useful because they govern a larger domain than simply prohibiting a particular action. These principles are not set out without context; instead they are put into the context of medicine's mission.

Beginning in #1 the tone is set that medicine is an art that is "given by the gods." It is an esoteric art that is to be reserved for those who are willing to commit to the provisions of the code. Thus, it is not open to everyone. This fulfills the condition of specialized knowledge mentioned earlier. It is for the sake of doing good to others and always avoiding harm. This fulfills the condition of providing a service for others.

Thirdly, the code ties itself to the larger moral tradition, "I will commit no intentional misdeeds." Whereas "harm" has a direct link to the manner in which medicine is practiced, "misdeeds" links the physician to the larger moral tradition. There is no possible hiding in the shared community perspective alone. These three factors are the basis of any good professional code.

A good professional code should contain:

1. A specific listing of common abuses.
2. A few general guidelines that tie behavior to the mission of the profession.
3. A link to general theories of morality.

Where codes of professional ethics fail is in emphasizing one of these elements too highly or in ignoring an element entirely. If codes of ethics exist in order to remedy the "inward perspective" problem described above, then they must create links to more general "shared worldviews." This would put them in the realm of common morality.

This is the most important point from my perspective. So often the "practice" of the profession defines its excellence in an introspective way such that the achievement of these functional requirements is all that matters—divorced from any other visions, namely, moral visions.

In the modern arena, many professional codes have evolved from a legal perspective. The practitioners of the profession do not want to go to jail or to be sued. Thus, they create certain codes that will make this possible situation less probable. These sorts of codes are defensive in nature and stand at the opposite end of the spectrum from the Hippocratic Oath. Their mission is not to set internal standards and link to common morality, rather they seek to "shave" as close as possible to maximizing an egoistic bottom line at the expense of the pillars of professionalism: one's specialized education and one's mission to serve others.

Any code that takes as its basis merely a negative approach designed to protect the practitioner from going to jail or being sued is fundamentally inadequate. This is not where one should set one's sights. Rather, we should dream about what the profession may be in the best of all possible worlds. The Oath of Hippocrates thus properly sets the mission that should drive all codes of ethics.

A. Paternalism and Autonomy

Overview: How much control should each of us have over our own healthcare choices? Most of us would reply that we should have as much control as possible. Who would turn over control of his or her life to another? Does autonomy not go hand in hand with the freedom and self-determination that are upheld by most moral theories?

This view has a twofold problem: First, to be autonomous (literally a self-lawmaker), an individual must have adequate knowledge to explore and examine all options and what risk and benefits are involved. This specialized knowledge is beyond the scope of most patients, so that they must rely on others to present the information they lack (often in a simplified version). The professional's judgment is generally superior to that of an enlightened layperson. Thus, the factual understanding along with the judgment of experience generally puts the physician/nurse into a paternalistic position from the outset. (*Paternalism* refers here to acting in the patient's best interests. It is especially troublesome when patients do not understand what is in their best interests so that physicians are in the position of ignoring the patients' wishes and acting as they, the physicians, see fit.)

In the practice of medicine, patients can (and should) be brought into the decision-making process, but they are rarely able to become full collaborators. Thus, their knowledge and judgment limit patient autonomy.

Second, the patient is often in an impaired state, which makes fully deliberative decision-making rather difficult at best. The patient is either in pain, emotionally traumatized, or in some way unable to make a fully unemotional, rational decision.

To burden a patient with the full weight of being an autonomous partner in the health-care decision-making process may be unfair to the patient.

Including the patient in the process as much as circumstances permit has advantages, although the time constraints involved in split-second life-and-death situations often prevent this. By including the patient in the process, the physician/nurse is recognizing and affirming the patient's dignity. Too often physicians have included only their more intelligent patients in the decision-making process. Also, paternalism can cloak racist or sexist predilections on the part of the physician/nurse. Thus, some form of autonomy seems absolutely necessary. If both autonomy (in some form) and paternalism (in some form) are inevitable, how should they be balanced? Are there any guiding principles that might be used to assist healthcare professionals?

To answer these questions, John-Stewart Gordon begins his essay by distinguishing between strong and weak paternalism. This distinction is then situated in Mill's understanding of liberty. Next, the birth of paternalism in the Western tradition is examined via the Hippocratic tradition. The various reasons for the rise of paternalism are set out and then contrasted to the rise of patient autonomy. All of these factors are developed into a current model of four types of physician-patient relationship. Using this model, the spin-off issues include human subject research, surrogate decision-making situations, and cost efficacy ratio along with futile treatment. In short, Gordon sets up most of the major questions into a current context.

Julian Savulescu argues that conventional defenders of patient autonomy are mistaken because they view the physician as merely a fact provider to the patient, who will then make the decision about what to do about the patient's health. He argues that the physician must be more than a fact provider and must become an "argument" provider. This means that physicians must first determine what they think is the best course of treatment and then engage patients in a Socratic-style dialogue to ensure that patients really understand what they are doing when they make choices about their own treatment. This scenario is rational because it engages physicians in a logical, ethical argument but is non-interventional because it does not have to seek overriding the patients' wishes as its ultimate goal.

B. Privacy and Confidentiality

Overview: Privacy and confidentiality find their source in the Hippocratic Oath. The underlying assumption is that a physician, nurse, or healthcare worker must know all the facts to be able to treat a patient effectively. If patients believe that some health facts are embarrassing or otherwise wish not to disclose them, they will not divulge them unless they know that these facts will be held in confidence. Failure to disclose pertinent information is a particular problem in the public health field. It affects not only the patient but also people with whom the patient has had contact and to whom the patient may have transferred the disease. Because these people may be denied information, they may not receive necessary treatment.

A threat to the privacy and confidentiality issue is the increasing number of data-bases that record our health information so that insurance companies can assess it to determine medical reimbursement. Although these databases strive to be accurate, anecdotal information leads me to believe that sometimes this information is misused. Obviously, the Internet has made the movement of information very easy. It has also created the possibility for "black-hat" hackers to steal medical information. This information can be used to discriminate against us in our work and threaten our status in society.

One way that such threats are meant to be addressed in the United States is by the Health Insurance Portability and Accountability Act (1996), also known as HIPAA. This act calls for certain safeguards of patient information and an informed consent procedure that requires the patient to authorize various form of dissemination of the information—for example, to a spouse or to a telephone answering machine. Even the transmission of test results is controlled by HIPAA.

However, despite HIPAA, all is not rosy on Main Street. The first of the two essays in this section explores the new biology and ownership of DNA information and privacy as it plays out in testing vulnerable populations. This new frontier of information privacy is examined by David Koepsel, who has written a book on the subject.[2] He explores first the idea of there being a legal zone of privacy. This was explored in the courts in *Griswold v. Connecticut* in 1965. But biomedical privacy is a little trickier (as indicated above because of the new information age). When it comes to genomic technologies a whole range of information about ourselves is at stake. If there are some genetic predispositions for phenotypic behavior that can be tested, then these tests can be used against an individual. Clearly, a firewall of some sort is necessary. Our genetic make-up is a part of our personhood so that our very identity is at stake in this timely instantiation of privacy.

In the second essay of the section, Katharine Smith and Jan Russell explore privacy issues from the point of view of African American women infected with the human immunodeficiency virus (HIV). How do the concerns of privacy affect these individuals in their day-to-day lives? Obviously, whether to disclose their HIV status is an ethical issue; embedded within it are the various personal factors that confront these women, such as the "unfairness" of being afflicted with HIV in general and aspects of their self-image. If the ethics of caring requires us to empathize with another's particular circumstance, then appreciation of the needs and concerns of actual people suffering is crucial in being able to treat their medical needs. Thus, gaining trust and building confidence in another is crucial so that the patient will reveal her or his true health condition.

C. Informed Consent

Overview: Informed consent is related to autonomy. The assumption is that a patient provided with all pertinent information will be able to deliberate and determine a course of treatment. The physician in this model acts as a fact provider, and the patient considers various options and then makes a free and unforced choice.

The model is perhaps flawed. To be fully informed, a patient would have to be a physician in that specialty. Obviously, most people cannot fully understand all the relevant information about their conditions. They can get some narrow sense of what is at stake, but this information may easily be contextually misunderstood.

This does not give license for complete paternalism. But one must recognize that "informed" is relative to the capability of the patient. A physician who waters down an explanation to the patient's level is paternalistically making choices in the way he or she presents alternatives.

Obviously, the choice of what to present can be affected by the physician's personal attitudes. In such cases, the physician or healthcare professional may decide that because of their race, religion, or gender, certain patients may or may not be capable of understanding their conditions. As a result, the healthcare provider engages in diagnosis-treatment discussions that may not engage patients at the highest level they can comprehend.

The last aspect of informed consent concerns clinical testing. For too long, researchers have not fully disclosed all known consequences that might befall a clinical test subject. From the Tuskegee experiment to various tests involving new pharmaceuticals, the history of informed consent in scientific research has not been good. We must determine how far we are willing to go to enforce strict standards.

Julian Savulescu and Richard Momeyer argue that for consent to be informed, it must be rational. They continue Savulescu's earlier argument by contending that the physician should be more than just a fact provider but also must be a Socratic agent who flushes out false beliefs. Obviously, this action causes the physician to create a set of acceptable beliefs. The authors of this essay use an example of a Jehovah's Witness to prove their point.

Ellen Agard, Daniel Finkelstein, and Edward Wallach present a case in which a woman's informed consent may be unduly influenced by her husband. Because the proposed operation will cause infertility, the hospital staff wants to be sure that "true" informed consent exists. The wild card is that this couple is from a culture in which the husband typically is allowed decision-making power over all the members of his household—including his wife! The issue is whether the hospital staff should determine the wife's true feelings and use those as the basis of informed consent or whether they should bend to the couple's cultural tradition and allow the husband to make the decision.

D. Gender, Culture, and Race

Overview: The practice of medicine concerns people interacting with each other in a vertically structured organizational scheme (much like the military). At the top are the head administrators. Then come the physicians, residents, nurses, and other support personnel. Whenever there is a strict chain-of-command organizational culture, power becomes critical. Those who are marginalized already in society because of gender, cultural heritage, or race will be even more put into the background of invisibility or else fired.

It is also the case that within this power structure, European-descent males are the most prevalent. This can lead to a disconnect between the healthcare provider and a diverse patient population. Ideally, the hospital staff should mirror the patient population by gender, cultural background, and race. This will lead to better communication and more effective care.

One developing philosophical tradition is that of feminist bioethics. In this tradition, these possible problems within the existing system are examined with the best interests of all at heart. This includes some emotive connection through the doctrine of care. However, emotive connection is a high hurdle for medicine. The history of doctor–patient interaction has traditionally been one in which the physician is a god who can do no wrong and is surrounded by an impersonal aura to *avoid* any emotional connections. If *Homo sapiens* are more than just rational animals, but are emotional, feeling people as well, then the traditional model is deficient. Just how this deficiency plays out is the subject of these essays.

Mary Mahowald begins the discussion by using the metaphor of nearsightedness to describe the present state of the medical community. Near-sighted people do not see certain realities because their vision extends only so far and they need glasses to allow them to see a wider range of phenomena that hitherto had been unclear. Mahowald argues that biomedical ethics should go beyond the narrow focus on groups and mere abstractions and focus on individuals as well. Individuals and their personal relationships are just as much the stuff of ethics as abstract concepts.

In making her argument, Mahowald refers to "standpoint" theory, which has some similarities to my own discussions of personal worldview. An extension of the feminist standpoint to medical ethics involves entering into the particularity of individual cases *for their own sake*, not merely for the generic description that they represent (as in the case of Al Brown). One way to integrate the feminist standpoint into the mainstream is to expand the range of voices heard and recognized. Such a prescription may well alter the ethos of biomedical practice.

In the second essay I take a look at a couple of ways in which cultural considerations can complicate the process of medical intervention. In much the same strategy as Agard *et al.*, I structure the essay around two key cases that involve patients with cultural backgrounds not of the United States, where care is being rendered. If the medical caregivers *ignore* culture altogether (under the assumption that the cultural standards of the United States are the only ones relevant), then the standard of care will suffer. The essay argues for increasing a standard of cultural competency to overcome this.

In the third essay, Richard E. Grant and I examine the reality of healthcare disparity, first from the perspective of ill served populations and then from the perspective of healthcare providers, who are often blind to this problem. It is the contention of the authors that one step toward addressing the first problem is to focus upon the second problem. This will benefit all segments of society. This essay then describes a pilot project to do just that at Case Western Reserve Hospitals that has been initiated by Grant and others.

Notes

1   Translation is mine.
2   David Koepsell, *Who Owns You?: The Corporate Gold Rush to Patent Your Genes*. Malden, MA, and Oxford: Wiley-Blackwell, 2009.

A. Paternalism and Autonomy

Medical Paternalism and Patient Autonomy

JOHN-STEWART GORDON

Introduction

According to Julian Savulescu and Richard W. Momeyer, it can be the case that patients suffer from irrational beliefs with regard to medical decisions they may be called upon to make. It may be that (1) their decisions are often based on ignorance, (2) patients do not devote enough attention to rational deliberation, or (3) patients may make mistakes in deliberation (Savulescu and Momeyer 2000, p. 129). With reference to such beliefs, the authors rightly argue that "it is the responsibility of physicians not only to provide relevant information (which addresses 1), but to improve the rationality of belief that grounds consent (2 and 3)" (Savulescu and Momeyer, 2000, p. 129). Admittedly, patients are not usually experts in either medicine or ethics and are therefore inexperienced in ethical reasoning and decision-making. Therefore, patients need the expertise and experience of physicians in order to make well-informed decisions. Given these circumstances it is to some extent understandable why physicians adhere to the idea of medical paternalism. However, the importance of patient autonomy needs to be stressed very strongly. It seems fair to say that, over the last 2500 years or so, physicians have adopted a disposition toward their patients based on the *Corpus Hippocraticum* (Hippocratic Corpus), which has made it almost impossible for them *not* to be paternalistic. The twentieth century has seen many atrocities conducted in the name of medicine and performed by physicians (e.g. during the Nazi era, the Tuskegee Syphilis Study, human radiation experiments). A general revulsion after the occurrence of such atrocities certainly contributed to the rise of patient autonomy and patients' rights. Nowadays, the idea of patient autonomy is highly influential and the right of a competent person to make autonomous decisions related to medical matters is acknowledged in many countries. This chapter gives an overview of some of the important issues related to medical paternalism and patient autonomy.

Preliminary Distinctions

According to Joel Feinberg, it is necessary to distinguish between two types of paternalism. The first type can be called "strong paternalism" and the second "weak paternalism" (Feinberg, 1971). Weak paternalism describes cases where a person's decision will be overruled because that person is deemed unable to make an autonomous and competent decision in his or her own best interest. Strong paternalism describes a situation in which someone is acting on another person's behalf without his or her consent when that person is competent and autonomous. The latter case is an instance of interfering with a person's civil rights and liberties. It was John Stuart Mill who famously set out the first systematic anti-paternalistic critique of (weak) paternalism in his important book *On Liberty* (Mill, 1859), where he argued that only in cases of a possible danger to third parties should a person's right to self-determination be limited. Medical paternalism is not only confined to weak paternalism but also covers strong paternalism. In addition, (medical) paternalism is not only about interfering with a patient's freedom of action, but also concerns either the withholding of vital information or the practice of misinforming the patient about his or her health condition, that is, undermining his or her right to freedom of information.

The Birth of Medical Paternalism

The Hippocratic Oath and the self-conception of the physician

The *Corpus Hippocraticum* (500 BC) was the first collection of important fragments of medical practice and medical ethics in early European history that could be seen as a general ethical guide for physicians. In this text, the physician is portrayed as a virtuous godlike healer with great authority and expertise that justifies paternalistic decision-making. The dominance of the approach of the *Corpus Hippocraticum* can be easily detected by its widespread use on a global level. All physicians are nowadays obligated to swear the Hippocratic Oath and to meet the demands stated in the *Corpus Hippocraticum*. The *Corpus Hippocraticum* contains the two leading principles of medical ethics, namely, the principle of non-maleficence (*primum nil nocere*) and the principle of beneficence (*salus aegroti suprema lex*). Furthermore, it prescribes—among other things—the principle of physician–patient confidentiality, it forbids taking sexual advantage of the patient, and it allows for acting against the declared patient's will, if it is for the sake of the patient.

Over the last 2500 years, the *Corpus Hippocraticum* has deeply influenced the self-conception of physicians as godlike[1] healers who deal with the most important human good, namely, the health of human beings. Good physicians, admittedly, have to be true experts in medicine in order to save lives and to defy death. Even with respect to less serious matters than life and death, most people tend to have a high degree of respect and honor for physicians. They are generally regarded as an outstanding group of people because it is thought that they perform such a difficult task in such a professional manner that it simply far exceeds their own capacities, knowledge, and intelligence to such a great extent that they cannot help but gaze in wonder, independently of whether this is always the case or not. Interestingly, however, many people not only see physicians as godlike healers but also think that they are (almost as) good at other tasks as well (as if they were also experts in other numerous fields), which is, of course, an absurd assumption. To put it in a nutshell, physicians have almost always been highly regarded and well respected, which, in turn, has influenced their self-conception accordingly. This is the background of medical paternalism as a kind of "natural disposition" of physicians.

Justifying medical paternalism

What are the reasons for medical paternalism? We have already seen that the amalgam of the complex physician-patient relationship in terms of praising the praiseworthy is rather an explanation for *why* there *is* medical paternalism but not a justification for *why* there *should be* medical paternalism. In other words, one should seek some valid arguments to justify this position. There are, at least, three main arguments—the physician knows best, the patient may be overwhelmed by the situation, and there may be a significant risk—in favour of medical paternalism, and these will be examined below.[2]

The physician knows best

The idea that the physician should decide what is in the best interest of his or her patient—even if it means that some decisions are made against the will of the patient—is derived from the physician's powerful standing as a great expert in matters of life and death related to human health, in addition to his or her great expertise in and knowledge of medicine. Against this background, the very idea to leave it up to the patient to decide which treatment plan should be followed seems almost ludicrous. The "normal" patient is usually incompetent in terms of medical knowledge and its application to specific cases (including his or her own case). If this is the case, why should the physician respect the will of the patient at all?

Doubtless, the physician is an expert and will be able to help the patient. However, it does not necessarily follow that a patient would definitely have no say with regard to the treatment plan. One might object that one must consider the particular circumstances of a given case (i.e., context-sensitivity). For example, it is certainly true that in emergency cases a patient will be unable to make a good decision—if he or she is still responsive—and hence the physician should make the decision for the sake of the patient in the patient's best interest. In other cases, however, a different strategy is more appropriate, for example, in non-extreme cases in which the patient's will and autonomy should be respected. All depends on the given circumstances of the particular case. Even in extreme cases such as end-of-life issues, and in particular euthanasia, it should not be entirely up to the physician to decide what the patient should do (Gordon *et al.*, 2011). Ethical reasoning and decision-making in extreme cases is strongly dependent on the personal worldview, idiosyncratic life history, cultural context, religious views, and value system of the particular patient, which have to be taken into account in order to make a good decision. Hence, it does not follow that the physician should, in general, decide what the patient must do. Physicians are morally obligated to respect the autonomy and the will of the patient, even if they disagree with the personal decision of the patient in question (see Mill's line of argumentation against anti-paternalism in *On Liberty*).

The patient is overwhelmed by the situation

Each diagnostic and therapeutic medical intervention can potentially present a problem for the patient's self-determination, because it limits his or her capacity to make good decisions—at least to some extent—because of the following factors: experiencing pain, physical and psychological distress, and ignorance / unknowingness (the list is not complete). Hence, medical paternalism is, in general, preferable since the damage to the patient's health in cases of non-compliance with the physician's decision may be a greater loss than the comparably smaller damage related to the limitation of patient autonomy.

If the patient is overwhelmed by the situation, for example, in emergency cases, then it seems appropriate to follow the physician's advice. But the idea that *each* medical intervention undermines the patient's self-determination and hence the physician should make the decisions in all cases is certainly exaggerated. Furthermore, in extreme cases where there is a living will while the patient is not responsive, the physician must consider the will of the patient and take it as seriously as possible. Otherwise, the physician should be held accountable for acting against the declared living will or current will of the patient. Patients are not little children who constantly need guidance and whose "decisions" can be easily overruled by their parents.

The significant risk

A good argument in favor of strong paternalism, according to its proponents, can be found in cases where either the non-action of the physician or the non-compliance of the patient directly leads to a significant risk of ill health with regard to the particular patient. Since the patient does not want to worsen his or her situation, he or she must accept a legitimate sense of medical paternalism.

The above-mentioned argument in support of strong paternalism presupposes that each patient is always interested in doing everything within his or her power to either remain healthy or to regain his or her strength. It can easily be the case that a particular person wants to commit suicide because of his or her ill health (or other reasons) and does not want to comply with the physician's decision to have more painful surgery, or such like. At some point the physician must accept that sometimes treatment is either futile or that the patient feels that his or her life is no longer worth living.

The Invention of Patient Autonomy

The notion(s) of autonomy

Generally speaking, a decision is autonomous if the person can be held accountable for his or her actions. The idea of patient autonomy, with particular regard to the notion of individual informed consent, is a modern invention and it is now standard practice for the patient's consent to be obtained with regard to a treatment plan if the patient is competent. In cases where the patient is incompetent, due to factors such as severe depression, mental disability, old age, or if they are suffering from Alzheimer's, a surrogate decision-maker—either a family member or a legal official—must be appointed to make decisions in the best interest of the patient.

Many authors wrongly assume that the notion of informed consent has its origin in the Nuremberg Code (1947). This resulted from the famous Nuremberg trial (1946–7) of German physicians who carried out research on human beings during the Nazi era without obtaining the consent of their guinea pigs (mostly Jews). Among the 10 universal moral principles of the Nuremberg Tribunal's judgment was one exclusively directed to the issue of research on human beings. This principle is the principle of autonomy, which contains the proposed "new" idea of informed consent. In fact, however, the idea of informed consent has a different historical origin. In particular, the idea of individual informed consent is due to the Prussian and German bureaucratic regulations of 1900/01 that appeal to the case of Dr Albert Neisser in 1896, who publicly announced his concern about the possible dangers to the experimental subjects whom he vaccinated with an experimental immunizing serum. Additionally, the investigation of the deaths of 75 German children caused by the use of experimental tuberculosis vaccines in 1931 revealed that the *mandatory* informed consent was not obtained. Robert Baker rightly states that "[t]he informed consent doctrine was thus originally a regulatory innovation created by Prussian bureaucrats. It was not an artefact of American legal or philosophical culture but of German bureaucratic culture. It was a German solution to problems created by the advances of German biomedical science" (Baker, 1998b, p. 250). Admittedly, Baker's following comment on this point is certainly true: "It is indeed ironic that the 1931 German position on *informed* consent to research on human subjects was considerably more advanced than anything in Anglo-American ethical or legal theory at the time of the Nuremberg Trial. Compounding the irony, the Nuremberg Tribunal may be the first *American* court to introduce the *German* idea of *informed* consent into American law and thus into American and international medical ethics" (Baker, 1998b, p. 269).[3]

The elements of (individual) informed consent are described clearly by Tom Beauchamp and James Childress in their influential book *Principles of Biomedical Ethics* (Beauchamp and Childress, 2009, pp. 99–148). The following brief and self-explanatory depiction is taken from their book (Beauchamp and Childress, 2009, pp. 120–1).

Elements of informed consent

- Threshold elements (preconditions):
  1. competence (to understand and decide);
  2. voluntariness (in deciding).
- Information elements:
  3. disclosure (of material information);
  4. recommendation (of a plan);
  5. understanding (of 3 and 4).
- Consent elements:
  6. decision (in favor of a plan);
  7. authorization (of the chosen plan).

In *Global Ethics and Principlism* (Gordon, 2011) I state that "Beauchamp and Childress propose that obtaining an individual's informed consent, which is, according to Western medical practice, an ethical and legal requirement (Agard *et al.*, 2000, p. 154) is a specification [of] the principle of autonomy (Beauchamp and Childress, 2009, pp. 117–35). However, non-Western countries such as China, Japan and most African countries do not share the idea of individual informed consent in biomedical ethics. Instead, they generally demand that either family- or community-informed consent should be obtained in cases such as life-threatening diseases, breaking bad news at the bedside of terminally ill patients, human research experimentation, and female circumcision/mutilation." (Gordon, 2011, p. 261). The implication of this is that patient autonomy is not only limited to individual-informed consent, but also includes family- or community-informed consent. This is an important observation, since the viewpoint of the family may clash with the family member's decision in, for example, end-of-life cases (e.g., euthanasia) or in cases where the family wants to withhold information from the sick family member for the sake of the person in question (bedside rationing, truth-telling).

What is *in* the best interest of the patient? The case of truth telling

A classic case in which patient autonomy and patient rights have been (and are still) neglected on a regular basis concerns terminally ill (cancer) patients and the common idea that one should not inform the patient in question about his or her bad prognosis. This policy was often carried out in many Western countries until very recently and is still common in some non-Western countries such as Japan (Macklin, 1999). The underlying assumption in support of this paternalistic reasoning is the idea that to inform the patient about his or her severe condition, that is, to tell the truth, would not be beneficial to the patient as the knowledge would be likely to harm the patient because he or she might, in addition, develop a severe (suicidal) depression, which would worsen the condition and most likely hasten death. Hence, it follows that one should not inform terminally ill patients about their true condition because it would not be in the best interest of the particular patient.[4] However, this line of argument not only obviously undermines the patient's autonomy (i.e., *individual* informed consent) and individual rights but also his or her dignity. Furthermore, it seems inappropriate not to give patients the opportunity to settle their affairs, for example, to say goodbye to their family (depending on who makes the decision to not inform the person), relatives, and close friends. Additionally, it also poses a problem in that patients are not given the chance to reconcile themselves with friends or relatives or some family members with whom they may have been in conflict. If one does not know that one will die (very) soon, then one cannot take appropriate steps to settle one's affairs in an appropriate manner. Of course, most patients might "feel" that they will most likely die soon but "to feel that one will die soon" is certainly not the same as "to know that one will die soon." The issue in question concerns this "small" but vital difference and there is no easy solution to the problem. To put it in a nutshell, one might cause patients some additional harm (e.g., depression), but helping them to settle their affairs certainly benefits patients. Ultimately, telling them the truth is now seen as the most ethical course and the most beneficial with regard to patients' peace of mind.[5]

The Four Models of the Physician-Patient Relationship

Ezekiel L. Emanuel and Linda L. Emanuel (1992) elaborated four different models to illustrate the dynamics of the physician-patient relationship: the informative, the interpretive, the deliberative, and the paternalistic model:

- **Informative Model**
  a. Patient values: Defined, fixed, and known to the patient.
  b. Physician's obligation: Providing relevant factual information and implementing patient's selected intervention.
  c. Conception of patient's autonomy: Choice of, and control over, medical care.
  d. Conception of physician's role: Competent technical expert.
- **Interpretive Model**
  a. Patient values: Inchoate and conflicting, requiring elucidation.
  b. Physician's obligation: Elucidation and interpreting relevant patient values as well as informing the patient and implementing the patient's selected intervention.
  c. Conception of patient's autonomy: Self-understanding relevant to medical care.
  d. Conception of physician's role: Counsellor or adviser.
- **Deliberative Model**
  a. Patient values: Open to development and revision through moral discussion.
  b. Physician's obligation: Articulating and persuading the patient of the most admirable values as well as informing the patient and implementing the patient's selected intervention.
  c. Conception of patient's autonomy: Moral self-development relevant to medical care.
  d. Conception of physician's role: Friend or teacher.
- **Paternalistic Model**
  a. Patient values: Objective and shared by the physician and patient.
  b. Physician's obligation: Promoting the patient's well-being independently of the patient's current preferences.
  c. Conception of patient's autonomy: Assenting to objective values.
  d. Conception of physician's role: Guardian.

Their important article, "Four models of the physician-patient relationship," has come to be regarded as authoritative and has been very influential in the field of medical ethics (Emanuel and Emanuel, 1992, pp. 2221–7). The traditional paternalistic model, in which the physician is seen as an unquestioned guardian, and the (extreme libertarian) informative model, where the physician is a mere handmaid with great expertise (e.g. in cosmetic surgery), can be seen as the two extremes of the physician-patient relationship. The interpretive and the deliberative models are moderate approaches. Against this background, it seems crystal clear that one should avoid the extreme models and try to adhere to moderate approaches in order to maintain patient autonomy and to limit the influence of paternalistic reasoning and decision-making in medical ethics. There is no good reason to simply accept the idea that there is no problem in undermining a competent person's autonomy and thereby to limit his or her self-determination (see "What is *in* the best interest of the patient? The case of truth telling" above). Strong and weak forms of paternalism need to be justified well and must only be applied to special cases, that is, in emergencies. They should not be regarded as the general way to proceed but should only be considered as exceptions.[6] In the following three cases, the ethical problems of medical paternalism are examined briefly within the context of the previous discussion.

Vital Issues Concerning Medical Paternalism

Research on human subjects

Medical experiments, for example, experiments on hypothermia, high-altitude studies in decompression chambers, forced sterilizations of women with X-rays, and experiments to make sea water drinkable, which were conducted on Jews by Nazi physicians in Germany, are only one example of (medical) research involving physicians (Annas and Grodin 1995). The Tuskegee Syphilis Study, in which US physicians studied the natural spread of syphilis among African-Americans between 1932 and 1972 in Tuskegee, Alabama, is another example (NCPHS, 1979). Finally, the Human Radiation Experiments conducted on prison inmates by physicians in the United States during the Cold War period, where some inmates and their food were contaminated with radioactivity, is yet another example of medical research on human subjects (Advisory Committee on Human Radiation Experiments, 1996). What all these cases have in common is that no individual informed consent was obtained, even though it was legally necessary to do so. It is fair to claim that no research subject would have given their consent if they had had any relevant information about the details of the given research in the above-mentioned cases. In this respect, medical paternalism and patient autonomy are—at least to some extent—mutually exclusive. It is a "golden rule" that physicians and researchers are obligated to obtain the individuals' informed consent when it involves research on human subjects—a rule articulated by the Nuremberg Code (Trials of War Criminals Before the Nuremberg Military Tribunals under Control Council Law, 1947), the Declaration of Helsinki (World Medical Association, 1964), and the Universal Declaration of Human Rights (United Nations, 1948). But even in our time, some pharmaceutical companies conduct research on human beings in developing countries because the requirements are less stringent than in their home countries (Macklin, 2004). The upshot is that medical paternalism is liable to abuse in a wide range of different cases. If this is the case, however, why not take *patient autonomy* seriously in order to avoid the slippery slope? Medical paternalism is based on or presupposes a trusting relationship between patients and physicians. This trust may become treacherous and misleading in cases of abuse where the research subject is harmed. In such cases, the physician uses the trust which has been established to conduct his or her research, not for the sake of the patient but for the sake of the research. This is one of the main reasons—among others—why the abuse is so abominable.

The incompetent patient and surrogate decision-making

There are quite a few cases where a person may suddenly lose his or her autonomy and hence become incompetent, by virtue of a severe accident, for example (other cases may include persons with a mental disability[7]). The patient, therefore, needs a surrogate decision-maker. If the accident was very bad and the patient is in coma and the prognosis means that recuperation is impossible, then the question of what to do remains. Sometimes people have made a living will that depicts the kind of circumstances under which they would, for example, wish to be unplugged from a respirator, and so on, and be left to die in peace and dignity, according to their personal beliefs, because they may have decided that such a life would simply not be worth living (e.g., the Terri Schiavo case; see Caplan *et al.*, 2006). If this coincides with the viewpoint of the surrogate decision-maker—who is either a family member or a legal official—then the patient in question might be unplugged from the respirator given that there is no probability of recuperation. This last step, however, could bring some great problems. Physicians, including members of the administration, working at a hospital are usually not very keen to comply with such demands and often opt out by claiming that such a procedure is against their professional ethos (i.e. the Hippocratic Oath), their conscience, personal and cultural values, or religious views. In such cases, the patient will have no opportunity get have his or her wish fulfilled, unless there is another physician who is willing to unplug the patient from the respirator. Even if a court decrees that unplugging the person from the respirator can be done, it still needs a person to unplug the patient. This means that since one cannot force a physician—and maybe rightly so—to act against his or her conscience, this kind of situation regularly poses problems for relatives. This is a case where medical paternalism may be in conflict with patient autonomy, since the very idea of the *living will* is to represent a person's autonomy in cases of incompetence. The physicians' negative attitude is a case of strong paternalism. There is, indeed, no easy way out in such cases.

The cost-efficacy ratio and futile treatment

The most straightforward case with regard to a clash between medical paternalism (physicians, hospital administration) and patient autonomy concerns cases in which a particular medical treatment is seen as futile, with a high cost-efficacy ratio (particularly important in times of great strain on the healthcare systems) and very limited benefit to the patient.[8] The treatment is, medically speaking, futile and the physician and the hospital administration deny that further action should be taken. The patient and his or her family want the medical treatment because they believe that it would be (very) beneficial to the patient. If the patient's decision is based on ignorance or on a failure in rational deliberation (Savulescu and Momeyer, 2000), then the physician should try everything in his or her power to clarify the facts (e.g., consult other physicians, discuss the issue with a clinical ethics consultant[9]). If it is not possible to come to a solution and the physician still denies further medical treatment, then the patient should have the opportunity to ask another physician and/or hospital. The physician, however, should not be forced to treat a person against his or her professional judgement (that it would be a futile treatment) concerning the case in question. Medical knowledge should be decisive in such cases, but one should, of course, acknowledge that such cases are not only about medical facts but also raise concerns about underlying values, and cultural and religious views, as well as substantive views of how one should live and die in dignity. The different views of the particular parties (i.e., physicians, patients) may make a simple solution very difficult and sometimes (almost) impossible. Hence, it follows that in some (rare) cases one should not fulfill all wishes and comply with all the ideas a patient has only because one is obligated to respect his or her patient autonomy and rights. Patient autonomy is no charter for everything that a patient wants in medical matters. Patient autonomy should be respected as long as it is reasonable. But what is reasonable? A medical decision about the reasonableness of a given treatment—whether it is futile or not—certainly involves medical facts, rational deliberation/practical wisdom, and the ability to put oneself in the position of the patient. If all the issues have been carefully considered and the particular case has been competently examined in great detail and effort, then one should accept and trust the physician's advice to forgo the medical treatment.

Conclusions

Medical paternalism—as a *general* strategy of ethical reasoning and decision-making in medicine—should be in retreat. Taking patient autonomy and patient rights seriously is not only a matter of taking competent adults seriously but also respecting them as rational human beings of equal moral standing. Physicians *must* obtain the informed consent of the patient so that there is an agreement with regard to the treatment plan. Otherwise, they act immorally. With regard to the disclosure of vital information concerning the health of the patient in question, it seems that the physician is obligated to reveal the truth under normal circumstances. In extreme cases, however, it seems reasonable to withhold the relevant information if and only if it is beneficial to the patient.

Notes

1   In the introduction to *A Companion to Bioethics* Helga Kuhse and Peter Singer cite M.B. Etziony (1973) in the following way: "A monument in the sanctuary of Asclepius, for example, tells doctors to be 'like God: saviour equally to slaves, of paupers, of rich men, of princes, and to all a brother, such help he would give'" (Etziony, 1973, in Kuhse and Singer, 2009, p. 4).

2   Bernard Gert, Charles M. Culver, and K. Danner Clouser thoroughly examine the notion of paternalism and its justification in the chapter 10 ("Paternalism and its justification") of their book *Bioethics. A Systematic Approach* (Gert et al., 2006, pp. 237–82). The general view is that "Although paternalism is often unjustified, it is not always morally unacceptable. On the contrary,

not only is paternalism often justified, it is sometimes even morally required so that in some situations not acting paternalistically can be immoral" (p. 237).

3   The answer of the main question, then, as to why the Germans did not practice "informed consent" on their subjects of experimentation, namely the Jews, is obvious. They did not regard the Jews as *human beings*. They were, rather, *Untermenschen* and, hence, according to the doctrines of Nazi Germany, were not protected by the legal regulations of informed consent of 1931 (see also Baker, 1998a, p. 211). Animals were better protected than those people who were guinea pigs of German research experimentation. These people were treated as non-humans and were

also regarded as standing below the animals—a detestable point of view.

4   A (still) valuable contribution is Donald Oken's influential study, first published in *JAMA* (Oken, 1976), of medical paternalism with regard to legally competent patients in "What to tell cancer patients: a study of medical attitudes", subsequently reprinted in *Moral Problems in Medicine* (eds. Samuel Gorovitz et al., 1976, pp. 109–16). Even though one has to acknowledge that there has been a great deal of change since that study, it is still fair to say that many physicians around the world do not inform their patients in cases of terminal cancer.

5   An interesting discussion with further compelling arguments in support of truth telling with regard to terminally ill cancer patients can be found in Allen Buchanan's article "Medical paternalism" (Buchanan, 1978).

6   Tom Beauchamp argues in his article "The concept of paternalism in biomedical ethics" (Beauchamp, 2009) that strong paternalism can be justified in some cases, despite the contemporary trend in biomedical ethics to question the strong paternalistic approach. His final conclusion is "It is clear that many paternalistic interventions are justified. It does not follow that they all are. I have argued that it is an open question whether reasonably minor offenses to autonomy such as withholding certain forms of information are justified in light of critical medical goals such as the administration of life-saving therapies and the prevention of suicide" (p. 92).

7   For this particular problem see, for example, Stephen Wear's article "Patient autonomy, paternalism, and the conscientious physician" (Wear, 1983).

8   Nancy S. Jecker, on the contrary, argues in her article "Is refusal of futile treatment unjustified paternalism?" (Jecker, 2000) that it is not the case that to refuse futile treatment is (always) an instance of unjustified paternalism, but instead may be consistent with patient autonomy and other positive values in medicine. It seems fair to say that, indeed, not all cases in which futile treatments are refused are due to medical paternalism, but that some cases can be plausibly conceived of in this way.

9   On the issue of clinical ethics consultation see the book *Clinical Ethics Consultation. Theories and Methods, Implementation, Evaluation* (Schildmann et al., 2010).

References

Advisory Committee on Human Radiation Experiments (1996) *The Human Radiation Experiments*. New York: Oxford University Press.

Agard, E., Finkelstein, D., and Wallach, E. (2000) Cultural diversity and informed consent. In: M. Boylan (ed.), *Medical Ethics. Basic Ethics in Action*. New Jersey: Prentice Hall; pp. 150–55.

Annas, G.J. and Grodin, M. (eds) (1995) *The Nazi Doctors and the Nuremberg Code: Human Rights in Human Experimentation*. New York: Oxford University Press.

Baker, R. (1998a) A theory of international bioethics: The negotiable and the non-negotiable. *Kennedy Institute of Ethics Journal* 8(3): 201–31.

Baker, R. (1998b) A theory of international bioethics: The negotiable and the non-negotiable. *Kennedy Institute of Ethics Journal* 8(3): 233–73.

Beauchamp, T.L. (2009) The concept of paternalism in biomedical ethics. *Jahrbuch für Wissenschaft und Ethik* 14: 77–92.

Beauchamp, T.L. and Childress, J.F. (2009) *Principles of Biomedical Ethics*. New York: Oxford University Press.

Buchanan, A. (1978) Medical paternalism. *Philosophy and Public Affairs* 7(4): 372–87.

Caplan, A.L., McCartney, J.J., and Sisti, D.A. (eds) (2006) *The Case of Terri Schiavo: Ethics at the End of Life*. New York: Prometheus Books.

Emanuel, E. and Emanuel, L. (1992) Four models of the physician-patient relationship, *Journal of the American Medical Association* 267(16): 2221–6.

Feinberg, J. (1971) Legal paternalism. *Canadian Journal of Philosophy* 1(1): 105–24.

Gert, B., Culver, M., and Danner Clouser, K. (2006) *Bioethics. A Systematic Approach*, 2nd edn. New York: Oxford University Press.

Gordon, J-S. (2011) Global ethics and principlism. *Kennedy Institute of Ethics Journal* 21(3): 251–76.

Gordon, J-S., Rauprich, O., and Vollmann, J. (2011) Applying the four-principle approach. *Bioethics* 25(6): 293–300.

Jecker, N. (2000) Is refusal of futile treatment unjustified paternalism? In: M. Boylan (ed.), *Medical Ethics. Basic Ethics in Action*. New Jersey: Prentice Hall; pp. 80–86.

Kuhse, H. and Singer, P. (2009) *A Companion to Bioethics*. Oxford: Blackwell.

Macklin, R. (1999) *Against Relativism. Cultural Diversity and the Search for Ethical Universal in Medicine*. New York and Oxford: Oxford University Press.

Macklin, R. (2004) *Double Standards in Medical Research in Developing Countries*. Cambridge: Cambridge University Press.

Mill, J.S. (1859) On liberty. In: J. Gray (ed.), *On Liberty and Other Essays*. Oxford World Classics (2009). Oxford: Oxford University Press.

NCPHS (National Commission for the Protection of Human Subjects of Biomedical and Behavioral Research) (1979) *The Belmont Report: Ethical Principles and Guidelines for the Protection of Human Subjects of Research*. Washington, DC: U.S. Government Printing Office.

Oken, D. (1961) What to tell cancer patients: A study of medical attitudes. *Journal of the American Medical Association* 175(13): 1120–8. Reprinted in:S. Gorovitz et al. (eds) (1976), *Moral Problems in Medicine*. Englewood Cliffs, NJ: Prentice Hall; pp. 109–16.

Savulescu, J. and Momeyer, R. (2000) Should informed consent be based on rational belief? In: M. Boylan (ed.), *Medical Ethics. Basic Ethics in Action*. New Jersey: Prentice Hall; pp. 128–40.

Schildmann, J., Gordon, J-S., and Vollmann, J. (2010) *Clinical Ethics Consultation: Theories and Methods, Implementation, Evaluation*. Farnham: Ashgate.

Trials of War Criminals Before the Nuremberg Military Tribunals under Control Council Law (1947) *The Nuremberg Code*. http://ohsr.od.nih.gov/guidelines/nuremberg.html [accessed February 21, 2013].

United Nations (1948) *The Universal Declaration of Human Rights*. www.un.org/en/documents/udhr/ [accessed February 21, 2013].

Wear, S. (1983) Patient autonomy, paternalism, and the conscientious physician. *Theoretical Medicine and Bioethics* 4(3): 253–74.

World Medical Association (1964) *The Declaration of Helsinki*. http://www.wma.net/en/30publications/10policies/b3/index.html [accessed February 21, 2013].

Rational Non-Interventional Paternalism

Why Doctors Ought to Make Judgments of What Is Best for Their Patients

JULIAN SAVULESCU

It is almost universally accepted that doctors ought to make judgments of what is medically best for their patients. However, the view that doctors ought to make judgments of what is, all things considered, best for their patients has fallen into serious disrepute. It is now widely believed that it is up to patients, not their doctors, to judge what they ought to do, all things considered. I will argue that doctors ought to make value judgments about what is best for their patients, not just in a medical sense, but in an overall sense.

In the bad old days of paternalism, doctors did make judgments about what patients ought to do, all things considered. They also compelled patients to adopt what they

"Rational Non-Interventional Paternalism: Why Doctors Ought to Make Judgments of What Is Best for Their Patients," by Julian Savulescu, originally published in the *Journal of Medical Ethics* 1995; 21: 327–31. Reprinted with permission of the BMJ Publishing Group.

judged to be the best course of action. Over the last twenty years, this approach has received much criticism. Liberal societies are founded upon a belief that we each have a fundamental interest in forming and acting on our own conception of what is good for us, what direction our lives should take, what is, all things considered, best for us. Forming a conception of what is best for oneself and acting on that conception is being an autonomous agent. By taking away from patients the ability to make and act on conceptions of what they judged was best, paternalists frustrated the autonomy of their patients.

There is a second problem with the old approach. Paternalists were making value judgments (often under the guise of what was 'medically or clinically indicated' [1]) which would have been more properly made by the patients who were going to be affected by the treatment. Consider one example. Joe is about to have an operation to remove a tumour from his diaphragm. An anaesthetist visits him preoperatively to discuss his anaesthetic. She then discusses post-operative analgesia. This, she explains, is very important because the major complication after his operation will be the development of lung collapse and pneumonia. If he does not receive adequate analgesia, and is unable to breathe deeply and cough comfortably, this will be much more likely. She informs him that there are two forms of analgesia available after his operation: thoracic epidural analgesia and intravenous narcotic infusion. The analgesic effectiveness of the thoracic epidural is greater. Joe will more easily be able to cough and breathe deeply, so better preventing the development of pneumonia. She explains that the risk of nerve damage from any epidural is around 1/15,000. There is an additional risk with thoracic epidurals in particular: a very small risk of spinal-cord damage from the procedure (damage from the needle) or complications that arise after it (epidural haematoma or abscess). In some of these cases, spinal-cord damage could result in paraplegia. There have only been isolated case reports of these complications so it is not possible to put a figure on how great the risk is but it is certainly very small. Overall, the risk of nerve damage is very small and the risk of developing pneumonia much greater. The anaesthetist explains the significance of developing pneumonia. In some cases, it results in respiratory failure requiring artificial ventilation. Such infections are sometimes very difficult to treat and patients stand a reasonable chance of dying if they develop respiratory failure. The overall risk of serious morbidity and mortality is greater if one has the narcotic infusion than if one has the epidural. She recommends having a thoracic epidural. (If she had been a paternalist, she would have simply inserted a thoracic epidural at operation.)

Joe, having understood all this information, chooses to have the narcotic infusion. He is an active sportsman and the risk of spinal-cord injury is very significant for him. He also claims that he is willing to put up with more pain, and still attempt to cough and breathe deeply, if in this way he will avoid the potential for harm to his spinal cord.

Two Reasons

In this case, which treatment Joe ought to have is not simply determined by facts related to Joe's health (the medical facts). There are two reasons why Joe's doctor ought not make a decision about what is, all things considered, best for Joe. Each has to do with a different sense of 'value'. Firstly, Joe's decision is based on his values, that is, what he is valuing. It is an essential element of self-determination that people construct a notion of what is important in their lives (their values) and act on these. Joe values independence and an active physical life. His choice reflects these values.

Secondly, the question of whether Joe ought to have the thoracic epidural is a value judgment, a judgment of what is of value. Judgments of what is of value, all things considered, are different from judgments of fact. It is a fact, let us assume, that a thoracic epidural is associated with better analgesia and a lower risk of developing pneumonia, but a greater risk of spinal-cord damage, than a narcotic infusion. However, it is not a fact that this makes thoracic epidural overall better for Joe. That is a value judgment. Value judgments must be based on all the relevant facts. These include the medical facts but also facts about the significance of the medical procedures for Joe's own life, and facts about his values. Since no one but Joe knows his plans, his hopes, his aspirations and his values, the argument goes, Joe is better placed than his doctor to evaluate the significance of the various benefits and complications of each treatment. Joe is in a privileged position to judge what is best, all things considered. Joe's doctor, ill-placed to know these other relevant facts, ought to stick to judgments about the medical facts.

For these reasons, medical practice has moved away from the old paternalistic model of 'Doctor knows best' or 'Doctor's orders' to the currently fashionable 'shared decision-making' model.

'Physicians bring their medical training, knowledge, and expertise—including understanding of the available treatment alternatives—to the diagnosis and management of the patients' conditions. Patients bring a knowledge of their own subjective aims and values, through which the risks and benefits of various options can be evaluated. With this approach, selection of the best treatment for a particular patient requires the contributions of both parties' [2].

On one widely held interpretation of this account, doctors bring medical knowledge, medical facts, to the patient who makes a judgment of what ought to be done on the basis of his or her values. Doctors give up making judgments of what is, all things considered, best for the patient and stick to providing medical facts. This approach has found considerable favour in the literature and in practice. Many informed general practitioners and medical students whom I have taught tell me that doctors ought not make tricky value judgments about their patients' lives.

This model of doctor as fact-provider has some serious shortcomings.

Firstly, it is not clear that doctors *can* avoid making value judgments about what patients ought to do, should do, or what it is best for them to do. Sometimes these value judgments are difficult to spot. Consider the oncologist whose patient has lung cancer. 'Chemotherapy is medically indicated', he says. This appears to be a purely descriptive, factual statement. But it is really also a prescription to have chemotherapy. If we were to ask this oncologist why chemotherapy was medically indicated, he might offer this argument: 1. chemotherapy will prolong your life; 2. longer life is better than shorter life; 3. so you ought to have chemotherapy. Premise 2 is clearly a value judgment.

It is difficult to see how doctors, as persons, could avoid making judgments like 2. The content of these value judgments varies from person to person, but it is difficult to imagine a person with no values. Most people have some norms which they apply to their behaviour. It is also difficult to imagine that these values do not come into play when a doctor is asked to perform a procedure on a patient.

'Framing Effect'

Perhaps doctors cannot avoid making value judgments, but they should keep these to themselves. According to the fact-provider model, doctors should just provide facts such as, 'Chemotherapy will prolong your life'.

However, it is not clear that facts can be communicated free of value. Psychologists have described how the way information is presented can determine the significance of that information for people. This is called the 'framing effect'. When choice is framed in terms of gain, we are risk-averse. When choice is framed in terms of loss, we are risk-taking [3]. For example, lung cancer can be treated by surgery or radiotherapy. Surgery is associated with greater immediate mortality (10 per cent v 0 per cent mortality), but better long term prospects (66 per cent v 78 per cent five-year mortality). The attractiveness of surgery to patients is substantially greater when the choice between surgery and radiotherapy is framed in terms of the probability of living rather than the probability of dying. This effect still occurs whether the evaluator is a physician or someone with statistical knowledge [4].

The manner in which physicians present information is influenced by their values. Surgeons present the probabilities of the outcome of surgery in terms of survival, not death. It is not clear that framing effects can easily be overcome. Even if we present probabilities in terms of both survival and mortality, people are 'loss averse'. They focus myopically on the loss associated with events [5]. Subtle nonverbal cues also influence the impact of information. Indeed, information seems ineluctably to bring with it a message. It is not difficult to recognise what someone values, even if they do not tell us. Far better, I think, to bring the practice out into the open, and argue explicitly for what we believe in.

But let's assume that doctors can give up either making value judgments or communicating them. Should they?

Medicine as a practice is founded on commitment to certain values: pain is bad, longer life is usually better than shorter life, and so on. A part of learning to practise medicine is learning to take on these values. These implicit evaluative assumptions rarely surface because they are a matter of consensus. 'Ethical dilemmas' arise when patient values diverge from medical values [6].

Should medicine give up a commitment to certain values? To be sure, we might believe that some of medicine's values are mistaken. Some ought to be changed or refined. But medicine should have a commitment to *some* values. Otherwise what would direct research effort, provide a standard of care or a framework for the organisation of practice? Mass consumer choice, a thin reed which bends to the prevailing winds, is sometimes irrational and even chaotic, at other times immovably apathetic, and seems ill-suited to provide such direction alone. This may be slightly hyperbolic, but it does seem true that medicine needs a set of values, no doubt shaped by informed public attitude, which guides practice. Those values must be more substantial than a commitment to do what every individual patient desires.

Moral Stakes

The second serious shortcoming of the doctor as fact-provider model is that medicine differs from many other professional practices in that the doctor is often called upon to do very serious things to his patient. In deciding to ablate a patient's bone marrow prior to bone-marrow transplantation, a doctor is going to make his patient very sick. There is unavoidable serious harm associated with medical practice that is far greater than in engineering or tax consultancy. The moral stakes are much higher. Since medical practice involves serious harm to others, as well as benefit, doctors ought to form a judgment of what ought to be done, all things considered. In the extreme case of assisted suicide, a patient asks her doctor to help her die. Should a person do this without making a decision whether it is for the best? Surely not. It is at least generally true that good moral agents reflect upon and form judgments concerning what they ought to do. The same applies to less spectacular, every-day instances of medical practice. Prescribing an antibiotic may cause renal failure. A good doctor must form a judgment about whether prescribing that antibiotic is really justified, even if the patient has an informed desire to have it.

Thirdly, and most importantly, patients can fail to make correct judgments of what is best, just as doctors can. Patients can fail to make choices which best satisfy their own values [7]. They can make choices which frustrate rather than express their own autonomy [8]. The mere fact that a competent patient makes an informed choice does not imply necessarily that that choice reflects what he values.

Patients can also make incorrect value judgments. They can fail to give sufficient weight to relevant facts, just as the old paternalists did when they concentrated on the medical facts. Consider an example.

Joan is 35 years old and has a one cm cancer of the breast without clinical evidence of lymph node metastasis. Her mother and sisters had cancer of the breast. Her surgeon argues, based on her history and the cytology of the tumour, that she has a very high chance of developing a second carcinoma. He recommends a bilateral mastectomy. This, he argues, will give her the best chance of survival. Joan replies that this will be very disfiguring. She would prefer to have a lumpectomy followed by yearly mammography. This, she argues, will give her a better quality of life.

Joan's surgeon inquires further. It turns out that by better quality of life, she means that she will retain her present physical appearance. Her husband would be shocked if she had a bilateral mastectomy, even if she were to have breast implants. 'He is very attached to my breasts', she says. Her marriage is difficult at present, and she does not believe that it would survive the shock of such operation.

These are of course relevant facts to which the surgeon was not originally privy. Previously, he believed she ought to have a mastectomy. Are these new facts of sufficient importance to cause him to change his judgment? In some cases, they might be. If survival with lumpectomy and mammography was roughly the same as that after mastectomy, then he might change his mind. If Joan's life was really going to be miserable after a mastectomy, and much happier after a lumpectomy, then this would be a good reason not to have the mastectomy.

However, in some cases, the surgeon might retain his original judgment. He might believe that, if the risk of dying from not having the mastectomy was significant, that it was not worth risking death to conform to her husband's and society's expectations of her physical appearance. Moreover, he might believe that if her relationship would be destroyed by her having a mastectomy, it was not likely to survive or was not worth dying for. He might believe, not necessarily without basis, that Joan will be unhappy in her marriage whether she has a lumpectomy or a mastectomy. He might believe that Joan is mistaken in attaching so much weight to her husband's attachment to her breasts. He might continue to believe that she ought to have the mastectomy, despite the revelation of new facts. Indeed, even in the presence of *all* relevant facts, if these could be discovered, he might believe that Joan ought to have a mastectomy. Despite having access to the same facts as Joan, such a doctor might continue to differ with her about what is best and he may continue to try to convince her that she is wrong.

Some value judgments are wrong. To claim that one's life is not worth living because one's bunion is painful is mistaken, no matter how well-informed the judgment. To be sure, doctors make wrong judgments of what is best. But so do patients at times.

It is of course easier to turn the decision over to Joan and just provide some medical facts. It is easier to avoid making an all-things-considered value judgment. It is difficult to discuss with a patient why she holds the views she does. It is difficult to provide an argument for why she is wrong which is convincing to her. But such discussion and argument can help patients to make better decisions for themselves. Good advice, which we should expect from our friends and doctors, consists in more than information.

Shared Decision-Making

There has been a movement away from paternalism. There are, however, two ways of responding to the problems which have thrown paternalism into disrepute. The first is for doctors to give up the practice of making judgments about what is, all things considered, best for their patients. They should stick to providing medical facts to competent patients who then make choices as to what is best based on their values. This is the model of 'shared decision-making'.

The second approach agrees that in the past doctors concentrated too much on medical facts. Other facts are also important in determining what is best. These include facts about the patient, his values, his circumstances and so on. But this approach denies that the patient has sovereign access to the relevant facts, though in many cases she knows them better than anyone else. Doctors can, and ought to, try to discover these other facts and form for themselves an all-things-considered judgment of what is best. Doctors need not give up making value judgments; they can try to make better value judgments. If a doctor's value judgment differs from that of her patient, she ought to engage her patient, find reasons for their differences, and revise her own views. Or, if her view still appears justified, she ought to continue to attempt to convince her patient that she is wrong.

Does attempting to convince a patient that he is wrong in choosing some course threaten his autonomy? It may. One can argue coercively or non-coercively. There are many ways in which a doctor might get a patient to come around to agreeing with him that do not involve rational convergence between the two parties. I am not discussing these ways of arguing. What I am discussing is attempting to convince a patient by rational argument that he is wrong. Far from frustrating a patient's autonomy, this enables a patient to act and choose more autonomously. There are at least three ways in which this is so.

1. To be autonomous, one must be informed. A doctor, in attempting to convince his patient, will appeal to reasons. Some of these reasons will draw attention to relevant facts. He will be asking his patient to reconsider the significance of these facts for her life. Thinking about these facts in a new light, her choice will become more active, more vivid and so more an expression of her autonomy [8].
2. The second point I cannot argue for in detail here. For a choice to be autonomous, one must be informed. But one must not only be informed of the facts, but also of what is of value. (Or, a relevant fact is what other people have rationally valued or thought to be of value.)
3. As a result of a patient rethinking her choice and giving reasons for that choice in the process of arguing for it, that choice will become a more rational choice and one which she really does value.

So a doctor ought not to be merely a fact-provider but also an argument-provider. In this way, he enables his patient to make a more autonomous choice.

Paternalists went wrong not in forming judgments about what was best for their patients, all things considered. They went wrong in concentrating too much on only medical facts. Moreover, they went wrong in *compelling* patients to live according to their, the doctors', evaluations of what was best. That often does violate patient autonomy. If Joan continues to want a lumpectomy despite her surgeon's attempts to convince her that she is wrong, he ought not to compel her to have a mastectomy (though in some cases, he might believe that her judgment is so wrong that he cannot provide what she asks and withdraws from the case). We ought not to compel competent people to do what is best, even if what they desire is substantially less than the best. However, allowing competent people to act on their judgment of what is best for their own lives does not imply that those judgments are right. Nor does it imply that doctors should not form for themselves judgments about what is best. Nor does it imply that doctors should not try to convince their patients by rational argument that what they are advocating is the best course. Indeed, a doctor ought to form such judgments for his own sake as a moral agent and the patient's sake as an autonomous agent. We can retain the old-style paternalist's commitment to making judgments of what is, all things considered, best for the patient (and improve it) but reject his commitment to compelling the patient to adopt that course. This practice can be called rational, non-interventional paternalism. It is 'rational' because it involves the use of rational argument. It is 'non-interventional' because it forswears doing what is best.

Medicine is entering a new era. Doctors are now required not only to have medical knowledge, but knowledge of ethics, of what constitutes a value judgment, of the fact/value distinction, of how to make value judgments and how to argue rationally about what ought to be done. This requires new skills. It is relatively easy to be a fact-provider (though how to present facts itself presents a problem). It is easy to turn decision-making over to patients and say: 'There are the facts—you decide'. It is difficult to find all the relevant facts, to form evaluative judgments, and critically examine them. It is even more difficult to engage a patient in rational argument and convince him that you are right. If doctors are to avoid the shortcomings of being mere fact-providers, if they are to function properly as moral agents, if they are to promote patient autonomy, they must learn these new skills. They must learn these skills for another reason: gone are the days when they could make uninformed judgments of what was best for their patients and act on these. Gone too are the days when they did not have to provide a justification for the position they were advocating. And that justification goes beyond the fiction of a 'purely medical' justification.

References

1. Hope T, Sprigings D, Crisp R. Not clinically indicated: patients' interests or resource allocation? *British Medical journal* 1993; 306: 379–381.
2. Brock D W, Wartman S A. When competent patients make irrational choices. *New England Journal of Medicine* 1990; 322: 1595–1599.
3. Tversky A, Kahneman D. The framing of decisions and the psychology of choice. *Science* 1981; 211: 453–458.
4. McNeil B J, Pauker S G, Sox Jr H C, Tversky A. On the elicitation of preferences for alternative therapies. *New England journal of Medicine* 1982; 306: 1259–1262.
5. Kahneman D, Varey C. Notes on the psychology of utility. In: Elster J, Roemer J E, eds. *Interpersonal comparisons of well-being*. Cambridge: Cambridge University Press, 1991: 127–163.
6. Thanks to one referee for expanding this point.
7. See reference (3), and also: Kahneman D, Tversky A. Choices, values, and frames. *American Psychologist* 1984; 39: 341–350.
8. Savulescu J. Rational desires and the limitation of life-sustaining treatment. *Bioethics* 1994; 8: 191–222. Savulescu J. *Good reasons to die* [doctoral dissertation]. Monash University, Jun, 1994.

B. Privacy and Confidentiality

Medical Privacy in the Age of Genomics

DAVID KOEPSELL

The idea of privacy in medicine emerged, as it did in the law, from the pragmatic need to ensure that patients shared their confidences willingly with those who would help them. Like attorney-client privilege, or that between a priest and confessor, without some guarantee that confidences divulged in the context of a special relationship would be immune to being pierced in other contexts (as in the law, or by governments) the full, beneficial nature of the special relationship would not be realized.[1] Modern notions of privacy, in both ethics and the law, only began to emerge in the twentieth century. The idea, for instance, that we have "spheres" or "zones" of privacy that govern what goes on behind closed doors, in our homes, or within our bodies, does not take shape in American law until the mid-twentieth century, with seminal Supreme Court cases like *Griswold v. Connecticut*, which introduced the idea that we have personal zones of privacy that prevent states from interfering with such basic, personal decisions such as contraception use.[2] Even now, however, states can and do regulate interpersonal, sexual conduct to varying degrees, and among the various nations of the world there are both more and less expansive views of the "right" of privacy.

Biomedical privacy, however, has become even more complicated of late due to the emergence of new technologies, such as electronic health records, and, as we will discuss in this essay more fully, due to the rapid development of genomics. Privacy, as an ethical or moral *right* is often confused with some related concepts, including the professional duty of confidentiality, which dates back in medicine to the Hippocratic Oath, and the legal notion of a "fiduciary relationship" that exists in certain circumstances.[3] Modern genomic technologies, and emerging potential technologies and practices, pose challenges to each of these concepts. Nonetheless, ironing out the problem of a moral basis for a personal right to privacy may hold the key to solving these new issues. The problem is that, given the promise of new genomics technologies, especially in light of their commercialization and direct delivery to consumers, old issues of medical confidentiality, or that of a fiduciary relationship, will not suffice to define the realm of personal privacy over potentially personal information. Let us first look at the emergence and role of medical confidentiality and related legal concepts of fiduciary duties, and then explore the potential for a new definition of a broad moral right to personal privacy.

Medical Privacy

Physicians have long recognized not only the pragmatic need to assure patients that their disclosures to them in the course of treatment or consultation will remain in confidence, but also a duty owed by physicians to keep those confidences. Arising out of Aristotelian virtue ethics, the professional virtue of a good physician includes fidelity to one's patients. Among the final promises in the Hippocratic Oath is "What I may see or hear in the course of the treatment or even outside of the treatment in regard to the life of men, which on no account one must spread abroad, I will keep to myself, holding such things shameful to be spoken about." What is striking about this pledge's notice of a duty to keep confidences is that it actually extends beyond more traditional notions of privacy in both ethics and the law, and has been pushed back in recent years in prominent legal cases. Specifically, a physician must keep secret not just confidences, but accidental displays or admissions about which one would ordinarily consider disclosure "shameful."[4]

The broad extent of this version of medical privacy was probably necessary in an age when physicians could, and were expected to, come into people's own homes to treat them. Even under modern law, homes are accorded special treatment as zones of expected privacy. Doors with locks and windows with shades are used to prevent prying eyes from intruding upon our most personal affairs and belongings. In order to allow for, and encourage house-calls without fear in case of dire needs, when personal effects and household business might be visible or transpiring within, a physician was to be expected to keep *everything* he might witness a secret. Physicians have a special duty, as spouses were long considered to have, to keep confidences within the realm of a special relationship that even the state cannot pierce.

This duty became more complicated in the modern era, as medical practices changed, and the nature of clinical research was altered. The growth of combined medical practices, hospitals, medical schools, and clinical studies of human subjects have all intruded upon the traditional physician-patient relationship and changed it irrevocably. The circle of those involved in medical care today typically involves multiple specialists, healthcare workers, technicians, researchers, and others in addition to primary care physicians. Moreover, medical records, many of which are now electronic, circulate among those involved and also insurers, sometimes physically, and often virtually, so that the chain of custody of any particular records could be quite long and complex. In sum, and as some have pointed out, there is no "privacy" of medical records anymore, although there is still a recognized duty of confidentiality in the physician-patient relationship.[5]

Medical records, however, are the least of patients' problems in the new age ushered in by genomics and its associated technologies and practices, at least inasmuch as our customary notions of privacy are threatened in new and troubling ways. The mapping of the human genome was supposed to bring us groundbreaking new ways to treat diseases, including targeted gene therapies for genetic diseases, and personalized medicines, adapted to our particular genetics. Gene therapies that work remain few and far between, and still in the early testing stages in the aftermath of the Jesse Gelsinger tragedy, and personalized medicines are such a niche market, promising only small returns on big investments, that except for the controversial BiDil®, well-known or successful examples remain few.

As with a number of other medical technologies, the *commercialization* of genomics and genetic data also threatens our privacy by completely circumventing the physician, and exposing our most personal data to previously unforeseen parties. Below, we will examine the rise of genomics and genetics in light of our notions and established "rights" of privacy, and examine how the concept of ownership and control over our genetic data must be re-examined.[6]

Genomics: A Revolution in Revelations

Much of the medical promise of genomics technologies has always hinged upon defining strict correlations between the presence of some genetic code and its expression as some definite phenotype. The theory is that with better understanding of the role of genes in our everyday and lifetime health, we will gain better control over our destinies. Over the past few decades, during the process of mapping the human genome and beyond, notions about the role of genes in phenotypes, health, and disease have been confirmed, even as the landscape has become more complex than originally conceived. While some diseases are indeed monogenic, relating to the presence, absence, or mutation of a single gene, others are apparently the results of combinations of genes, or mutations involving numerous genes or even single nucleotide polymorphisms (SNPs, variations of a single nucleotide) or combinations of SNPs across the genomes. Epigenetic factors are also being discovered to play greater roles in our health, and the *expression* of certain genetic tendencies, but overall, the correlation between genetic information and medically important knowledge of propensities or presence of diseases has been strengthened.[7]

As we learn more about the roles of genes in health, we continue to strive toward ways of directing that knowledge for medical interventions. In the process, through studies, clinical trials, and increased access to tools that enable the discovery of individual genetic data, a backlog of information about patients and human subjects has built up, with no corresponding legal or moral determination about the status of that information in relation to those individuals. In fact, because of disparity of treatment of genetic data among nations, and within the laws of single nations, there remains unfortunate moral ambiguity about our rights over the information contained in our own genomes. Complicating this is the fact that until now we have not needed to maintain control over our tissues in the way that modern access to genetic technologies now requires. Simply put, in the past there was little one could discover about another person by tissue samples alone, excepting perhaps blood type, gender, or the presence of known pathogens. Now, with expanding knowledge about the role of genomics in health, disease, and phenotypes, our tissues reveal a great deal more about us than we might wish others to know.

Genomic technologies that can now help us to understand ourselves much more completely, and provide guidance as never before for maintaining our health and treating disease, reveal a great deal more about ourselves, and threaten in the future to reveal even more than we could now conceive. Yet who will be the curators of our personal genetic data now and in the future? We have ceded much of the control of this data already to third parties. Studies involving human subjects have routinely involved the taking of tissue samples, with consent documents that reserve the ability of researchers to warehouse samples, do supplementary genetic studies, and although typically de-identified, samples long stockpiled are being revisited for their potential store of genetic information useful for further study. Large biobanks are currently growing, holding potentially valuable new data as technologies for revealing that data become more inexpensive and accessible.[8] A vast storehouse of potentially useful tissue samples and genetic data continues to expand daily, through national initiatives, criminal justice procedures, research trials of human subjects, and medical interventions. The evolving legal and moral question remains: who has claims to *owning* such data properly?

DNA, Genes, and Information About Persons

The special problem posed by increasing knowledge about the genome is exacerbated by the ambiguity in both the law and ethics regarding our individual relationships to our own particular genomes. Recent legal attempts to protect medical consumers and study participants from discrimination in health insurance and employment based upon information in their genomes may be a step forward for utility, but the fundamental issue remains unanswered: who owns our personal genomic data? This is complicated in part by the mess created by intellectual property law, specifically patents, which have granted a form of ownership rights to genomic data that exists, in many cases, in millions of individuals. Patents over naturally occurring genes have been granted now for almost two decades. Companies and universities have filed for and been granted patents, most notably for genes found to be related to genetic diseases. Patents confer not an ordinary property right (so those holding patents over disease genes do not have a right, for instance, to "take" their (your) genes from you or demand some sort of payment (rent) from you), but rather an *exclusionary* right over certain reproductions and uses of those genes. Thus, the owner of a disease gene patent can exclude you from *knowing* about the presence of a gene in your body without you paying some royalty to them. Because testing for the presence of genes in your genome requires processes that often involve reproducing the sought after gene, and because gene patents often cover the method of comparison of the patented gene against genes in your genome, gene patents often work to monopolize the testing for certain, known, monogenic disease genes.[9] If these genes are *part* of us, the information encoded in our genomes being largely the same from person to person, gene patents clearly complicate the landscape for medical privacy.

It is a strange sort of privacy that excludes us from knowing even about ourselves unless we enlist help and pay someone else who has monopolized various genes. Patent genes are kept private, in a sense, from ourselves. In order to discover something unique, personal, and potentially revealing about our personal genomes, we *must*, in many cases, reveal that information to others. While this seems to be not terribly unexpected in the present era, when genetic testing is expensive, complicated, and rare, it poses real questions about the nature of our ownership of our personal genomic data in a future in which such testing might, for instance, be done by ourselves as easily and cheaply as having our blood pressure taken at the corner pharmacy.

Questions about the extent of our ownership of our "own" personal genome and the genes it contains are complicated not just by the law of patent, but also by the relationships between our bodies, our tissues, and our "selves." There are many ways in which we might question whether we may rightfully exert exclusion of information about ourselves over others. Modern notions of privacy conflict, in some ways, with reality. After all, people can generally learn much about ourselves by observing us, our actions, our bodies, and the items we carelessly leave in our wake. Most of our privacy notions emerged (in the West, at least) from concerns about the reach of the state into our personal lives. The famous *Griswold* case regarded the state of Connecticut's attempt to criminalize the use of contraceptives. Subsequent cases have expanded the notion of "zones" of privacy that are supposedly implicit in the US Constitution, but generally also relate to the reach of the state into our homes, bedrooms, families, and to some degree, our bodies. But while privacy against intrusions of the state has been bolstered, there is grave ambiguity about the nature and extent of personal privacy against intrusions by our neighbors. This should be hardly surprising, especially since we reveal so much about ourselves in our everyday lives. The extent to which we now reveal our lives to the public has only increased with modern technologies. We may put up curtains over our windows, put locks on our doors, and fence our yards, but we publicize much of what goes on behind those curtains, doors, and fences through modern social media.

The central question surrounding whether we have "privacy" in genomic data comes down to this: is privacy a personal right, or a personal duty? The answer to this question may well have changed with the introduction of new genomic technologies, as we will discuss below.

What May Once Have Been a Duty Must Now Become a Right

The idea that we have autonomy, and thus some sort of privacy, over our own bodies is an essential element of liberal philosophy. Our minds, our bodies, and some "zones" surrounding our persons are ours, to be free from intrusion, and to do with (with some minor exceptions) as we please. But the rights we exert over our minds, bodies, and personal space, which must be respected by others, do not extend to that which is publicly accessible. Our faces, for instance, reveal ourselves in often very personal ways. Yet we have no right to keep others from looking at our faces, or seeing whether we walk with a limp, or have some sort of publicly visible disfigurement, despite our urgent wishes that others know only what we wish them to know. In other words, while we have rights to be free from any intrusion into our minds, bodies, and to some degree, our personal space, we have no right to not be seen, heard, or otherwise observed in our public meanderings. Rather, if we wish to keep things private that others can otherwise observe without causing us harm, then we have a *duty* to keep those things private.

In the medical context, this means that we have a duty to keep private confidences divulged to our physicians if we wish those confidences to remain private. If we publish our medical records, or publicize information about our health, we have no right to expect privacy about that information. The special relationships that have evolved in the medical sphere have helped ensure that the expectation of privacy over medical data is maintained, but it does not create an impenetrable sphere of privacy over medical information against personal, intentional divulgence by patients themselves. Nor should it. Even while physicians have a professional duty to maintain confidences revealed as part of the physician-patient relationship, patients have a duty to maintain secret that which they wish to remain private. Once published, a secret becomes public domain.

Genomic technologies, both present and future, impose a heavy burden on would be curators of their own medical information, one that may require rethinking the nature of medical privacy, or establishing a previously non-existent *right*. Namely: outstanding tissue samples, and even the everyday detritus of our bodies, may reveal sensitive health and other data about us that we had previously expected would remain private, or more likely, that we never even knew existed. It is not inconceivable that in the near future, with minimal or no intrusion into our *geographic* zones of privacy (our minds, bodies, or personal space) bits of tissue (like skin flakes, eyelashes, hairs, etc.) could be easily scanned by anyone happening to find them to reveal countless potentially valuable bits of information of a very personal nature. This sort of detritus is already used for finding out who has been at a crime scene through "DNA fingerprinting."

It is the ubiquity and uncontainability of this sort of "evidence" about us that will require rethinking our notions about the rights of privacy we have begun to develop, or duties to be expected from us as curators of our private information. Simply put: we cannot contain this information in any reasonable way. Unlike the information we keep behind closed doors, or share with our trusted advisors, counselors, confidants, and others with professional duties to keep secrets, our genetic data will literally be subject to revelation upon the winds. In the meantime commercially available conduits by which we are now enticed to reveal our genetic data, for the sake of our own self-education about ourselves, attract consumers to bypass the traditional physician-patient relationship to gain insight into their health. Services like 23 and Me, and other private gene-scanning companies, offer to test self-collected samples through the mail; in so doing we entrust our genetic information to companies lacking the professional duty of privacy that has traditionally constrained physicians. As they often do with social networking on the Internet, many consumers may be revealing far more about themselves, and expanding the potential universe of abuses of personal information, far beyond what they know or might reasonably expect.

To combat the possibility that new technologies have developed far quicker than consumer knowledge or responsibility about their uses and abuses, two paths must be pursued. One is education. If we are to be expected to responsibly curate the information contained in our DNA, and oversee its spread and use, then we must have some basic knowledge about DNA and genetics. The second path is ethical. We need to develop a consistent notion about what the nature of the relationship between ourselves and our genetic data is and should be. Since enclosure and containment cannot define this relationship in satisfying ways, we need to found an expanded right to genetic privacy upon something more.

One promising approach to the question of *ownership* or *dominion* over our own personal genomic data requires first invalidating claims by others over it (such as by patent, or through contractual releases submitted through consent procedures in previous studies), and then linking a foundational right of privacy in genomic data to existing notions of identity or personhood. "Persons" have rights. Humanity as a whole is defined by our common genome, and our individual identities as *persons* must be to some degree, strong or weak, linked to our *personal* genomes. As rights-bearing entities, we might argue, our genetic identities are in part responsible for imbuing us with our personal identities as well as our identities as *persons* having rights. Thus, our rights to our genetic identities ought to be as strong, or perhaps stronger, than our rights over our bodies, since our existence in our bodies is ontologically dependent upon the existence of our genes in certain permutations.[10]

This approach is partly founded upon a theory of personhood that views its essential attributes in part as genetically determined, which is itself a controversial approach. Genetic determinism is largely rejected now as environment is increasingly viewed as playing a large role in how genetic traits are expressed. But it is indisputable that we make decisions about who holds rights based upon (i) belonging to a species, which is genetically determined, and (ii) possessing certain attributes, some of which are genetically determined. Genetic material, unlike the other physical components of our being, is also an information carrier, and that information is the ontological *cause* of the physical components with which we are familiar. If we are willing to grant that we *own* our bodies, derive our personal autonomy over that ownership and occupation, then ought we not also to look at the bases for that ownership and occupation and ask whether that information ought also to be inviolable? If it is not as a matter of course (we cannot defend it as we do our other forms of property) then this may suggest we need to create some *positive* right to that information if we are to respect the rights that derive from our DNA-dependent personhood.

Of course this sort of massive reconfiguring of our notions of privacy would be disruptive. The ownership of genetic data in databanks around the world would be undone if we recognized that, for instance, like our freedom and other essential attributes of personhood, our genetic identities cannot be bargained away. But that is an argument based upon utility, not justice. Justice may demand massive reconfiguring of our notions of rights to privacy over our genes, just as it demanded reconsidering the extent to which states could insert themselves into decisions about our bodies, reproductive decisions, medical decisions, or our homes.

The Right to Your Genes

I have argued that the human genome, and the commonly shared elements that define our humanity and that comprise it, are part of a "commons by necessity" that cannot justly be monopolized by anyone. This argument is predicated upon a theory of property that "grounds" just claims of ownership in the encloseability or possessability of some thing (like land, moveables, etc.).[11] Because the human genome is an inherently uncloseable, distributed object, like the laws of nature, ideas, axioms of math, and so on, there is no just way to establish some monopoly over parts of it. But what of our *personal* genomes?

There is a very real sense in which our personal genomes are a part of our bodies, and thus susceptible to dominion under liberal theories of autonomy over our bodies and minds. But DNA poses a special problem of *containability*. We literally shed samples of our DNA wherever we go, in our hairs, dead skins cells, and other bodily detritus that we leave in our wakes. Moreover, through the hundreds of tissue samples we willingly give in common medical procedures, treatments, and studies, our DNA almost inevitably becomes widely spread, with few of us really knowing the outcome or fate of each sample, nor thinking twice about the potential uses of them. Our personal genomes are not logically uncontainable or uncloseable (since we could envision radical ways to ensure that they remain in our control, as with the Ethan Hawke character in the 1997 movie *Gattaca*) but they are certainly *practically* uncloseable. Like sunlight, which cannot be actually monopolized short of some evil genius with unlimited resources devising some Monty Burns-like device to block all sunlight, it is a practically uncontainable resource. It is also closely linked to our individual existence as persons, and reveals a great deal of information about ourselves that we would often like to be able to control. The question is: could we justly create norms and institutions that would make private and inviolate our personal genetic data? I think, for the reasons described above, we could. In doing so, we would deprive no one of any grounded rights, and would go a long way to ensuring that consumers would be protected from the unknown and unknowable consequences of ordinary medical care, study participation, and the unavoidable consequences of engaging in our daily lives in public.

Notes

1 Leo J. Cass and William J. Curran, "Rights of privacy in medical practice," *Lancet* 1965; 286(7416): Oct. 16.

2 *Griswold v. Connecticut*, 381 U.S. 479 (1965).

3 Robert J. Levine, *Ethics and Regulation of Clinical Research*, 2nd edn. New Haven: Yale University Press, 1986; p. 163.

4 See S.G. Marketos, A.A. Diamandopoulos, C.S. Bartsocas, E. Poulakou-Rebelakou, and D.A. Koutras, "The Hippocratic Oath," *Lancet* 1996; 347(8994): 101–2; doi: 10.1016/S0140-6736(96)90216-0.

5 See, e.g., Mark Siegler, "Confidentiality in medicine—a decrepit concept," in Tom L. Beauchamp and LeRoy Walters (eds), *Contemporary Issues in Bioethics*, 3rd edn. Belmont, CA: Wadsworth Publishing Co., 1982; pp. 405–7.

6 R.M. Berry, "Genetic information and research: emerging legal issues," *HealthCare Ethics Committee Forum* 2003; 15(1): 70–99.

7 See D.L. Wiesenthal and N.I. Weiner, "Privacy and the human genome project," *Ethics and Behavior* 1996; 6(3): 189–201.

8 H.T. Tavani, "Genomic research and data-mining technology: implications for personal privacy and informed consent," *Ethics and Information Technology* 2004; 6: 15–28.

9 P.J. Whitehouse, "The evolution of gene patenting," *American Journal of Bioethics* 2002; 2(3): 23–4.

10 I suggest this argument in D. Keopsell, *Who Owns You? The Corporate Gold Rush to Patent Your Genes*. Chichester: Wiley-Blackwell, 2009; pp. 80, 162.

11 Koepsell (2009), pp. 11, 119.

Ethical Issues Experienced by HIV-Infected African-American Women

Katharine V. Smith and Jan Russell

Introduction

Human immunodeficiency virus (HIV) and acquired immunodeficiency syndrome (AIDS) have given rise to a variety of ethical problems about 'what is right or what ought to be done'[1] for those infected with the virus, their loved ones, their health care providers, and society. For example, do persons with AIDS (PWA) have the right not to inform past sexual partners of the diagnosis? Do those past sexual partners have a right to be told the diagnosis? Although many authors have addressed such ethical problems on a theoretical level, few have addressed these issues through research. Most research that has addressed HIV-related ethical issues has

"Ethical Issues Experienced by HIV-Infected African-American Women," by Katharine V. Smith and Jan Russell, originally published in *Nursing Ethics* 1997; 4: 394–402. Reprinted with permission of Edward Arnold Permissions.

investigated the ethical problems and/or the attitudes of nurses rather than those encountered by the infected persons themselves.[2-15]

Method

Sample

This study was part of a larger project exploring the lives of HIV-infected African-American women; a purposive sample of five women participated. Two were 23 years old, and the others were aged 26, 40 and 42. Two were married. Of the three single participants, two had current partners and one did not. One participant had completed the 11th grade; two had passed the General Education Diploma (GED); one had completed high school and some vocational training; and the fifth had completed two years of college. Only one participant had health insurance; the other four had only Medicare. All of the participants had children. One had two children, one of whom had been killed. Two women each had three living children, ranging from six months old to six years old in one, and from one to nine years old in the other. Another participant had three grown children, one of whom had also been killed. The fifth participant had four children, ranging from 18 months to five years of age. Among the five participants, there was therefore a total of 13 living children and two deceased.

Procedure

To explore the ethical issues faced by these women, each was asked in an audiotaped interview to describe her 'experience as a black woman infected with HIV/AIDS'. No other prompts were given; rather, each woman's story was allowed to unfold in her own words. In a follow-up interview, data from the first interview were validated, and more directed, but again open-ended, questions derived from the literature were asked. Questions focused on their exposure to HIV/AIDS, its effects on their lifestyle, its effects on their family, and the ethical issues (if any) that they dealt with regarding their diagnosis. The data were analysed using Giorgi et al.'s[16] method of phenomenological analysis.

Findings

The findings of this study indicate that four broad categories of ethical issues are faced by HIV-infected African-American women, revolving around issues of: diagnosis; disclosure; treatment by, and of, others; and future pregnancies.

Diagnosis

One issue that participants had faced in relation to their diagnosis was the need to be tested. One had learned from friends that a previous partner had died of AIDS. She said:

> I took the tests because someone that I had been with had died from AIDS, a guy I had been with prior to me getting married ... I came to the clinic and I talked to my doctor

and told him that I was told a previous lover had died from AIDS and that I wanted to be tested. So I was and two weeks later I came back for the results and sure enough, I was positive.

Another was tested because she was suspicious of her current partner:

… because I had a good idea that my mate was positive … that was another reason I got tested, because he wasn't telling me, you know, the full detail of why he was in the hospital.

Participants discussed the fear associated with being tested for, and potentially being diagnosed with, HIV/AIDS:

[Other people] don't want to get tested because they're scared they are going to say yes. I didn't want to get tested either, but I did. I could still be walking around, right now, today and not be tested. I was scared then, but I still laughed 'cause I didn't think it could happen to me. But it wasn't funny then and it wasn't funny before I laughed. It is serious.

Despite their fears, each woman did make the decision to be tested:

I went down there and I got tested, and I was six months pregnant. They told me that the test that I took was negative and to come back in three months. Well, I delivered in February, February 14, 1993, and I went down there February of 1993 and they told me that my test came back and was positive.

Once the women were tested, they faced ethical issues about the way they were informed of their positive HIV/AIDS status. One participant said:

I Went into the treatment centre and I came in, I was laughing and joking. She said, 'Your test results are back.' Well I told her, 'I know I ain't got AIDS.' She said, 'Sit down, you're HIV.' Then I didn't hear anything else she said, I busted down, broke down …

Disclosure

Several aspects of disclosure presented ethical issues for these women. The first issue was their partner's disclosure (or lack of disclosure) of his HIV status. Three of the five participants had specifically asked their partners about their status, and all three were assured the partners did not have HIV. These three women later found that their partners had not been honest about their status, and subsequently found themselves to be HIV positive, too, despite their efforts to the contrary. This aspect of disclosure, or the lack of it, illustrates the dilemma of their own right of disclosure versus their partner's right to privacy. One woman stated:

I asked him why he didn't tell me before we did something, you know, and he said, 'Well, I thought you was going to tell somebody.' I told him: 'Well, you put my life in your hands and the kids.' I had three kids when I met him and he didn't tell me until I told him I might be pregnant, we'd been together about six months then and I didn't know nothing about it. He died before I had my baby.

Although these three women did not believe their partners' lack of disclosure was right, none of them expressed anger about it. One woman believed most HIV positive people would not disclose, but she believed she both should and would:

But nine times out of 10, 90%, you know, of the world, they would not tell anybody: 'Hey, I got HIV', but I would, because I don't want nobody to go down that road.

Another said:

Right, we talked about it, and that's when I told him that if he had it to let me know, that we could work something out. But he says that he felt that I would of, you know, he really cared about me, but it was just something that he wasn't ready to tell me because so many people have rejected him … and he didn't want that. So, and I guess I would have felt the same way.

Perhaps the participants' own experiences with HIV enabled them to understand their partners' fear of rejection, although all three maintained that they would choose to deal with this issue differently:

But see, if it was me, I would tell somebody and if they didn't want to be bothered, well, you know, I would kind of feel lost behind too. But, I think every person has a right, in this world, to make that decision upon themselves. Because, that is like taking a life.

Deciding that they would deal with this issue of disclosure differently from their partners was one thing, but actually doing it was another. The women who had not contracted HIV/AIDS from their current partners had to decide if they would inform their present partners of their diagnosis. Invariably, these women did. One woman said:

The first day I was diagnosed he was at the clinic with me and I came out and on the way home I told him. I had prepared for a divorce that day after I left the clinic, I got in the car and I had already made up my mind that we would be divorced so he could go on because his came back negative. His is negative and that's okay you know and I just, I couldn't pay him to leave, he has always been there.

Another ethical aspect of disclosing their HIV/AIDS status was *how* to disclose:

It is not something that you can just tell somebody, you know, somebody that you are with 'cause you're going to feel like they're going to kick you off to the side. You know, like kicking you to the curb, you know, not wanting to be bothered. And, it is something that you can't really tell someone: 'Hey, I'm infected with HIV.' I mean it is a hard thing to deal with … it depends on the individual.

Although it was hard, these women told their partners in the best way they could; one woman said:

Well, it was right after I had my baby and before I got off the drugs and stopped drinking. I had got, I had already set myself up to tell him, but we'd never been, we hadn't had sex at all ... because I was pregnant. So, I went and got me some beer and liquor. So I drank it and I drank a fifth, about ten cans of beer, because I wanted to be really, really, really drunk when I told him. And, so I said man, I told him, and it was like he just sat there, like I didn't tell him nothing at all. He really didn't take it too hard and I told him the next morning, well: 'If you want to leave you can leave, you know. I'll understand and everything. I love you ... and everything'. We've been together ever since.

Besides the issue of disclosure to partners, there was the issue of disclosure to others with whom the participants had sex. Two women specifically stated that they sometimes divulged their diagnosis to sexual partners, but at other times chose not to. They felt no need to disclose if proper precautions were taken, although one woman took those precautions to protect herself:

Some of them I tell that I got it [HIV/AIDS] and some of them I don't. But I'm not only protecting them, I'm protecting myself too from getting another sexually transmitted disease.

The other woman, however, took those precautions to protect her partner:

'Cause, my motto is: You are going to put on everything I tell you or we won't have sex. And if you ask me why I'm doing this and you're serious about this I will tell you. But if you don't ask me why, I won't as long as I know I'm protecting you.

The final disclosure issue for these women was the disclosure of their diagnosis to others, including family, friends and employers. Sometimes the women had a choice about whether to disclose or not:

A guy that I worked with, that I really cared about, we had an affair and so I told him. I felt like, well I found out and my husband has to have it and this guy has to have it too; these are the only people I have been with.

Sometimes, however, the diagnosis was disclosed by others, against the women's wishes:

He called my mother and told my mother that I have AIDs and it set my mother through such a shock she went through. Anyway when I called my mother and she told me that he said that I was, I was devastated, so I came over to her house and sat down and talked to her.

Perhaps one of the most important ethical issues these women faced was whether to disclose their positive HIV/AIDS status to their children. They struggled with this issue ('... it was just really hard for me to decide if I wanted, you know, to tell them, you know ...'), and chose to deal with it in different ways. One woman said:

> I tell them that I have HIV and they know and I tell them don't tell everyone, don't discuss this with no one, but I want you two to know that.

In fact, this particular woman said:

> Right now today they are nine and eight, and I'll tell them. I tell them that I'm HIV and I tell them what condoms are, I tell them about AIDS, I try to get tapes. I want them to see them because I don't want them to grow up like that.

Another participant, however, chose not to inform her children:

> I don't want to tell my family what I have, because I don't want my family to tell them [her children] that I'm died of AIDS ... because it's going to be really hard on them, something that they probably won't be able to accept.

Discussion

This was a particularly difficult area of ethical decision-making because the women did not have to make one decision: to disclose or not to disclose. Rather, they had to make multiple decisions about whether to disclose to this person, or that group, or this employer. Also, when deciding about disclosure, they seemed very cognizant of other people's feelings, needs and rights. This was different to, for example, issues of diagnosis, where the women made one definitive decision either to be tested or not. The decision to be tested, at least in an immediate sense, affected the woman only. After all, she might test negative, in which case the issue stopped with her; it was only after she tested positive that she had to begin to consider others and their need to know of her diagnosis. She then moved into the complex arena of disclosure decisions.

Conclusion

This study suggests that HIV-infected African-American women deal with many daily decisions regarding what is right or what ought to be done. As these women described their experiences, they expressed concern regarding diagnosis, disclosure, treatment of and by others, and pregnancies. Perhaps the most fundamental truth of their experience, however, was the conviction that HIV/AIDS, itself, is 'not fair': 'It's [HIV/AIDS] not fair to the kids that are being born; it's not fair to the people who get it; it's not fair to the people who have it.'

Further research must be conducted regarding this most 'unfair' disease, and the ethical issues that its African-American female victims deal with on a daily basis.

References

1. Davis A, Aroskar M. *Ethical dilemmas and nursing practice*. Norwalk, CT: Appleton and Lange, 1991.
2. Alexander R, Fitzpatrick J. Variables influencing nurses' attitudes toward AIDS and AIDS patients. *AIDS Patient Care* 1991; 5: 315–20.
3. Chubon SJ. Ethical dilemmas encountered by home care nurses. *Home Healthcare Nurse* 1994; 12(5): 12–17.
4. Forrester DA, Murphy PA. Nurses' attitudes toward patients with AIDS and AIDS-related risk factors. *J Adv Nurs* 1992; 17: 1260–66.
5. Jemmott JB, Freleicher J, Jemmott LS. Perceived risk of infection and attitudes toward risk groups: determinants of nurses' behavioral intentions regarding AIDS patients. *Res Nurs Health* 1992; 15: 295–301.
6. Martin DA. Effects of ethical dilemmas on stress felt by nurses providing care to AIDS patients. *Crit Care Nurs Q* 1990; 12(4): 53–62.
7. Murphy JM, Famolare NE. Caring for pediatric patients with HIV: personal concerns and ethical dilemmas. *Pediatr Nurs* 1994; 20: 171–76.
8. Prince NA, Beard BJ, Ivey SL, Lester L. Perinatal nurses' knowledge and attitudes about AIDS. *J Obstet Gynecol Neonatal Nurs* 1989; 18: 363–69.
9. Scherer YK, Haughey BP. Nurses' experiences in caring for patients with AIDS in Erie County. *J NY State Nurs Assoc* 1988; 19(2): 4–8.
10. Scherer YK, Haughey BP, Wu YB. AIDS: what are nurses' concerns? *Clin Nurse Specialist* 1989; 3 (1): 48–54.
11. Scherer YK, Haughey BP, Wu YB, Kuhn MM. AIDS: what are critical care nurses' concerns? *Critical Care Nurse* 1992; 12(7): 23–29.
12. Scherer YK, Haughey BP, Wu YB, Miller CM. A longitudinal study of nurses' attitudes toward caring for patients with AIDS in Erie County. *J NY State Nurs Assoc* 1992; 23(3): 10–15.
13. Scherer YK, Wu YB, Haughey BP. AIDS and homophobia among nurses. *J Homosex* 1991; 21(4): 17–27.
14. van Servellen GM, Lewis CE, Leake B. Nurses' responses to the AIDS crisis: implications for continuing education programs. *J Continuing Educ Nurs* 1988; 19(1): 4–8.
15. Webb AA, Bunting S. Ethical decision making by nurses in HIV/AIDS situations. *J Assoc Nurses AIDS Care* 1992; 3(2): 15–18.
16. Giorgi A, Fischer C, Murray E eds. *Duquesne studies in phenomenological psychology*. Pittsburgh, PA: Duquesne University Press, 1975.

C. Informed Consent

Should Informed Consent Be Based on Rational Beliefs?

Julian Savulescu and Richard W. Momeyer

I. Introduction

Medical ethics places great emphasis on physicians respecting patient autonomy. It encourages tolerance even towards harmful choices patients make on the basis of their own values. This ethic has been defended by consequentialists and deontologists.

"Should Informed Consent Be Based on Rational Beliefs?" by Julian Savulescu and Richard W. Momeyer, originally published in the *Journal of Medical Ethics*, 1997; 23: 282–8. Reprinted with permission of the BMJ Publishing Group.

Respect for autonomy finds expression in the doctrine of informed consent. According to that doctrine, no medical procedure may be performed upon a competent patient unless that patient has consented to have that procedure, after having been provided with the relevant facts.

We have no quarrel with these principles. We do, however, question their interpretation and application. Our contention is that being autonomous requires that a person hold rational beliefs. We distinguish between rational choice and rational belief. Being autonomous may not require that one's choices and actions are rational. But it does require that one's beliefs which ground those choices are rational. If this is right, what passes for respecting autonomy sometimes consists of little more than providing information, and stops short of assessing whether this information is rationally processed. Some of what purports to be medical deference to a patient's values is not this at all: rather, it is acquiescence to irrationality. Some of what passes for respecting patient autonomy may turn out to be less respect than abandonment. Abandonment of patients has never been regarded as a morally admirable practice.

We will outline three ways in which patients hold irrational beliefs: (1) ignorance, (2) not caring enough about rational deliberation, and (3) making mistakes in deliberation. We argue that it is the responsibility of physicians not only to provide relevant information (which addresses 1), but to improve the rationality of belief that grounds consent (2 and 3).

II. Rationality and Autonomy

II.I True belief and autonomy

The word, "autonomy", comes from the Greek: autos (self) and nomos (rule or law).[1] Autonomy is self-government or self-determination. Being autonomous involves freely and actively making one's own evaluative choices about how one's life should go.

It is a familiar idea that it is necessary to hold true beliefs if we are to get what we want. For example, John loves Northern Indian dishes and loathes Southern Indian dishes. Yet he is very confused about which dishes belong to which area. He consistently orders Southern Indian dishes thinking he is ordering Northern Indian dishes. His false beliefs cause him to fail to get what he wants.

However, true beliefs are important for evaluative choice in a more fundamental way: we cannot form an idea of *what* we want without knowing what the options on offer are *like*. Consider a person with gangrene of the foot. She is offered an amputation. In evaluating "having an amputation" she is attempting to evaluate a complete state of affairs: how much pain she will experience, whether she will be able to live by herself, visit her grandchildren, and so on. (Importantly, knowing the name of one's disease and the nature of the operation are less important facts.)

II.II True belief and practical rationality

Practical rationality is concerned with what we have reason to care about and do. Let's distinguish between what there is good reason to do and what it is rational to do. Paul sits down after work to have a relaxing evening with his wife. She gives him a glass of what he believes is wine, but is in fact poison. There is a good reason for Paul not to drink it, even if this is not known to Paul. However, if he believes that it is wine, it is rational for him to drink it.[2] Thus:

> It is rational for a person to perform some act if there would be a good reason to perform that act if the facts were as he/she believes them to be.

Thus holding true beliefs is important in two ways: (1) it promotes our autonomy and (2) allows us to see that there is good reason to do. This does not collapse autonomous choice with rational choice. Even holding all the relevant true beliefs, a person may autonomously choose some course which he or she has no good reason to choose. For example, assume that the harms of smoking outweigh the benefits. Jim has good reason to give up smoking. However, he may choose to smoke knowing all the good and bad effects of smoking. His choice is then irrational but his beliefs may be rational and he may be autonomous. His choice is not an expression of his autonomy if he believes that smoking is not only pleasurable, but good for your health.

II.III Coming to hold true beliefs

One important way to hold true beliefs is via access to relevant information. For example, one way to get Paul to believe that the wine is poisoned is to provide him with evidence that it is poisoned.

We can never know for certain that our beliefs are true. We can only be confident of their truth. Confidence is the likelihood that a belief is true. Beliefs which are based on evidence (rational beliefs) are more likely to be true than unfounded (irrational) beliefs. The likelihood that our beliefs are true is a function both of how informed they are and of how we think about that information.

Theoretical rationality is concerned with what it is rational to believe.

> It is rational for a person to believe some proposition if he/she ought to believe that proposition if he/she were deliberating rationally about the evidence available and his/her present beliefs, and those beliefs are not themselves irrational.

Let's say that a person is "deliberating rationally" if[3]:

1. She holds a degree of belief in a proposition which is responsive to the evidence supporting that proposition. For example, the firmer the evidence, the greater the degree of belief ought to be.
2. She examines her beliefs for consistency. If she detects inconsistency, she ought appropriately to contract her set of beliefs or adjust her degree of belief in the relevantly inconsistent beliefs.
3. She exposes her reasoning to the norms of inductive and deductive logic. Valid logic is important because it helps us to have the broadest range of true beliefs.

Consider the following example. Peter is trying to decide whether to have an operation. Suppose that he is provided with certain information and reasons in the following way.

1. There is a risk of dying from anaesthesia. (true)
2. I will require an anaesthetic if I am to have this operation. (true)

Therefore, if I have this operation, I will probably die.

The conclusion does not follow from the premises. Peter comes to hold an irrational belief because he commits a logical error. Irrational beliefs are less likely to be true than rational beliefs. Since knowledge of truth is elusive for subjective beings like us, the best we can hope for is informed, rational belief.

If we are right that information is important to evaluative choice because of its contribution to a person holding the relevant true beliefs necessary for evaluation, then deliberating rationally is as important as being informed, since this also affects the likelihood that one's beliefs are true. Being fully autonomous requires not only that we are informed, but that we exercise our theoretical rationality.

III. An Example of Irrational Belief: Jehovah's Witnesses and Blood

Jehovah's Witnesses (JWs) who refuse life-saving blood transfusions for themselves are often taken to be paradigm cases of autonomous, informed choice based on different (non-medically shared) values that require respect and deference.

Jehovah's Witnessess refuse life-saving blood transfusions because they believe that if they die and have received blood, they will turn to dust. But if they refuse blood (and keep Jehovah's other laws) and die, they will enjoy eternal life in Paradise.[4]

Jehovah's Witnesses interpret *The Bible* as forbidding the sustaining of life with blood in any manner. They base this belief on passages such as:

> "Every creature that lives and moves shall be food for you ... But you must not eat the flesh with the life, which is the blood, still in it".[5]

Anyone eating the blood of an animal would be "cut off" or executed.[6] The only legitimate use of animal blood was as a sacrifice to God. Leviticus 17: 11 states:

> "... the life of the creature is the blood, and I appoint it to make expiation on the altar for yourselves: it is the blood, that is the life, that makes expiation"[7]

Jehovah's Witnesses believe these views concerning blood were important to the early Christian Church. At a meeting of the apostles and older men of Jerusalem to determine which laws would continue to be upheld in the new Church, blood was again proscribed:

> "... you are to abstain from meat that has been offered to idols, from blood, from anything that has been strangled, and from fornication".[8]

Jehovah's Witnesses believe that these passages imply more than a dietary proscription. They attach great symbolic significance to blood: it represents the life or soul. Thus they claim that the exhortation "abstain from blood" applies to all forms of blood, at all times. They argue that there is no moral difference between sustaining life by taking blood by mouth ("eating blood") and taking blood directly into the veins.

Relative to their beliefs, JWs are practically rational. Any (practically) rational person would choose to forgo earthly life if this ensured that one would enjoy a blissful eternal existence in the presence of God. If JWs are irrational, it is because their beliefs are irrational. A failure of theoretical rationality causes them to do what there is good reason not to do and frustrates their autonomy.

We believe that the beliefs of JWs are irrational. One way to show this is to question the rationality of belief in the existence of God or in the truth of some religious version of morality. For argument's sake, we will accept theism. However, the vast majority of those in the Judaeo-Christian tradition have not interpreted these passages from *The Bible* as proscribing blood transfusion. The beliefs of JWs are irrational on at least two counts: their particular beliefs are not responsive to evidence nor are their interpretations of Biblical text consistent. These failures of rationality are shared with other forms of religious "fundamentalism" and so-called "literal" interpretations of religious texts. It is worth noting that many JWs are also Creationists, believing all of Genesis to be literally true. Ignorance of historical context, the diverse intentions and circumstances of Biblical peoples and authors, oral and written traditions in the Middle East, other religious traditions and interpretations of Biblical texts, inconsistencies between different canonised works and the like all help ground an unduly simplistic interpretation of *The Bible*.

Mere ignorance, however, is not to be equated with irrationality. Wilful ignorance is. And wilful ignorance is what lies behind grounding understanding of *The Bible* on faith rather than the kinds of knowledge suggested above. This sort of wilful ignorance cuts across educational levels as it is rooted in dogmatism and closed-mindedness rather than degrees of education.

However, we believe that JWs' beliefs are irrational even in terms that should be acceptable to JWs.

Firstly, their interpretation is inconsistent with other passages of *The Bible* and Christian practices. It is inconsistent with the Christian practice of communion. Communion is the holy ceremony of the Last Supper. At the Last Supper

> "Jesus took bread, and having said the blessing he broke it ... with these words: 'Take this and eat; this is my body.' Then he took a cup [of wine], and having offered thanks to God ... [said] ... 'Drink from it ... For this is my blood, the blood of the covenant, shed for many, for the forgiveness of sins'".[9]

Secondly, Paul warns against slavish obedience to law:

> "... those who rely on obedience to the law are under a curse ...".[10] "Christ bought us freedom from the curse of the law by becoming ... an accursed thing".[11]

The answer is not obedience to law but faith.

> "... the law was a kind of tutor in charge of us until Christ should come, when we should be justified through faith; and now that faith has come, the tutor's charge is at an end".[12]

Paul himself does not understand *The Bible* to be literally true, as evidenced when he speaks of the story of the origin of Abraham's sons being "an allegory".[13] He goes on to say:

> "Mark my words: I, Paul, say to you that if you receive circumcision Christ will do you no good at all ... [E]very man who receives circumcision is under obligation to keep the entire law. When you seek to be justified by way of law, your relation with Christ is completely severed ... [O]ur hope of attaining that righteousness ... is the work of the Spirit through faith ... the only thing that counts is faith active in love".[14]

If the beliefs of JWs are irrational, why are they irrational?

IV. Three Examples of Holding a False Belief

In all three of the following cases, the person lacks a true belief which is relevant to choice. We describe how to help a person come to hold true beliefs, drawing out the parallels with patients and JWs.

Case 1. Lack of information

Arthur 1 is burning rubbish in the garden. The fire grows rapidly. It begins to threaten surrounding buildings. They are not in imminent danger but Arthur wants to douse the fire with water before it gets out of hand. He goes to the shed where he keeps a jerry can of water for just such a situation. He has a high degree of belief that this can contains water. Unbeknownst to him, someone has substituted petrol for water in the can. He throws the liquid on the fire and the petrol ignites, causing an explosion. He is badly burnt. Was Arthur irrational?

We need a more complete description of the state of affairs.

Arthur always locks the shed. There had been no signs of forced entry. There was only one jerry can in the shed. It was in the position where Arthur always kept it, next to the shovel. He had only the previous weekend refilled it with water after using it to put out another garden fire. If Arthur simply had no reason to suspect that the can contained anything but water, it was rational to believe that it contained water. A person who unavoidably lacks relevant information is neither theoretically nor practically irrational.

What should we do if we see Arthur about to throw the liquid onto the fire?

Arthur is rational, but he lacks a relevant true belief that he could have. In this case, the solution is simple. Provide information. Tell him, "Stop. The can contains petrol." If there were no time to provide this information, we ought to grab the can from his hands.

Many patients who hold false beliefs are like Arthur 1: uninformed. What we ought to do is provide them with information. If this is not possible, we should do what is best for them.

Are there any JWs like Arthur 1? Jehovah's Witnesses are remarkably well informed about blood transfusion, the effects of refusing it, and the Biblical context of their belief. But some may be unaware of the conflicting Biblical passages. These ought to be treated like Arthur 1. However, many are not like him. The provision of information is not alone an adequate response. What is required is rational argument.

Case 2. Not engaging in rational deliberation

Arthur 2 is the same as Arthur 1, but in this case Arthur goes to the shed and finds it unlocked. He is not sure whether he left it locked last weekend. He thinks he probably did. The jerry can is next to the lawn mower. Arthur thinks that he normally keeps it next to the shovel. But, again, he is not sure. Is he irrational if he believes the can contains water?

Arthur clearly ought to believe that the door is open and the can is next to the lawn-mower. But for these propositions to constitute evidence for the conclusion that the contents of the can are not water, Arthur must believe that the position of the can and door have changed. Should Arthur believe that he left the jerry can next to the shovel? This depends on the degree of belief Arthur has in his recollection of how things were. If he is vague, then there is no evidence.

Arthur may not lack information as much as a context for that information because he fails to remember relevant facts. This may be beyond control. In this case, Arthur 2 is like Arthur 1. But in some cases, a person fails to remember because he fails to think about the issue. And he may fail to think about the issue because he fails to care enough about the truth of his beliefs or the consequences of his actions.

Arthur could be directed to think more carefully about what he sees and of the possible implications of his actions. There may be other evidence he would find, if he looked, for believing the propositions that the door was locked and the can was next to the shovel. He may notice other items in the shed have been moved.

It is often thought that consultation in medicine involves presenting information so that it is understood. But even understanding is not enough. Facts must be assembled to tell a story or to construct an argument which stands in the foreground of deliberation. The arrangement and form of the facts is as important as their content.

Are there any JWs who are like Arthur 2? There is, we are assuming, evidence that their beliefs are false. However, being informed of these facts is not sufficient to cause them to hold the relevant true beliefs. They also need to care about thinking about that information in a rational way. The hallmark of faith is a stubbornness to respond to the evidence for a proposition. While this may be necessary for belief in God, it cannot be the appropriate paradigm for interpretation of God's word. *The Bible*, as a guide to how to live, aims to sanction some ways of living and proscribe others. Faith *in any interpretation* of God's word cannot be acceptable.[15] When interpreting Biblical text, the appropriate paradigm for theists is rationality and not faith. Indeed, the efforts of JWs to argue for their interpretation of *The Bible* indicates that they subscribe to this paradigm. What they are required to do by that paradigm is to care more about the proper exercise of rationality.

Intervention in this case would include trying to persuade JWs to care more about rationality by showing how they themselves appeal to rational argument and why *The Bible* must be interpreted rationally.

We are often like Arthur 2 and some JWs: we fail to care enough about what we believe and what we commit to memory. This failing is at the interface of practical and theoretical rationality: we fail to care enough (a practical failing) about the rationality of our beliefs (a theoretical failing).

Case 3. Theoretical irrationality

Arthur 3 is the same as Arthur 2 but in this case, Arthur is sure he left the door to the shed locked and sure that the jerry can is in a different position from where he left it. On entering the shed, he smells petrol. He doesn't normally keep petrol in the shed. None the less, he throws the fluid on the fire.

As the evidence mounts up, Arthur becomes more theoretically irrational if he fails to consider the possibility that the can contains petrol. At the limit, if the evidence is overwhelming, he is like a person who believes that p, and that if p then q, but fails to believe that q.

Why might Arthur be theoretically irrational?

He may simply fail to believe that what he smells is petrol. This would be an error of perception.

He may fail to examine his beliefs for inconsistency. He may fail to compare what he believes to what the evidence suggests is the case.

Most importantly of all, Arthur may not be very talented at theoretical reasoning. He may not be good at assembling the evidence and drawing conclusions from it. It is not enough for a person to throw up *any* explanation for evidence presented to him. To move from "I saw a light on the water" to "I saw a ghost at Dead Man's Bluff" is to make an unjustified and irrational leap. Ideally, we should infer to the best explanation.[16]

Physicians, concerned to promote theoretical rationality, may assemble facts in a way which together suggest a conclusion. But patients may still fail to draw the right conclusion. Telling a patient that he has "advanced cancer" may imply that he will die. But the patient may not conclude this. Indeed, even telling a patient that he will die may not convey "the message" that the physician intends to give: perhaps that the patient ought to sort out his affairs, that he will not offer any more curative treatments, and so on.

How would a person who is in a similar epistemic position to Arthur, but who is more theoretically rational than Arthur 3, convince him that the can contains petrol? He would engage Arthur in argument. He would provide reasons. He might say something like, "The can seems to be in a different position from how you left it. That might suggest that someone has used it. I can smell petrol. Perhaps someone has used the can to carry petrol."

The reason why most JWs hold an irrational belief is because they make mistakes in their theoretical reasoning. What is the best way to correct these mistakes? For many, it is a matter of someone versed in the relevant texts taking them through the argument.

In other cases, the route may be more indirect. A JW may be presented with some information, call it, I, which should or would cause him to conclude that C if he also held other beliefs, B. However, he may fail to believe B or utilise B. He may have forgotten B in the urgent search for salvation, or had it drummed out of his head, or failed to see any longer its relevance. Intervention requires that we tap into these other beliefs. For an argument to be convincing for him may require the construction of the appropriate context: to show him that his belief should be rejected in his own terms.

Our object is the beliefs of JWs, not necessarily their choices. In some circumstances, JWs might autonomously choose to reject blood. We can autonomously adopt a course of action with a low probability of success, provided that we hold the relevant rational beliefs. Neither risk-takers nor the exceedingly cautious are necessarily non-autonomous, nor are they necessarily doing what there is good reason not to do.[17]

If JWs were to hold the relevant informed, rational beliefs, they might then autonomously choose to reject blood. But from their revised epistemic position, many would no doubt accept blood.

V. Summary and Implications

Where most rational agents differ from JWs is that they do not hold all of the following beliefs:

1. There is a God.
2. Divinely conferred immortality is possible for human beings after death.
3. God forbids eating blood.
4. Accepting a blood transfusion is no different from eating blood.
5. If one eats blood when alive, one turns to dust upon death.
6. We know 3–5 to be true based on faith that a (selectively) literal interpretation of *The Bible* reveals God's will.
7. If one lives a faithful life in accord with Jehovah's laws, eternal life is assured.

Many health care workers no doubt believe 1 and 2 and some variation on 7; it is 3, 4, 5, or especially 6 that is rejected. But this is a difference not in moral beliefs or values but about the structure of reality. This is a difference of opinion about metaphysics.

Hence if we are to respect JWs' refusals of life-prolonging blood transfusions, it is not on the grounds that we are obliged to respect decision-making that is based on a different value system from ours. Their values are the same as many other theists and atheists. They value earthly life and immortality as much as others do.

We often hear that we should allow people to do what there is no good reason to do out of respect for their nature as autonomous beings, as ends in themselves. But many such instances are something else entirely. They are cases in which people hold irrational beliefs. They are cases of theoretical irrationality. We do not respect autonomy when we encourage people to act on irrational beliefs. Rather, such beliefs limit a person's autonomy.

Rational Deliberation

Our aim has been to expand the regulative ideal governing consent. We have argued that true beliefs are necessary for evaluation. Information is important to choice insofar as it helps a person to hold the relevant true beliefs. But in order to hold the relevant true beliefs, competent people must also think rationally. Insofar as information is important, rational deliberation is important. Just as physicians should aim to provide relevant information regarding the medical procedures prior to patients consenting to have those procedures, they should also assist patients to think more clearly and rationally. They should care more about the rationality of patients'' beliefs.

Since holding true beliefs is necessary to be autonomous, we do not respect autonomy when we allow patients to act on irrational beliefs. Should physicians override choices based on irrational beliefs? Should life-saving blood transfusions be given to JWs against their wishes?

When we look at to how informed medical decisions must be, we see that a requirement of informedness functions as an ideal to be striven for, and not as a requirement to be enforced. Society generally accepts that patients should be informed of all the relevant facts, but not that they must be compelled to accept information which they do not want. To force information on a person would be coercive.

The requirements of theoretical rationality should be on a par with requirements of informedness. This raises the question whether we should override both choices made in ignorance of relevant information or on the basis of irrational beliefs. We believe that there are reasons against taking this radical departure from the notion of informed consent as a regulative ideal.

The first reason is consequentialist: if we allow doctors to override choices based on some species of irrationality, then other JWs will be distressed at the thought their decisions will be overridden. The general misery and distrust of medicine that would result would reduce the value of such a policy. In the vast majority of cases, JWs' refusal of blood does not compromise their care. In fact, many may receive better care. Given the small numbers of people who would be saved by such a policy, it is not clear that it would be for the best. As is usually the case, education is better than compulsion.

Secondly, though a practice of allowing people to act out of wilful ignorance or irrationality may not promote their autonomy in the short term, respect for autonomy is not the only ground for non-interference in another person's life. It is surely enough that it is his life, and that he ought to be allowed to do what there is no good reason to do, if he chooses. Respect for persons is not restricted to respect for wholly rational persons.

In some cases, irrationality is so gross that it calls into question a person's competence. In these cases, intervention may be justified. But at lesser degrees of irrationality, we encourage the development of autonomy for all people in the long term by adopting a policy of empowering people to make their own choices.

Thirdly, *requiring* that choice be grounded on rational beliefs before it is respected is fraught with dangers. Those who claim to know Truth with certainty are at least as dangerous as those who claim to know Right and Good with certainty. Dogmatic ideologues of either sort show a lamentable propensity to use their "knowledge" to oppress others, sometimes "benignly" as paternalists, more often tyrannically as authoritarians. Hence a measure of epistemic scepticism about our own rationality or the lack of rationality in others is highly desirable.

In the end, deferral to irrationality, to partial autonomy, to imperfect consent and to unexplored values and metaphysical beliefs in patients may be necessary, even morally required. But before reaching this point, a physician committed to the highest standard of care will exercise her talents as an educator to promote greater rationality in patients. Not to make the effort to promote rational, critical deliberation is to risk a very contemporary form of patient abandonment: abandonment to human irrationality.

Duties as Educators

In important ways, physicians have always been expected to be educators: about how bodies work, do not work, and go awry; about how to care for our bodies in sickness and health; about, in the end, how to live a mortal embodied existence. Our discussion suggests, however, that physician duties as educators are more extensive. For in order genuinely to respect autonomy and patients' values, physicians must be prepared to do more than provide patients with information relevant to making evaluative choices. They must attend to how that information is received, understood and used. Good education is not restricted to providing information. It requires encouraging in others the requisite skills for dealing with information rationally.

If an ethic of respect for persons in contemporary medicine rules out—except in the most extreme cases—coercion as a response to patient irrationality, it also makes more imperative a "critical educator" response to patient irrationality. One caveat, however: effective educators know when to promote critical enquiry. Physicians, whose primary obligations are to the medical wellbeing of patients, will do well to resist the secondary obligation to promote rational criticism of deeply held beliefs at a time when their patients are impaired and suffering greatly. Thus the time to engage a hypothetically irrational JW in a critical enquiry about her convictions on "eating blood" is not the time at which she might benefit from an immediate blood transfusion because her life is in jeopardy.

It may be a very contemporary form of physician abandonment of patients in need to accept wilfulness as autonomy, the mere provision of information as adequate for informed consent, and acceptance of any morally or metaphysically bizarre view held by patients as grounds for not pursuing a medically beneficial course of treatment. But if physicians are to promote autonomy, if they are to respect patients as persons, if they are to help patients to choose and do what there is good reason to do, they should care more about the rationality of their patients' beliefs. Physicians must concern themselves with helping patients to deliberate more effectively and, ultimately, must themselves learn to care more about theoretical rationality. To do any less is to abandon patients to autonomy-destroying theoretical irrationality.

Acknowledgement

Thanks to Derek Parfit, Michael Lockwood and David Malyon for many helpful comments.

Notes and References

1. Dworkin G. *The theory and practice of autonomy.* Cambridge: Cambridge University Press, 1988: 12.
2. Adapted from Parfit D. *Reasons and persons.* Oxford: Clarendon Press, 1984: 153.
3. Forrest P. *The dynamics of belief: a normative logic.* Oxford: Basil Blackwell, 1986.
4. Watch Tower Bible and Tract Society of Pennsylvania. *Family care and medical management for Jehovah's Witnesses.* New York: Watch Tower Bible and Tract Society of New York, 1995.
5. *The new English Bible*: Genesis 9: 3–4.
6. *The new English Bible*: Leviticus 17: 10, 13, 14; 7: 26, 7; Numbers 15: 30, 31; Deuteronomy 12: 23–5.
7. *The new English Bible*: Leviticus 17: 11.
8. *The new English Bible*: Acts 15: 29.
9. *The new English Bible*: Matthew 26: 26–9.
10. *The new English Bible*: Galatians 3: 10.
11. *The new English Bible*: Galatians 3:13.
12. *The new English Bible*: Galatians 3: 24 5.
13. *The new English Bible*: Galatians 4: 24.
14. *The new English Bible*: Galatians 5: 2–6.
15. Belief in God may be a basic belief: a belief which does not rest on other beliefs. (Swinburne R. *Faith and reason.* Oxford: Clarendon Press, 1981: 33.) A basic rational belief is a belief in a proposition that is (1) self-evident or fundamental, (2) evident to the senses or memory, or (3) defensible by argument, inquiry or performance (Kenny A. *Faith and reason.* New York: Columbia University Press, 1983: 27). Beliefs about eating blood are secondary beliefs. They must be justified in terms of other beliefs. It is precisely this that cannot be rationally done.
16. Armstrong DM. *What is a law of nature?* Cambridge: Cambridge University Press, 1983: 59.
17. Pascal gave a rationalist argument for belief in God: we have more to lose if we do not believe in God, and we are wrong (eternal torment), than we have to lose if we do believe in God, and we are wrong (living under an illusion). So we ought to believe that God exists (Pascal B. *Pensées.* Geneve: Pierre Cailler, 1947: fragment 223). Theoretically rational JWs could give a similar justification for refusing blood.

Cultural Diversity and Informed Consent

ELLEN AGARD, DANIEL FINKELSTEIN,
AND EDWARD WALLACH

Case

Mr. and Mrs. R have recently come to the United States from Eastern Europe for medical care. They are a professional couple in their mid-thirties: educated, fluent in English, and financially comfortable. They have no children.

Mrs. R has a history of chronic pelvic inflammatory disease that has not responded well to conservative treatment. A year ago, she had a ruptured ectopic pregnancy that resulted in surgical removal of one ovary and fallopian tube. Since then, she has completed three courses of intravenous (IV) antibiotic therapy. She is admitted to the hospital for further diagnosis and treatment.

In consultation with her attending physician, Mr. R expresses great concern about his wife's pain and poor health. Mrs. R is concerned primarily about her ability to have children. Mr. R wants everything possible done to cure his wife, and asks for a surgical consultation.

The surgeon explains to Mr. and Mrs. R that although surgery might help to clear the infection, he does not recommend it at this time because it might well involve removing Mrs. R's second ovary, leaving her infertile. The couple requests that the surgery be done; Mrs. R signs the consent form, and surgery is scheduled.

On the evening before surgery, Mrs. R says to one of the nurses: "I have always wanted to have children, but my husband says that this has gone on too long; that we must do whatever is necessary for my health, so we can get back to our home and our jobs. He says I have been too sick to be a good wife to him." The nurse offers to talk with Mrs. R about her decision, or to arrange for her to talk it over with her physicians or a social worker. Mrs. R says, "My husband is sure that this is the right thing to do."

The nurse understands that in Mr. and Mrs. R's culture, it is customary for the wife to accede to her husband's wishes, and for the husband to make decisions about his wife's medical treatment. However, based on her conversation with Mrs. R, she is concerned that Mrs. R's decision to have surgery may represent her husband's wishes more than her own. The nurse discusses this concern with the attending physician, and they decide to seek guidance from the hospital ethics committee before proceeding with surgery.

Discussion

A clinical perspective

It would be preferable not to proceed with surgery until the options for medical treatment have been exhausted. Continued treatment with IV antibiotics offers the possibility of preserving Mrs. R's remaining ovary, maintaining her normal ovarian function and her fertility. However, if Mr. and Mrs. R understand the implications of this procedure, reach their decision together, and give consent, it is acceptable to proceed with surgery.

A legal perspective

Informed consent requires that the physician explain to the patient the nature of her ailment, the procedure to be performed, and its risks, benefits, and alternatives. The discussion with Mrs. R should include information about her chances of conceiving and having a normal pregnancy if the surgery is not done.

Mrs. R has been informed of the proposed procedure and has consented to it. She can always revoke her consent. Because she has expressed concern about the surgery, another discussion with her physician is indicated. In an attempt to keep the consent process free of coercion, this discussion should take place only between Mrs. R and her physician.

A cultural perspective

We are told that in Mr. and Mrs. R's culture, the wife accedes to the husband's authority in decisions about medical treatment and having children. However, we cannot determine on the basis of the limited information we have, if Mrs. R is being coerced. In fact, we do not know how the couple has arrived at their decision, or what meaning fertility has for them. Perhaps Mr. R is genuinely concerned about his wife's health. Perhaps Mrs. R is genuinely willing to forgo having children.

We must avoid making assumptions based on our own cultural values or our limited understanding of Mr. and Mrs. R's values. Mrs. R is better able than we are to understand the implications of her decision for her marriage and her future. If we interfere, we are assuming that we can make a better decision for her than she can make for herself.

Analysis

This case and commentary were developed by the authors to foster discussion about the impact of cultural diversity on ethical deliberation. As a composite, the case lacks some of the rich depth and detail that emerge during full ethics committee deliberation. First, Mrs. R's desire for children is made known only in a passing comment to one of the nurses. We do not know how to evaluate the strength or durability of this desire, or how to weigh it against the other preferences, desires, and goals in Mrs. R's life. Second, we do not know what efforts have been made to foster communication among Mr. and Mrs. R and the staff—whether they have talked with a social worker, obtained religious guidance (if appropriate), or talked with a representative from the hospital's international office. Finally, we do not have a final resolution for this case. Instead, we struggle to think through the issues that this case raises within these complex, unsatisfactory, and "real world" limitations.

This case presents a real ethical dilemma. Different decisions, choices, and courses of action are open to the couple and to the staff. These different options are supported by strong but conflicting ethical arguments. When it comes to choosing among them, we must decide which ethical arguments are the more compelling.

The dilemma that the staff confronts is this: is it appropriate to proceed with surgery when (1) Mrs. R's consent appears to reflect her husband's wishes rather than her own, and (2) the procedure to which she has consented places her reproductive capacity at risk? We need to consider whether and/or how to explore the decision for surgery further with this couple.

Respect for cultural diversity

In this case, Mrs. R has given written consent for surgery. The staff feels that Mr. R has unduly influenced her decision, and that the decision to proceed with surgery goes against her own desire for children. However, it is not clear whether or not it is appropriate for the staff to "second guess" the couple's decision-making process.

In Mr. and Mrs. R's culture, we are told, the husband traditionally takes a dominant role in making major decisions. If this is so, then Mrs. R's decision represents a decision that is consistent with her own social and cultural context. Furthermore, it represents her own understanding of her relationship with her husband, the options that are available to her, and the value of her fertility relative to other life plans and values. As outsiders to this culture, and to the couple's relationship, we are not in a position to evaluate or judge Mrs. R's own reading of her situation. By overriding her decision, the staff risks imposing their own cultural values on Mrs. R, values that may not be relevant or appropriate for her situation. Such interference would be paternalistic; it would assume that the staff can make a better decision for Mrs. R than she can make for herself.

Over time, our society has developed greater awareness, respect, and tolerance for cultural diversity. We recognize that customs, practices, and values vary greatly among cultures. We respect cultural diversity when, for example, we learn to appreciate various styles of art or cuisine, or learn to understand differing religious beliefs and practices. Occasionally such differences may be confusing or unappealing to us. Even so, it is generally appropriate to respond with tolerance and respect.

In the clinical setting, respecting cultural difference may require us to make accommodation in our ordinary practice. Efforts regularly are and should be made to respect dietary restrictions, religious commitments, and different standards of privacy, particularly between genders. Usually these accommodations can be made without compromising professional ethics or personal integrity. Occasionally, however, cultural differences engage our deeply held moral values, and threaten our deepest personal and professional commitments. When this occurs, it is difficult to discern how we ought to proceed.

Although we are obligated to be respectful and tolerant of values and customs that differ from our own, here we confront a cultural tradition that appears to undermine Mrs. R's choice and consent on a fundamental level. In this case, the stakes are so high that we need to consider our respect for cultural differences in the light of our concern for Mrs. R's right to make her own choices.

Respect for human rights and dignity

The validity of Mrs. R's consent, and the significance of the procedure for which she has given consent, are separate but inter-related concerns. We might be less concerned about the consent process if Mrs. R were undergoing a simple appendectomy or low-risk diagnostic test. In general, our scrutiny of the consent process is influenced by the invasiveness or risks of the procedure involved.

The risk to Mrs. R's fertility is not a critical issue in and of itself; for example, if Mrs. R herself did not desire children, and preferred surgery and a quick recovery, her decision would be far less troublesome. However, we do know that fertility and reproduction have profound meaning across cultures. Without necessarily knowing what they may mean to any particular individual, the risk that this surgery poses to Mrs. R's fertility is a matter for concern.

Although we do not know what value childbearing has for Mrs. R, she has made it known that her fertility is important to her, and that she does not want to lose it. The proposed surgery places at risk something she values. Thus the risk to her fertility raises our scrutiny of the consent process to a very high level, and highlights her lack of full consent as a critical issue.

In Western medical practice, obtaining an individual's informed consent is both an ethical and legal requirement. In requiring that consent for a procedure be fully informed, one ensures that patients make their own decisions about medical interventions that affect their health and well-being. Because this surgery affects Mrs. R in a way that is profoundly important to her, it cannot proceed without her full consent.

A commitment to the fundamental dignity and worth of all human beings provides the foundation for the perspective of human rights. From this perspective, fundamental human rights are universally applicable to all human beings, by virtue of each person's unique and intrinsic moral dignity and worth. As this perspective has gained recognition across cultures, it has been widely recognized that the right to make basic life decisions constitutes such a fundamental human right.

Cultural differences do not provide sufficient grounds for overriding what appears to be Mrs. R's deep desire to preserve her fertility. Knowing that gender inequities diminish the rights of women in many cultural settings, we would choose to question rather than reinforce such inequities in the clinical setting. Thus our reluctance to proceed with surgery represents a reluctance to participate in what can be viewed as a violation of Mrs. R's basic human rights.

Recommendations

A first step in addressing this case is to pursue further discussion with Mr. and Mrs. R, separately and together. Social services, the chaplain's department, and the services for international patients that are offered by many hospitals are significant resources for facilitating such discussion. Every effort should be made to understand and respect the decision-making process of Mrs. R and her husband, as well as the concerns of the clinicians involved in Mrs. R's case. An atmosphere of respect offers an opportunity to explore Mrs. R's decision in light of her own values and preferences, as well as those of her husband.

Such a discussion is needed because the details of this case, as we relate them here, do not allow us to make a clear choice for the claims of human rights over the claims of cultural difference. We argue against interpreting this dilemma too readily as a simple case of cultural difference. If we do this, we run the risk of proceeding with surgery that deprives Mrs. R of her fertility, against her wishes. At the same time, we recognize the risk of undue interference in this couple's decision-making process and final decision.

A discussion with Mr. and Mrs. R needs to include a review of the risks of morbidity and mortality associated with surgery, as well as an exploration of their values and how they make decisions. It is possible that after further exploration, Mr. R will place a different value on his wife's desire to have children. If he persists in preferring surgery, then Mrs. R's clinical team must consider how best to preserve her rights and dignity within the constraints of her culture and her relationship with her husband. It is of paramount importance that the medical team avoid generating conflict within the couple's relationship. An imperfect resolution may be to proceed with surgery, but only after making sure that Mrs. R has every opportunity to act according to her own wishes.

As our healthcare system cares for more and more patients from different health-care backgrounds, our moral obligation to respond to conflicting value judgments will become increasingly apparent. Our duty to respect each individual's human dignity and worth can be as challenging as the case presented here. Recognizing and responding to such conflicts challenges clinicians to obtain all the consultation available to them in situations where cross-cultural differences raise concerns about human rights.

D. Gender, Culture, and Race

On Treatment of Myopia
Feminist Standpoint Theory and Bioethics

MARY B. MAHOWALD

The insights of feminist standpoint theory provide a corrective to the near-sightedness, unselfconsciousness, and arrogance that arise in health care and in bioethics, as in other areas of life and work. A *feminist standpoint* is one that reflects the perspectives of women while challenging the social dominance of men's perspectives. Feminist standpoint *theory* refers to the rationale that supports that standpoint and strategies for implementing it.[1] Although my account focuses on sexism, similar arguments apply to racism and classism, and there is obvious overlap in these applications. The common element is that the differences between groups are the grounds by which one group obtains or maintains advantages or power over another. In defense of inequality or injustice, irrelevant differences may be invoked or relevant differences overlooked. From a feminist standpoint,[2] the ethical criterion for determining the relevance of differences between women and men is gender justice or equality.[3]

In what follows I point out flaws in contemporary health care and bioethics that indicate the need for a feminist standpoint.... I argue for a view of care and justice as compatible. The ethical and epistemological strengths of standpoint theory are illustrated through a case that reveals one physician's view of her relationship with patients. As a means of promoting gender justice in health care and bioethics, I conclude with a proposal for utilizing feminist standpoint theory on an ongoing basis.

Some Flaws in Contemporary Health Care and Bioethics

Nearsightedness, unselfconsciousness, and arrogance are related flaws, each reinforcing a natural tendency to construe one's partial perspective as the full picture. By nearsightedness, I mean that none of us, as finite, situated individuals, can see all of the parameters of the decisions we make. This limitation says something positive as well as negative. It allows that we at least see what is near, even though we cannot see what is beyond our range of vision, including the long-range implications of our decisions.

To some degree, nearsightedness is encouraged within health care. Medical specialization and hierarchical (usually patriarchal) distribution of roles increase the propensity to limited vision. Beyond the maximization of health expertise that specialization facilitates, the choice of specialties is often motivated by the higher status of those who focus narrowly on a particular area of medicine. Generalists tend to be less rewarded by income and prestige than their specialist counterparts. Nearsightedness is also encouraged whenever the practitioner's obligations are defined exclusively in terms of the patient or client, ignoring the ripple effect that such decisions have on others.

Bioethicists are nearsighted too. Some view bioethical issues solely from their offices, classrooms, and lecture halls, maintaining their distance from the clinical settings in which the actual issues arise. While some are experts in areas on which their work relies, such as metaethics, ethical theory, medical science, clinical skills, and social science, they cannot be experts in all of these areas. Nearsightedness is also evident in the overall failure of bioethicists to attend to the ethical problems raised by racism, classism, and sexism, including heterosexism. Moreover, those who work in medical schools and hospitals may be co-opted by the values and priorities of the institutions that employ them. Such co-optation suggests the nearsightedness that William James referred to as "a certain blindness" regarding other values and priorities.[4]

Unselfconsciousness is used here to mean the lack of a sense of one's limitations. Some unselfconscious persons assume themselves capable of "point-of-viewlessness," defining their particular views as universal.[5] In contrast, a self-conscious person acknowledges her weaknesses as well as strengths, and acts accordingly. Like Socrates in the *Apology*,[6] the self-conscious person is anxious to avoid having others falsely attribute expertise to her. Socratic wisdom, and the imparting of that wisdom, necessarily includes knowledge of one's own ignorance. In areas of health care that emphasize treating the whole person or even the entire family, such as primary care medicine, family practice, nursing, and social work, there is sometimes a tendency to ignore or forget one's limitations. The clinician may then attempt the god-like feat of single-handedly providing for all of her patient's needs, without drawing on the more focused expertise of others whose involvement might improve her care.

Similarly, health care specialists sometimes pass judgment unselfconsciously on areas of health care about which they have relatively little knowledge in comparison with those practicing in those areas—for example, doctors vis-à-vis nurses, or surgeons vis-à-vis psychiatrists. One group may assert authority over the other, while ignoring the fact that they lack the experience and training of the other. This point applies also to clinicians who are ethicists. Although they may provide ethics consultations at the bedside, their clinical specialization limits the extent to which their clinical advice is appropriate for patients who require treatment by other specialists. Patient care, in all of its complex clinical, social, and ethical dimensions, cannot be optimized without the collaboration of those who are optimally qualified for different aspects of its provision.

Titles, positions, social attitudes, and publicity often promote unselfconsciousness. The public sometimes associates leadership in any area of medicine or philosophy with expertise on ethical issues relevant to medicine. Accordingly, a leader in a particular area of medicine or philosophy may be invited to speak or write on ethical issues about which others have broader and more critical knowledge. If she is selfconscious about her limitation, she will defer to those others, or at least call on them and credit them for their input. If she is unselfconscious, she may accept such invitations under false pretenses regarding her expertise. . . .

While unselfconsciousness ignores limitations, arrogance exaggerates strengths. To some, medicine presents a context in which arrogance serves a useful purpose. Consider, for example, the routine behavior of surgeons. To cut into a human body, to manipulate and remove organs, to place other organs and devices into the body—possibly these procedures could only be done by someone who is arrogant. Moreover, just because invasiveness is overt does not mean that it is more drastic than covert interventions. Psychotherapy, for example, may be more invasive than surgery because it affects people's minds rather than their bodies.[7] In both contexts, arrogance may be necessary for therapeutic effectiveness. Arrogance may also be both essential and problematic in nonmedical specialties or professions such as teaching and politics. Rightly or wrongly, bioethicists who are not clinicians may be just as arrogant as those who are.

The dictionary offers "pride" as a synonym for "arrogance." Pride is sometimes construed as a good thing, and only bad if it constitutes a false assessment of the facts. When it is construed in the latter way, pride is purportedly the principal sin of humankind. As Valerie Saiving maintains, however, the principal sin of women is not pride but "underdevelopment or negation of the self."[8] To be truthful about one's strengths along with one's weaknesses is a form of humility. The arrogance to be avoided involves denial of one's limitations, leading to expressions of power that place others at risk. It is not only possible but crucial for health care practitioners and bioethicists to avoid this kind of arrogance.

To some extent, nearsightedness, unselfconsciousness, and arrogance are inevitable in human life. It is possible and desirable, however, to reduce their negative implications through standpoint theory. Standpoint theory is based on recognition that each one's point of view, expertise, and authority are situated and partial. It implies the need for attention to views that are often neglected, such as those of women. A feminist standpoint serves as a corrective to the overall neglect of women's interests, experience, and insights in contemporary health care and bioethics. . . .

Feminist Standpoint and Attention to Relationships and Context

An expanded version of feminist standpoint theory is reinforced by the attention that contemporary bioethics has directed to relationships and context. In health care as in other areas, relationships are often discussed in the context of roles. The dominant and dominating role of the paternalistic physician is often cited, but dominant and dominated roles abound within the health care hierarchy. Historically, nurses have been seen and have even viewed themselves as handmaids of physicians, reflecting gender stereotypes.[9] To the extent that standpoint theory has been incorporated into the health care system, nurses have enriched the epistemological base of clinical judgments. Nonetheless, hierarchical arrangements remain evident not only among the different health care professions, but also within each profession. Like society in general, health care reflects a patriarchal system.

In various models of the physician–patient relationship, the doctor's dominant role is the vantage point from which the relationship is explained and assessed. Obviously, patients also play a role in the relationship, but they are often considered only as the assumed object of beneficence, or in the context of *permitting* them to exercise autonomy. Because patients are generally dominated by doctors, standpoint theory is indispensable to the reduction of nearsightedness, unselfconsciousness, and arrogance on the part of physicians. From a feminist standpoint, this is doubly important because the majority of patients are women and the majority of physicians are still men.[10]

None of the prevailing models of the physician–patient relationship[11] reflects a feminist standpoint, that is, one that considers the experiences of women—whether as individuals, women in general, or members of other nondominant groups—as crucial to the analysis and assessment of that relationship. A feminist standpoint is crucial because it takes account of the embeddedness of the doctor–patient relationship in other relationships, whether these involve dominance or not. When feminist standpoint theory applies to individuals as well as groups, it also takes account, as traditional models of the physician–patient relationship do not, of the mutuality of that relationship, acknowledging that physicians and patients alike have rights and responsibilities vis-à-vis each other.

In their critique of traditional ethics, various versions of feminism insist on considerations of context, that is, the situatedness on which feminist standpoint theory relies. In health care, the consideration of context mainly takes the form of case based analysis. The clinician's thinking and decision making are usually precipitated by an actual case that raises questions about treatment or nontreatment. The health caregiver attempts to optimize care of a particular patient with whom she has a special relationship that involves a special responsibility. Although the term "care" is often identified with treatment, the caregiver knows that this is sometimes a mistaken identity, that optimal care sometimes means that treatment should be foregone or withdrawn.

Recently, Albert Jonsen and Stephen Toulmin have proposed a revival of casuistry as a method by which case-based analyses may be applied to bioethics. They affirm an extended version of feminist standpoint theory (without calling it that) when they write that *"moral knowledge is essentially particular."*[12] Not surprisingly, this method is broadly supported by clinical ethicists. Except for its neglect of broader social issues, it is also supported by feminist bioethicists.[13] The feminist reservation about the adequacy of casuistry for clinical ethics is that its emphasis on cases provides too limited a sense of context.

The Meaning of Care and the Pitfalls of Care-Based Reasoning

Taking account of the particularity of individual relationships through an extension of feminist standpoint theory not only shows consistency with the case-based reasoning of clinicians and clinical ethicists, but also with the care-based models of moral reasoning recently developed by Carol Gilligan and Nel Noddings. Both derive their understanding of care from an analysis of women's experience; both insist on the centrality of women's standpoint in women's own ethical judgment, but argue for its relevance to men as well. Gilligan, drawing on her studies of women facing unwanted pregnancy, defines a care ethic as concerned primarily with responsibilities that arise from attachment or ties to others, disregarding the impartiality that traditional ethics demands.[14] Noddings distinguishes between natural and ethical caring, claiming the experience of motherhood as the paradigm for ethical behavior. Ethical caring means deliberate expression of the natural inclination of mothers to be engrossed in concerns about their children and to identify their children's interests with their own.[15]

Despite the emphasis on relationships and women's experience that Gilligan and Noddings elaborate, many feminists have been uneasy about the implications of their views. Women's standpoints, after all, are not always identical with a feminist standpoint. Just as nurses who define their primary responsibility as care for patients experience gender injustice in a patriarchal health care system, mothers who naturally and ethically define their primary responsibility as care for their children are often exploited by being deprived of opportunities equal to their male counterparts. The same is true for women who are the predominant caregivers of the disabled, the sick, and the elderly. Feminists are therefore concerned that those who champion a care-based ethic may reinforce the long-standing practice of exploiting women's natural propensity to care. Through its insistence on critique of the dominant standpoint, feminist standpoint theory attempts to preempt this injustice. It thus argues that considerations of gender justice be joined to those of a care ethic.

One feminist who has argued persuasively for a necessary connection between care and justice is Marilyn Friedman. Her account further illustrates how feminist standpoint contributes to ethical theory and practice.[16] Acknowledging that a gender difference in moral reasoning is empirically disputed, Friedman analyzes the implications of gender differences that are not in dispute. "Even if actual statistical differences in the moral reasoning of women and men cannot be confirmed," she writes, "there is nevertheless a real difference in the moral norms and values culturally associated with gender."[17] This "real difference" leads to what Friedman calls a gender-based "division of moral labor," supported by stereotypically defined differences that may or may not be present in individuals.

According to Friedman, the two categories of care and justice overlap, and if care is morally adequate, it involves justice in personal as well as professional relationships. Similarly, if justice means giving people their due, it demands determination of what constitutes due care for each. The application of this concept to health care is obvious: the health practitioner must recognize and respond to the different health needs of each patient. Discovery and treatment of such needs are impossible without attunement to the patient's standpoint as privileged epistemologically and ethically. . . .

If care is defined broadly enough to encompass justice, it is care in either domain, and if justice is defined broadly enough to accommodate the uniqueness of interpersonal and professional relationships, it is justice in either domain. Defining either locus more narrowly requires recognition that human beings live and act in both contexts, with different roles to play in each. The political context mainly involves the narrower concept of justice, while professional and personal contexts mainly involve the narrower concept of care. Only if the concepts of justice and care are construed broadly are they equally applicable to either context. At that point, neither care nor justice has priority; the two are interchangeable because each entails the other. To the feminist position that the personal is political, we might then add that the political is personal.

Friedman proposes a model of friendship for ethical care.[18] If friendship includes both justice and care, it may serve as an ethical ideal for familial as well as for other interpersonal and professional relationships. Developmentally, we learn to care from those who care for us, and in most instances that means friends as well as relatives. The "caring work" that predominates in women's lives occurs in situations in which relatives or nonrelatives regard each other as friends. According to Ruddick, this "caring work" underlies a feminist standpoint.[19]

But is care in the health setting equivalent to the caring described by Gilligan, Noddings, and Ruddick? For all three authors the meaning of care derives from women's experience of caring. Maternal thinking is care-based because its defining feature is a natural inclination to care for one's child. The thinking involved in this process is particular, partial, and practical.[20] It aims to foster the development of another as a unique individual. Just as a woman first becomes a biological mother by pushing her baby out of her body, so the caring labor of maternal thinking (no matter who undertakes it) consists of pushing people toward independence through fulfillment of their own potential. Similarly, the goal of health care is to render the caregiver unnecessary. If the care provided in the health setting has this goal, it is consistent with the care described by Gilligan, Noddings, and Ruddick.

Unfortunately, however, care in the health setting is often equated with treatment, and treatment is not necessarily caring. It is not caring if it ignores or impedes the thrust toward self-differentiation epitomized in childbirth, which is biologically and psychologically natural in human beings. It is not caring if it fails to respect and support the uniqueness of the other that a loving parental relationship exemplifies. In other words, caring essentially involves attention to differences, whether these apply to groups or individuals.[21] An extension of feminist standpoint theory obviously supports this interpretation of caring.

An Illustrative Case

As already suggested, the reasons for extending standpoint theory to individuals are epistemological and ethical. To illustrate this in the context of health care, consider the following case:[22]

Al Brown is a seventy-three-year-old man with cerebral palsy and severe spastic paralysis in all four limbs. He was admitted to a dependent care facility forty years ago and has lived there ever since. Despite his significant physical impairment and need for assistance with basic life functions, he is cognitively intact.

Several years ago, Mr. Brown was given phenobarbitol for treatment of a seizure disorder. When the threat of seizures subsided, he continued to receive 60 milligrams of phenobarbitol four times a day. Now, each time a new pharmacist or physician is assigned to his unit, phenobarbitol levels are drawn. These invariably run in the 50s in micrograms per milliliter, suggesting to clinicians that his dosage should be reduced. Mr. Brown objects to the reduction, stating that he is doing fine, has not had any seizures, and "always gets messed up when people fool around with my medications."

Dr. Ann Joseph, the attending physician for the unit, has a somewhat novel view of her patients and their claims on her. She calls them "customers," and assumes that "the customer is always right" when there is any medical doubt about treatment or nontreatment. Although Dr. Joseph has explained to Mr. Brown the risks reported in the medical literature regarding his level of phenobarbitol, he insists, and she agrees, that these are statistical risks that may not apply to him. He says he feels well with the 60 milligram dosage and poorly whenever the dosage is lowered. Dr. Joseph regards his view as privileged and instructs the house staff not to reduce the "customer's" phenobarbitol level.

Although clinical texts do not support Mr. Brown's phenobarbitol dosage, Dr. Joseph recognizes that her patient has a uniquely valid standpoint from which to judge whether its administration hurts or helps him. She thus not only respects his autonomy but credits him with knowledge about his own condition that textbooks, articles, or even experience with other patients cannot provide. In other words, she recognizes her own nearsightedness, even when her vision is improved by input from colleagues; self-conscious about her own limitations, she avoids arrogance. As a patient, Mr. Brown belongs to a dominated group. By gender Dr. Joseph belongs to a dominated group, but by profession she belongs to a dominant group. While dominant in her relationship with Mr. Brown, she realizes that his standpoint constitutes "an engaged vision of the world opposed and superior to dominant ways of thinking."[23]

Perhaps it is no accident that Dr. Joseph (whose name I have changed here) is a woman. Recent studies indicate that female physicians spend more time than their male counterparts listening to patients.[24] With Ruddick, I believe it is possible and preferable for men as well as women to be "maternal thinkers," and with Gilligan and Noddings I believe it possible and preferable for men as well as women to be both care-reasoners and justice-reasoners. But if care for others involves attention to individual differences, the data obtained by Gilligan and her colleagues suggest that women are more likely than men to incorporate an extended version of standpoint theory into their moral, political, and professional judgments. Care as defined by Dr. Joseph goes beyond the maxim of clinical practice: "When in doubt, look at the patient." She recognizes not only the limitations of theoretical knowledge but also the privileged status of patients' experience and knowledge of their own illness. Care of patients, for Dr. Joseph, involves the dictum: "Listen to the customer."

Standpoint-based judgments may be more prevalent among women than men because women already belong to a group whose standpoint has been neglected throughout history. They are therefore more likely to challenge what Catharine MacKinnon calls "masculine partiality," the presumption of objectivity and universality that men have generally attributed to their limited knowledge and experience of the world.[25] Sometimes the presumption is overt; sometimes it is covert. Women themselves often support the presumption.

It is not difficult to understand why many women accept masculine partiality as definitive. Having been socialized in a sexist culture, the wonder is that there are so many women and men who challenge it. Even among those who reject the presumption, the self-consciousness implicit in feminist standpoint theory is sometimes lacking. Consider, for example, the current tendency to use gender-neutral language in addressing various topics in health care and bioethics. Even beyond reproduction, many issues are not gender-neutral. These include the health implications of the feminization of poverty, the problem of battered women, the high incidence of women who suffer from eating disorders and of those who subject themselves to health risks for the sake of appearance.[26] Recent articles on the Human Genome Project address the entire range of ethical and social questions raised by the project in gender-neutral language.[27] Yet it is women alone who supply ova, gestate, and give birth, and who undergo prenatal diagnosis, pregnancy termination, and fetal therapies. It is mainly women, but need not be mainly women, who are targeted for genetic screening, who are primary caregivers of those who are genetically disabled, and who work in those areas of clinical genetics that are least rewarded.[28] Clearly, then, the Human Genome Project is not gender-neutral in its implications.

Such examples call for attention to differences between the genders rather than gender-neutrality. Inattention to gender differences allows the dominant group, whether deliberately or not, to exclude the nondominant group from the advantages that it enjoys. To promote equality in heath care, which presumably is a goal of bioethics as well as feminism, attention to non-dominant standpoints is thus not only useful but necessary. But how can such attention be ensured or promoted? In closing I propose a modest strategy for implementing feminist standpoint theory.

Proportionate Representation as a Remedial Strategy

In American society we are familiar with the concept and strategy of proportionate representation. Despite failures in implementing this strategy, it is potentially a means by which each individual exerts some influence in policy decisions that apply to everyone. At an earlier point in history, direct participation of citizens in town meetings offered a purer form of democracy than we have now; that model ceased to be operable when society became too large and complex for every competent adult to be directly involved in its governance. Proportionate representation remains a mechanism intended to ensure as much democracy as possible under the circumstances.

Democratic process is considered a good not only because it maximizes the participation of individuals, but also because it manifests equal regard for each one's participation. Even within a system of equal voting rights, however, it is hardly true that each one's participation is, or is even considered, equal to everyone else's. A similar discrepancy is observable in health care, where the traditional paternalistic relationship of inequality between practitioner and patient prevails, and the income, prestige, and power of physicians is greater than those of other health practitioners.[29] Since most physicians are white men, their dominance involves the dominance of race and gender as well.

Feminist standpoint theory suggests that a means of countering the inevitable nearsightedness of the dominant class is to ensure that those who are not part of that class are included among the decision or policy makers. If such a strategy were implemented, the voices of women and minorities who disagree with those who are dominant would be heard in Institutional Review Boards and ethics committees at the local level, and in state and national commissions addressing health needs and health care ethics. They would also be heard as teachers of health practitioners, especially physicians and thus members of the dominant group, and as leaders or experts in health care and bioethical decision making. Recent meetings sponsored separately by the National Institutes of Health and The Hastings Center are steps in the direction of expanding the range of voices heard.[30]

Proportionate representation means inviting the input of people with whom members of the dominant class do not themselves identify, whose presence may reduce their level of comfort and whose views may challenge theirs. It also means that tokenism, such as having one woman or minority person on the committee, is not enough, particularly when the group's decisions disproportionately affect those who are not dominant. Truly proportionate representation extends beyond gender, race, and class to differences in sexual orientation, political orientation, physical abilities, and mental abilities. It extends beyond the decision making of formally established groups such as academic committees and centers to the informal contexts of health care teams and clinic management.[31] Ideally, proportional representation also takes account of the fact that the same individual many belong to both dominant and nondominant groups. For example, while I belong to the nondominant gender, I represent the dominant class, race, and sexual orientation. To be fully reflective of the engaged vision of the world that standpoint theory offers requires participation of all the nondominant counterparts to dominance. Accordingly, I ought to be self-conscious about the limitation of vision occasioned by my participation in dominant groups. Moreover, the requirement of proportionate representation is not satisfied by having a single individual represent several nondominant groups—unless her voice and vote are counted additionally for each of the groups she represents.

Unfortunately, situations arise in which too few nondominant persons are available to provide proportionate representation. Sometimes the claim that there are too few is refutable, but sometimes it is not. Self-consciousness is then especially demanded of the dominant individuals who render the representation disproportionate. Minimally, such self-consciousness means acknowledgment of differences between dominant and dominated perspectives and efforts to learn about the latter. With regard to gender differences, it means acknowledgment of a possible sexist bias even by those who consider themselves free of such bias. As Virginia Warren observes, "Sexist ethics would never appear sexist [even to the person practicing it]. It would be clothed in a cloak of neutrality because favoring some group or position would be unthinkable."[32] A similar observation applies to groups distinguishable by race and class, and often to those distinguishable by their mental or physical ability or sexual orientation.

The postmodern insight regarding the inadequacy of categorizations is an important reminder that proportionate representation cannot entirely eliminate nearsightedness because nondominant persons are nearsighted also. Those of us who belong to the nondominant gender need to be self-conscious about this limitation, thereby avoiding or at least reducing arrogance. When we make decisions and formulate policies, our judgments remain fallible. Accordingly, from time to time we need to reconsider and revise our judgments in response to changing circumstances and new insights or critique.

In health care and bioethics as in other areas of life, decisions and policies need to be developed by democratic means, inviting the standpoint of diverse individuals in order to maximize their ethical and epistemological validity. Because feminism is committed to equality and to the moral significance of women's experience, both collectively and individually, it supports this strategy for reducing the flaws of nearsightedness, unselfconsciousness, and arrogance. Because care involves ongoing recognition of the dynamic character of individuals and groups, and the complexity of their relationships, it demands attention to differences. The crucial contribution of feminist standpoint theory to bioethics is the egalitarian critique that it adds to that attention.

Notes

I wish to thank Elizabeth Guonjian, Laura Purdy, Mary Solberg, and Susan Wolf for their helpful comments on earlier versions of this chapter. Thanks too to Rosie Tong for her counsel and encouragement during its final revision.

1 Most of those who have written about feminist standpoint do not use the term "theory" in referring to its rationale or methodology. Some sources represent different versions of feminism, some write from and about a feminist perspective but do not use the term "standpoint," and some write about women's experience or perspective but not about feminism. For examples of all of these approaches, see Donna Haraway, "Situated Knowledges: The Science Question in Feminism and the Privilege of Partial Perspective," *Feminist Studies* 14 (1988): 575–99; Nancy C. M. Hartsock, *Money, Sex, and Power: Toward a Feminist Historical Materialism* (Boston, MA: Northeastern University Press, 1985), 232, and "The Feminist Standpoint: Devloping the Ground for a Specifically Feminist Historical Materialism," in Sandra Harding, ed., *Feminism and Methodology: Social Science Issues* (Bloomington, IN: Indiana University Press, 1987), 136–62; Dorothy E. Smith, "Women's Perspective as a Radical Critique of Sociology," in Harding, ed., *Feminism and Methodology*, 85–96; Sara Ruddick, *Maternal Thinking: Toward a Politics of Peace* (New York, NY: Ballantine Books, 1989), 127–39; Nel Noddings, "Ethics from the Standpoint of Women," in Deborah L. Rhode, ed., *Theoretical Perspectives on Sexual Difference* (New Haven, CT: Yale University Press, 1990), 160–293; Catharine A. MacKinnon, "Feminism, Marxism, Method, and the State," in Harding, ed., *Feminism and Methodology*, 136–56; Terry Winant, "The Feminist Standpoint: A Matter of Language," *Hypatia* 2 (Winter 1987): 123–48; Alison M. Jaggar, *Feminist Politics and Human Nature* (Totowa, NJ: Rowman and Allanheld, 1983), 369–71, 377–89.

2 Consider "*a* feminist standpoint" as equivalent to "*the* feminist standpoint" described by Hartsock and Winant, note 1, above. I prefer the indefinite article because it suggests that there is more than one feminist standpoint. While different versions of feminism concur in their opposition to the oppression of women, they offer different ways of explaining and rectifying the oppression. This leads to different feminist standpoints. To use a visual image, different feminist standpoints are different points of view located within the common locus in which all feminists stand.

3 I have developed a meaning of "equality" essential to a feminist standpoint in *Women and Children in Health Care: An Unequal Majority* (New York, NY: Oxford University Press, 1993).

4 See William James, in John J. McDermott, ed., *The Writings of William James* (New York, NY: Modern Library, 1968), 629–45.

5 Catharine MacKinnon used the term "point-of-viewlessness" to identify the standard that men have erroneously imputed to their view of the world. See MacKinnon, "Feminism, Marxism, Method, and the State," 137.

6 Recall Socrates's discovery of why the oracle of Delphi considered him wiser than the statesman, who instead was reputed to be wiser: "I am wiser than he is by only this trifle, that what I do not know I don't think I do." See W. H. D. Rouse, trans., *Great Dialogues of Plato* (New York, NY: Mentor Books, 1956), 427.

7 While some surgical procedures affect the brain, even those *may* not affect the mind.

8 Valerie Saiving, "The Human Situation: A Feminine View," *Journal of Religion* 40 (1960): 100–12,108. See also Judith Plaskow, *Sex, Sin and Grace* (Lanham, MD: University Press of America, 1980).

9 Mary B. Mahowald, "Sex-Role Stereotypes in Medicine," *Hypatia* 2 (Summer 1987): 21–38. Thankfully, this view is rarely supported today.

10 Charlotte F. Muller, *Health Care and Gender* (New York, NY: Russell Sage Foundation, 1992), 7–10.

11   Various labels used for different models include pater-
     nalism, covenant, contract, business, beneficence-in-
     trust, friendship, and collaboration. See, for example,
     Edmund D. Pellegrino and David C. Thomasma, *For
     the Patient's Good: The Restoration of Beneficence in
     Health Care* (New York, NY: Oxford University Press,
     1988), 101–06; Melvin Konner, *Medicine at the
     Crossroads* (New York, NY: Pantheon, 1993), 3–27;
     Sherwin, *No Longer Patient*, 137–57; and Mahowald,
     Women and Children in Health Care, 28–32. The prevail-
     ing models include those that give priority to patient
     autonomy, to physician beneficence toward the
     patient, or to some combination of respect for patient
     autonomy and beneficence toward the patient.

12   Albert R. Jonsen and Stephen Toulmin, *The Abuse of
     Casuistry: A History of Moral Reasoning* (Berkeley, CA:
     University of California Press, 1988), 330 (italics
     theirs).

13   For example, Sherwin, *No Longer Patient*, 78–80.

14   Carol Gilligan, *In a Different Voice: Psychological Theory
     and Women's Development* (Cambridge, MA: Harvard
     University Press, 1982), and "Moral Orientation and
     Moral Development," in Eva Feder Kittay and Diana
     T. Meyers, eds., *Women and Moral Theory* (Totowa,
     NJ: Rowman & Littlefield, 1987), 19–33.

15   Nel Noddings, *Caring: A Feminine Approach to Ethics
     and Moral Education* (Berkeley, CA: University of
     California Press, 1984), 16.

16   Marilyn Friedman, "Beyond Caring: The
     De-moralization of Gender," in Marsha Hanen and
     Kai Nielson, eds., *Science, Morality and Feminist
     Theory* (Calgary, Canada: University of Calgary
     Press, 1987), 87–110. See also Michael Stocker,
     "Duty and Friendship: Toward a Synthesis of
     Gilligan's Contrastive Moral Concepts," in Kittay
     and Meyers, eds., *Women and Moral Theory*, 56–58.

17   Friedman, "Beyond Caring," 89.

18   Marilyn Friedman, "Feminism and Modern
     Friendship: Dislocating the Community," *Ethics* 99
     (1989): 275–90.

19   Ruddick, *Maternal Thinking*, 130.

20   I cannot here develop the relationship between par-
     ticularism and partiality, but see Alan Gewirth,
     "Ethical Universalism and Particularism," *Journal of
     Philosophy* 85 (1988): 283–302, and Marilyn Friedman,
     "Partiality," in Lawrence C. Becker and Charlotte B.
     Becker, eds., *Encyclopedia of Ethics*, vol. 2 (New York,
     NY: Garland, 1992), 932–35.

21   Martha Minow, among others, has delineated the
     importance of attending to gender differences as a
     means of ensuring that care is maximized on a soci-
     etal level. For example, see her *Making All the
     Difference: Inclusion, Exclusion, and American Law*
     (Ithaca, NY: Cornell University Press, 1990), 216–19.
     But Minow does not elaborate the import of paying
     attention to individual differences among women.

22   While the clinical details of this case are accurate, I
     have changed irrelevant details (including names) to
     ensure confidentiality.

23   Ruddick, *Maternal Thinking*, 129.

24   Natalie Angier, "Bedside Manners Improve as More
     Women Enter Medicine," *New York Times*, June 21,
     1992, sec. 4, p. 18.

25   Catharine A. MacKinnon, "Feminism, Marxism,
     Method, and the State: An Agenda for Theory,"
     Signs 7 (1982): 515–44, 537.

26   *Diagnostic and Statistical Manual of Mental Disorders*,
     3d ed. (Washington, DC: American Psychiatric
     Association, 1987), 66; Kathryn Morgan, "Women
     and the Knife, Cosmetic Surgery and the
     Colonization of Women's Bodies," *Hypatia* 6 (Fall
     1991): 30; Ruth Sidel, *Women and Children Last* (New
     York, NY: Penguin Viking Books, 1986), 158.

27   Consider, for example, Andrea Bonnicksen's descrip-
     tion of the options available after prenatal screening
     has detected an affected fetus: "the *couple* will either
     terminate the pregnancy ... or bear a child with the
     disease." See her "Genetic Diagnosis of Human
     Embryos," *Hastings Center Report* 22 (July–Aug. 1992):
     S5–11, S6 (my italics). But see also James D. Watson,
     "The Human Genome Project: Past, Present, and
     Future," *Science* 248 (1990): 44–48; Francis S. Collins,
     "Medical and Ethical Consequences of the Human
     Genome Project," *Journal of Clinical Ethics* 2 (1991):
     260–67; and Thomas H. Murray, "The Human
     Genome Project and Genetic Testing: Ethical
     Implications," in *The Genome, Ethics and the Law: A
     Report of a Conference on the Ethical and Legal Implications
     of Genetic Testing*, Coolfont Conference Center,
     Berkeley Springs, West Virginia, June 14–16, 1991,
     AAAS Publication No. 92–115 (Washington, DC:
     American Association for the Advancement of
     Science, 1992), 49–78.

28   For example, women constitute 93.5 percent of
     masters' prepared genetic counselors. See Deborah
     F. Pencarinha, Nora K. Bell, Janice G. Edwards, and
     Robert G. Best, "Ethical Issues in Genetic
     Counseling: A Comparison of M.S. Counselor and
     Medical Geneticist Perspectives," *Journal of Genetic
     Counseling* 1 (1992): 19–30, 22.

29 Mahowald, "Sex-Role Stereotypes in Medicine," 22.

30 For example, in September 1991, NIH sponsored a meeting to plan an agenda for the study of women's health during the coming decade; in November 1991, NIH sponsored a meeting on reproductive genetics. Both meetings were predominantly attended by, and led by, women. Participants in the Hastings Center Project on Feminism and Bioethics were also predominantly women.

31 Although the term "health care team" refers to all of those involved in patient care, the team coach or captain is the attending physician, whose dominance, while justified in terms of his medical expertise, may be influenced also by other dominant but irrelevant factors such as race, gender, and class.

32 Virginia L. Warren, "Feminist Directions in Medical Ethics," *Hypatia* 4 (Summer 1989): 73–87, 74.

Culture and Medical Intervention

MICHAEL BOYLAN

This essay examines two ways in which cultural considerations can complicate the process of medical intervention. In each case there are aspects of cultural literacy that should be appreciated and respected and other such aspects that may not trump more basic ethical concerns.

To facilitate this examination, two cases are set forward concerning two different societies: Guatemalan and Chinese. In each, an individual from the non-American society is seeking medical attention in an American hospital. In the process the patient interacts with an American physician. The same principles set out would apply to any native physician confronting a representative of another culture.[1]

This essay offers a dialectical presentation of opposing worldview perspectives, along with criticisms of each to heighten the awareness of how these dynamics may operate in clinical situations, and suggestions at finding a defensible direction for action.[2] This essay understands *cultural competency* as use of this dialectical method in cases dealing with competing cultural values.

Case 1

You are an emergency room physician at an inner city hospital. Mrs Lopez, a poor, first-generation immigrant from Guatemala,[3] comes to see you since she has no

"Culture and Medical Intervention," by Michael Boylan, was originally published in the *Journal of Clinical Ethics* 2004; 15(2, Summer): 187–99.

regular doctor. She has a bronchial infection that can be treated with antibiotics. In the course of your examination of Mrs Lopez, you discover a lump within her right breast. This lump concerns you and you suggest some tests. Through the hospital's interpreter, you inform her of your plan.

The translator relays to you that Mrs Lopez does not want tests. She just wants to get her medicine and leave. You ask the interpreter to inquire whether she knows her social service options—such as Medicaid. By the way Mrs Lopez answers the question put to her by the translator, you feel that she may not be here legally, but the translator assures you rather testily that Mrs Lopez has her Green Card, Medicaid coverage, and has been here for at least three years.

You fear that the lump within her breast may be malignant and that only by prompt treatment can you save her life. Mrs Lopez tells the hospital's female translator that she does not like talking about her breasts with strangers and that her husband would never allow anyone to cut her in that area of her body.

As a result of the information the hospital translator has given you, you feel it necessary to detain Mrs Lopez for a few more minutes while you discuss her situation with a senior Latina[4] nurse who is on duty. (There are no Latino/Latina physicians at your hospital.) Although the nurse is not from Guatemala, her general understanding of Central American cultures[5] gives you an assurance that she might understand Mrs Lopez's motivations. You tell the nurse that Mrs Lopez wants to leave and forgo any tests and that Mrs Lopez does not fully appreciate the danger she is in. The nurse nods her head at you with a little attitude (much like the translator did) and informs you that Mrs Lopez comes from a cultural tradition in which the husband's likes or dislikes (concerning the appearance of his wife's breasts) are decisive. The nurse tells you further that many Hispanics believe that breast cancer is the result of sinful behavior (such as alcohol and drug use) and that this belief might further make the husband upset with his wife should she be diagnosed with breast cancer.[6]

Now it's your turn to nod your head as you contemplate what you will do. In this instance, the question of proper medical intervention depends on several points. First, there is the issue of whether Mrs Lopez really understands what is happening to her. To simplify the case, let us assume that Medicaid will cover Mrs Lopez's treatment. In this case, money is not the issue.[7] Therefore, at least two possible descriptions of the problem are possible.

Dialectical Worldview Positions

Description 1: "There is a problem with my body that may kill me." Mrs Lopez may or may not understand enough medical science to know that the lump within her right breast may metastasize and kill her. Does she know the time frame involved? Does she know the different procedures that can be performed (for example, lumpectomy, radical mastectomy)? Does she understand the effectiveness of these treatments?[8] Does she understand the cosmetic repercussions of each? These questions and others like them are necessary to constitute an appraisal of the risk and reward from a medical health perspective. In the end, all people value living over dying. It is the physician's ethical duty to do no harm and to act to promote the health of the patient; therefore, the physician must do everything possible to make the woman submit to the biopsy. To do less would be to become an accomplice in her death.[9]

Description 2: "There is a problem with my body that affects my living a valuable life." Mrs Lopez believes that if she allows doctors to "mutilate" her breast her husband will abandon her. He might think her unattractive or he might think that she acquired the breast cancer from using drugs or by "loose" behavior. If her husband shuns her, her community will also shun her. As a recent immigrant who does not fluently speak the majority language, English, she feels very dependent upon her community. For Mrs Lopez, life is worthwhile so long as she is a respected wife and mother within a supportive community of people with similar values. "Mutilation" of her breast may possibly save her life, but what sort of life is it to live apart from those verities that give it meaning? The physician should recognize and be sensitive to these cultural dynamics and allow the woman to leave the hospital. Some portion of life consonant with one's quality-of-life principles is better than more life without them.

A Critical Examination of the Worldview Positions

Many physicians see case one only in terms of problem description 1. For these individuals, it is clear that the physician must assist the patient while doing no harm. This is a transcultural truth. But "doing no harm" from this perspective has a purely physical meaning. What about the psychological harm that may be incurred through disrupting the worldview in which the patient lives and finds life meaningful? The cultural components of a person's life situate it and define happiness. Although "doing no harm" may be a universal truth in the abstract, any actual understanding of the term must encompass the situated reality of the patient. Without knowing this cultural context, the physician runs great risk of negligently doing harm. Although the harm is not bodily harm, to most of us our bodies are only one component in a psychosocial mosaic that situates us in the world via a particular worldview. To help adjudicate some of these competing concerns, let's examine some of the presuppositions upon which each description rests.

On the face of it, problem description 1 has several suppressed assumptions that are important.

- Continuing to live is always the most rational decision a patient can make (A-1).
- Physicians are committed to carrying out expressions of patients' autonomy so long as they are the most rational decision (A-2).
- Informed consent that is not based on the most rational decision is not properly "informed," and therefore is no consent at all (A-3).

In some contexts, these points make perfect sense and can legitimately guide one's actions. However, it does not take too much imagination to find other contexts in which these assumptions are patently false. For example, there are many instances in which continuing to live may not be the most rational decision, challenging assumption A-1. A counter example is presented here: You are a spy for the Allies before the Normandy Invasion in World War Two (commonly called D-Day) and you are captured by the Nazis. You believe that the Nazis could make you disclose the real invasion site through a combination of torture and sodium pentothal. The consequence of your disclosing the real invasion site would be an increase in casualties by 10 000 Allied men (and threaten the success of the mission). Swallowing the lethal cyanide capsule issued to you would save 10 000 men and maintain the viability of the mission. In this counter example, it seems to this author, that continuing to live is not demanded by reason.[10] Who would say that the spy who took his cyanide capsule was irrational? Rather, we'd rightly call him a hero.

There are other such cases (such as Captain Oates in the Robert Scott expedition) that are generally agreed to exhibit heroism and honor even though suicide (for the sake of saving others) was the result. If this counter example is accepted as a rational (and moral) action, then A-1 is not absolute.

A second counter example to A-1 refers to maintaining dignity as judged by the integrity of a cultural tradition. Martin Luther King, Jr, saw the transplanted African community in America as being exploited and denied certain basic freedoms because (at least in part) they didn't fit into the "melting pot" of American society. Gandhi saw the indigenous population of India as being exploited and denied certain basic freedoms because (at least in part) they were not transplanted Britons. Being an exploited people who are denied certain basic freedoms is ethically unacceptable. The only way to alleviate the conditions of African-Americans in the United States and Indians under British Colonial control is to put one's life on the line in nonviolent protest exhibiting a moral superiority over one's oppressors. Putting one's life on the line in the circumstances cited above will most probably result in one's assassination.

In this counter example, few would criticize Martin Luther King, Jr, or Mahatma Gandhi for living a life that could easily be foreseen to result in their deaths. If living one's life at all costs were an absolute maxim, then they would be violators of the maxim.

Both counter examples illustrate that the value of continuing to live one's life is tempered by other values that infuse the life we live with meaning.

Assumptions A-2 and A-3 are also problematic. Should physicians only honor patients' claims that they consider to be rational?[11] Such a question would be easier, were reason and value always so neatly segregated. However, it has been this author's position that fact and value have many overlaps.[12] Because of this, physicians must realize that their determination that a patient's request is irrational may be colored by their own value system. For example, say the patient were a Jehovah's Witness who abjured a blood transfusion on the grounds that his religion forbids the "eating of blood" and that blood transfusions are interpreted as "eating blood." If the physician were an atheist, then all religious claims might appear to be total nonsense. If the physician had a religious viewpoint (though not Jehovah's Witness), she probably would feel some worldview dissonance between honoring someone's religious beliefs and, at the same time, feeling that those beliefs were false. Finally, if the physician were a Jehovah's Witness herself, she might view the patient's wishes as quite rational indeed. The point here is that it is no easy matter to determine rationality once one has overcome the hurdle of judging that your patient is uttering coherent statements that logically work together to form a conclusion.

For the purposes of clinical practice, a definition of rationality that is grounded in pragmatic coherence (no contradictions between the propositions put forth from within a working, established cultural context) is probably better than a theory of rationality that is based on correspondence to a single universal set of behaviors— behaviors often strikingly similar to those of the practicing physician![13] The physician must therefore create a working theory of rationality that is grounded in pragmatic coherentism, rather than a theory of rationality that corresponds to the physician's own cultural tradition. If a patient has a belief system that is coherent and is grounded in a working, established cultural context, physicians must accept consequential judgments derived from such a system as rational and indicative of informed consent (even if they disagree with it and think the system from whence it came is not as good as others—especially their own).

Problem description 1, by itself, has serious drawbacks to its claim of exclusively describing case one. Problem description 2 also has drawbacks, which can be seen through an examination of some of its key premises:

- There is an inherent dignity in all cultures that legitimates all of their customs and practices (A-4).
- Going along with a cultural practice that is entrenched is always the best course to take (A-5).
- The family bond between husband and wife is such that no physician should attempt to breech it by questioning the relative power dynamics (A-6).

Assumption A-4 is problematic because it implies moral relativism. This author (along with most moral philosophers) has taken the position that moral relativism implies the demise of ethics altogether.[14] If ethics is the science of the right and wrong of human action, and if science means that which can be known by all people at all times and places, then clearly ethical relativism means that morality is mistaken. If ethical relativism were correct, then no one could properly criticize Hitler, Stalin, or others for their murderous behaviors. They were simply acting out cultural traditions! However, on the other hand, the understanding of universal moral rules must always exist within a situated context. Thus one set of actions may be subsumed under different universal moral rules, depending on the cultural meaning of those actions.[15]

Assumption A-5 is equally problematic. It implies that "entrenched practices" equal "good practices." This is patently wrong.[16] The American tradition of slavery was well entrenched over 300 years. If A-5 were correct, there should have never been a reason to change slavery. Upon what principle would change be justified? However, most of us agree that slavery was wrong, is wrong, and will be forever wrong. This is based on the moral prohibition against exploitation of another for one's personal betterment. There can be no greater example of exploitation than literal slavery. Therefore, the fact that a cultural practice is entrenched is not cogent to its being ethically justified.

Finally, assumption A-6 asserts some sort of absolute bond between husband and wife, such that, if either party is comfortable with a certain state of affairs, then it is not up to outsiders to interfere. But this is problematic, as well. In my own experience working in shelters for battered women, I saw women who showed demonstrable signs of physical abuse who, after a stay at the shelter, went back to their husbands because they felt that they had no other real alternative. The dependence of the "slave" (in this case the abused wife) on the "master" (in this case the brutish husband) has fascinated philosophers over the years. Hegel writes influentially on this such that it affected Marx and later writers.[17] Whereas Hegel believes that there is always a freedom for the slave to free herself, it is unclear whether this sort of bondage is readily severed. Similarly, the so-called Stockholm syndrome among captive groups and battered women indicates that those in bondage may not act in their best interests because they become involved in trying to please their captors.[18]

These several examples serve to illustrate that the situation is not as simple as A-6 implies. The wife may say that she wants her husband to make the decision for her (or other coded versions of the same), but this may not be her real desire. The culture from which she comes may encourage the subjugation of women. Mrs Lopez may not really want to be dominated, but perhaps she has been beaten into submission in just the same way as those who suffer from the Stockholm syndrome. In this case, the physician has a difficult choice to make.

What should the physician do?[19] Problem descriptions 1 and 2 both seem flawed. The dialectical method (cultural competency) has revealed that neither is correctly action-guiding in all cases. This author's approach to dialectical dissonance is that the physician must understand and then make an assessment of the worldviews of all the relevant parties using the method above. After the positions and their opposites are set out with reasons for each, the physician needs to make a judgment based on principles of well-wrought ethical theory (such as virtue ethics, utilitarianism, deontology), respecting the cultural context as much as possible without violating morality.[20] In this case, since the author holds a de-ontological rights-based theory, I would find the relationship of the woman with her husband as the key to providing her with adequate care. On the face of it, the cultural practice that allows a husband to view his wife's unscarred body as being of more importance than her life itself is ethically flawed. It does not fully acknowledge the wife's autonomy and moral agency. Since autonomy and the fundamental conditions of moral agency are crucial to being human, and since those conditions of agency are what we will claim first above all else, all agents may properly claim the basic goods of agency as moral rights.[21]

Second, the culturally held misconception that breast cancer is contracted via immoral behavior must be addressed head-on. The most effective spokesperson for this may be the senior Latina nurse, because the ethnicity of the physician may be a barrier in communicating certain messages. For example, many commonly held beliefs in certain racial/cultural groups are influenced by the presence of the dominant majority population. If it is the case that urban Hispanics believe that breast cancer comes from immoral behavior and that the dominant culture will try to deform them in a futile medical gesture, and if this belief is partially based on an assumption of exploitative power dynamics, then a physician of European descent may be a poor communicator of a contrary message. The sort of trust and acceptance necessary to convey these medical facts may only be present in a person from that cultural community (even widely understood). Since the hospital has no Latino physicians, the next best person to deliver these facts may be the senior Hispanic nurse.

In general, if this author were in the place of the physician, I would try to think about the cultural overlay to the problem both through descriptions 1 and 2. Then, sensitive that neither description is always the right, I'd seek to discern which of the crucial suppressed assumptions (A-1 through A-6) seemed to be most relevant in this case. If I am correct about the husband-wife relationship, then bringing in the intervention of a hospital family psychologist might allow a discussion to occur in which the husband could be brought into the process in a manner that is sensitive both to possible interpersonal exploitation and to the medical facts of the case. The goal of this strategy is to engage the husband in a discussion and attempt to bring him around to the position of supporting a treatment that may save his wife's life, over and against the attitude that sets as supreme the physical appearance of her breasts or superstitions about the etiology of breast cancer (via an appropriate messenger as per above). This conversation may also require a member of the ethnic community, priest, or social worker, so that the power of the argument might be conveyed in a nonthreatening, cooperative manner.

Through such a procedure, the physician may demonstrate sensitivity to cultural worldviews and yet be true to the physician's own cultural lens that seeks to reveal the overriding dictates of universal morality.

The second case concerns an elderly Chinese man.[22]

Case 2

You are a cardiologist in a teaching hospital. You have a patient, Mr Shin, who is 74 years old and is suffering from angina. Your tests have determined that he has a severe narrowing of the coronary artery. The condition is potentially life threatening. There are three possible treatments: drug therapy (cholesterol-lowering medication, anti-hypertensives, vasodilators, and antiplatelet therapy, which aims to thin the blood and help prevent a clot, the final event that closes a narrowed artery), angioplasty (to dilate the narrowed artery and place a stent to keep it open), and coronary artery bypass surgery (which may offer the best long-term solution). If you, as the physician, were to assess the risks and benefits of each therapy (on a scale of 10) as well as no therapy at all, it would look like this.[23]

A. No therapy: risk of treatment = 0 / resultant risk[24] = 9.5 / Total Risk = 9.5
B. Drug Therapy: risk of treatment = 0.5 / resultant risk = 8.0 / Total Risk = 8.5
C. Angioplasty: risk of treatment = 1.5 / resultant risk = 6.0 / Total Risk = 7.5
D. Bypass surgery: risk of treatment = 5.0 / resultant risk = 1.0 / Total Risk = 6.0

Obviously, all procedures (except for doing nothing) entail some risk. And each therapy has projected resultant risks (prognosis). Not all patients in the identical situation will balance risk and reward in the same way. This is why it is essential to understand what Mr Shin wants for his treatment. The problem here is that Mr Shin's extended family does not want the information about "risk-reward" to go directly to

Mr Shin, but instead to be funneled through Mr Shin's son, who is next in line in the hierarchical order of the clan. Mr Shin was born in China and emigrated to the United States in 1948, when Communists took over. He became a US citizen in 1958 so that others of his family might come over from Taiwan (the other place of refuge for this particular family). Mr Shin brought much of his clan to America over the years. Representatives from this clan are with him and want to screen any information and present it to Mr Shin in a way they think best. The problem for you, the physician, is that the consequences of this surgery are substantial (life or death). The consequences of not acting are also substantial (life or death). Can you trust such an important decision to a cabal of relatives hovering around at bedside?

Just as in Case 1, Case 2 can be given (at least) two problem descriptions.

Dialectical Worldview Positions

Description 1: "*It is my body and I should be the one to determine whether to intervene surgically or to employ some other (less invasive) choice of therapy.*" Mr Shin may not get adequate information if everything is filtered through his son (who is not a physician). Under the principles of autonomy and informed consent, it would seem that a physician should be able to approach a patient directly and not through a messenger service. To ensure that Mr Shin receives all of the information needed to make an intelligent choice, the physician should talk with Mr Shin in person.

Description 2: "*I exist most authentically within my clan. We have an ordering for decisions of importance. The traditional order should make this decision.*" Each society has its strategy of discourse. Some are more direct; others are more indirect. There is also an accepted way that information is transmitted. If the physician were to short-circuit either of these routes, there is a strong possibility that the patient would receive less and not more information. This is because information coming via an unknown format in an unaccustomed manner (that is, direct instead of indirect) may confuse Mr Shin and even make him suspicious. The best course of action is to go through the son.

A Critical Examination of the Worldview Positions

Underlying problem description 1 are the following assumptions:

- Principles of autonomy and informed consent trump cultural traditions (B-1).
- Since the therapy is being contemplated in the United States, the Shin family should adapt to our customs and not we to theirs (B-2).
- Too many interventions can be smokescreens for other (sometimes exploitative or nefarious) purposes (B-3).

Assumption B-1 takes as its argument the notion that principles of morality are international across time and space. This belief holds that such principles are grounded in the features of human action that are not particular to any single culture. Thus, any cultural tradition that seems to get in the way of the execution of a legitimate moral principle should be rejected. Whereas, on the face of it, this is a principle on which most ethicists would agree, it is not altogether clear that facilitating a different information flow would subvert the principles of autonomy and informed consent. These principles are satisfied through a decision-making process in which the patient is an active part. However, what better way to elicit the patient's true feelings than through a process with which he is familiar and trusts?

Assumption B-2 can be said to be true in one sense: that sovereign nations have the legal right to set conditions of care in their own country so long as they do not violate other principles of morality. But in this instance, is exercising such a right the most compassionate thing to do? It may not be an ethical requirement to treat others with compassion and care, but it certainly seems to be a requirement of medical professional ethics. Accommodation for cultural worldviews, all things being equal, breaks down artificial barriers that often make discussion across worldviews difficult (if not impossible).

Assumption B-3 works on the idea that when a single message goes through many translators, there is an increased probability of distortion with each screening of the message. If one of the translators (or perhaps the central translator) is himself an interested party, there is the potential for his conversation to be tainted by this self-interest. He might twist the communication and the presentation of the alternatives so that the alternative that seemed best for him might be the one communicated. For example, if the son were the translator and he was the sole or primary heir to the father's estate (assuming there is an estate), he might present the alternative he thought to be worst for his father so that he (the son), instead, might prosper.

On the other hand, it is just as likely that the son really does have the best interests of his father at heart. In such a case, the father may feel most comfortable discussing the various alternatives with the people he trusts most.

This last point is a segue to a discussion of problem description 2, which asserts that the clan (rather than the individual) is the primary unit, so that it is socially unacceptable to address one person (in a life-and-death decision) divorced from his clan.

Problem description 2 rests on the following key assumptions:

- We are born into a milieu whose primary element is the family/clan on which we depend for meaning: before all else we are members of a family/clan (B-4).
- Whatever is primary must be dealt with before all else (B-5).
- There is a sociologically based authority to the family/clan (B-6).
- There is a natural authority to the family/clan (B-7).

Assumption B-4 can be understood within the context of a sociologic causal framework (B-6) or within the context of evolutionary biology (B-7). The argument for cultural causation might set out the family as a critical center of authority and meaning for each family member.[25] (B-5 is merely a logical intensifier of this.) If B-6 is correct, then to deny the role of the family in such an important decision is to deny the father the fullness of the most meaningful context of his life and thereby raise the chance of creating an artificial choice situation that does not resonate with his considered personal convictions (thus undermining true informed consent and autonomy).

On the other hand, B-7 depends on a notion of kinship theory in which our biological/social bonds supervene all (B-5 is merely a logical intensifier of this). In individually oriented theories of evolutionary biology, kin selection is often set forth as a very plausible account.[26] If B-7 is correct, then to peel away one individual from the clan might create a biologically unnatural context that will force an already impaired patient into a choice situation that is bereft of the sort of support the agent has every biologically natural right to expect. Again, the outcome of ignoring the natural authority of the family will likely entail less than informed consent and impaired autonomy.

In either event, it might be the case that failure to recognize and utilize the family structure might undermine the very principles the physician is striving to maintain.

If one were to take a contrary view to assumptions B-4 through B-7, however, one could point to the real possibility that the family/clan relationship does not necessarily work according to plan. For example, a family/clan that is transplanted into a new environment may not receive the cultural nurturing requisite for it to survive. In fact, this particular family/clan may be suffering and thus be somewhat dysfunctional. In this event, the unit may actually cease to maintain the sort of causal efficacy described in assumptions B-4 through B-7. Such a situation might transform the family/clan from a supportive structure to one full of strife and contention. This sort of family/clan might actually do more harm than good.

So what's a physician to do? In this situation the real issue is whether there is an authentic family that is operating effectively in the patient's best interests and whether the patient acknowledges the family's necessary role in his decision making. When confronted with a foreign worldview, a physician should first seek a disinterested party who understands the worldview (like the senior Latina nurse in Case 1). This individual may bring a physician into an understanding of the cultural issues that may be involved. Second, the physician should take a moment alone with the patient to ascertain just how invested he is in the foreign worldview purported by the clan. There certainly exists the possibility that Mr Shin has rejected the worldview that includes clan decision making, but he may be reluctant to state this in the presence of his clan. Therefore, if the physician feels the patient is renouncing the worldview of his clan, this must be witnessed, documented, and accepted as the patient's autonomous desire. (An ethnic consultant familiar with this sort of decision-making process would also be useful here.)

If the patient wants to work through the clan process, every accommodation should be made to allow this to occur. Sometimes, this may require a mixing of the two traditions—such as the patient executing a durable power of attorney naming one or more clan members. In this way, the customs of our system can be maintained, while allowing for the cultural demands of another worldview. However, even if this approach is taken, the medical team must be sensitive to the apparent dynamics of the clan's behavior. The medical team does not want to aid and abet the exploitation of a clan member for the personal enrichment of another clan member. Such a situation would surely work against Mr Shin's best interests.

A third option might also be undertaken, a combination of the first two. It would dictate using the clan decision-making system but also periodically checking with Mr Shin about whether he is really comfortable with the manner in which information is reaching him—and checking for the accuracy of this information.

Even well-intentioned family members may get some of the details wrong. And some of the details are critical.

This third option is particularly important in those instances in which a patient shows some signs of embracing the worldview of his clan, but also shows signs of retaining control of his medical decisions. In cases of doubt about the sincerity of the patient's declaration of fidelity to the clan's worldview, this third option allows a middle course that can be modified toward either extreme as events unfold about the social dynamics vis-à-vis the patient's best interests in treatment and in fulfilling his needs for autonomy and informed consent.

Conclusion

This essay began with a question about worldview and how it affected medical intervention. The method of investigation was dialectical, assessing the argument from the worldview perspective of each party (the patient from a different culture and the physician working within established norms of ethical behavior) and then examining objections to these worldviews. The purpose of such a methodology was to engage the reader in seeing the issue from a multifaceted approach, suggesting that depending on the situation there may be different appropriate responses.

In the first case, the woman with a lump on her breast must be assessed both inside and outside her cultural milieu. The physician needs to protect the moral rights of the woman while at the same time being aware of the necessity to bring her culture (via the positive incorporation of the husband) into the support network that will be necessary for the possible postoperative adjustment period. This approach recognizes that there is more to treating a breast cancer patient than merely removing malignant tissue.

Likewise, in the second case the physician needs to ascertain the dynamics of the cultural decision-making process as well as to discover how committed his patient is to that cultural practice. It is only after these two sets of facts are understood that the physician is in a position to properly treat the patient.

In each case the physician needs to expand the purview of the process of medical intervention that is normally taught in medical schools. The practicing physician needs to be better equipped to deal with these issues than merely learning "medical Spanish." Cultural literacy requires more than this. At its heart, it requires the physician to be sensitive to the dialectical dynamics of worldview epistemology. The way a person views reality affects the way he or she understands facts and values and how they are interrelated. Thus, if a physician really wants to communicate with patients (a necessity for treatment in nonemergency situations), it is necessary to establish an understanding of and sensitivity to the structure of cultural worldviews and their adherents. Not all worldviews are alike. Not all worldviews are good.[27] However, if it is a goal for all sincere interpersonal interaction to require reciprocity of acknowledgment of who and what we are, and if medical intervention ought to be an instance of sincere interpersonal interaction, and if the acknowledgment of who and what we are is an instance of cultural literacy, then physicians must make themselves culturally literate in this fashion.

Sensitivity alone is not a silver bullet (as was shown by the dialectically analyzed cases). Cultural sensitivity should never lead the physician to unethical behavior: ethics trumps culture. However, the act of understanding certain acts as falling under the domain of certain moral institutions is affected by culture. This means that the manner in which physicians execute their ethical and professional duties is certainly enhanced by cultural literacy. And though it may not be a sufficient condition on which to base an entire theory of action in medicine, it is certainly a necessary condition for the maintenance of sound, ethical medical practice.

Acknowledgment

I would like to thank the two anonymous referees for their comments as well as William Mullins, MD, for practical insights and suggestions.

Notes

1 This depiction of the cultural frame is intentionally geared toward the patient. It is true that it is also important to examine the cultural background of the physician and other healthcare workers. However, this essay takes an intentionally bland position concerning the physician because when one sets out a variable (the patient) and a control (the physician), the dynamics of the variable are more apparent. In this case the variable is meant to be a patient whose cultural background can have clinical implications. If I were to set a frame of analysis for the physician as well, I am afraid that by creating two variables I would rob the force of the exposition of its clarity. As Jacques Derrida has said, the creation of interpretative frames is like going into a hall of mirrors. There is really no true stopping point. One could talk about the ethnicity of the narrator, and then of the author-as-narrator, and so on. Though there is some merit to also examining the physician's ethnic assumptions, such a treatment would be more appropriate to a book-length study than to an essay such as this.

2 The exploration of multicultural literacy in clinical practice is a developing area of research. Recent work includes K.K. Kundhal, "Cultural Diversity: An Evolving Challenge to Physician-Patient Communication," *Journal of the American Medical Association* 289, no. 1 (January 2003): 94; J.H. Tanne, "U.S. Medical Schools Should Consider Race in Admitting Students," *British Medical Journal* 325, no.

7364 (September 2002): 565; V. Tolo, "The Challenges of Change: Is Orthopaedics Ready?" *Journal of Bone and Joint Surgery* 84-A, no. 9 (September 2002): 1707–13; the special theme issue of *Academic Medicine* 77, no. 3 (2002), especially K. Fuller, "Eradicating Essentialism from Cultural Competency Education," A.R. Green, J.R. Betancourt, and J.E. Carrilo, "Integrating Social Factors into Cross-cultural Medical Education," and J. Drouin and P. Jean, "Educating Future Physicians for a Minority Population: A French-language Stream at the University of Ottawa"; the November/December 2001 issue of the *Park Ridge Center Bulletin*, especially L.M. Hunt, "Beyond Cultural Competence," D.B. McCurdy, "A 'Competence' We Can't do Without," and L. Barnes and G. Harris, "Changing Medical Landscape"; A.E. Núñez, "Transforming Cultural Competence into Cross-Cultural Efficacy in Women's Health Education," *Academic Medicine* 75 (2000): 1071–80; C. Brach and I. Fraser, "Can Cultural Competency Reduce Racial and Ethnic Health Disparities?" *Medical Care and Research Review* 57, supp. 1 (2000): 181–217; R.M. Mayberry, F. Mili, and E. Ofili, "Racial and Ethnic Differences in Access to Medical Care," *Medical Care and Research Review* 57, supp. 1 (2000): 108–45; J.E. Carillo, A.R. Green, and J.R. Betancourt, "Cross-Cultural Primary Care: A Patient-Based Approach," *Annals of Internal Medicine* 130 (1999): 829–34; P.M. Lantz et al., "Socioeconomic Factor, Health

Behaviors, and Mortality: Results from a Nationally Representative Prospective Study of U.S. Adults," *Journal of the American Medical Association* 279 (1998): 1703–08; and K.A. Culhane-Pera et al., "A Curriculum for Multicultural Education in Family Practice," *Family Medicine* 28 (1997): 719–23. Readers may look to note 22 for a discussion of issues regarding Asian cultures. The question of Guatemala is discussed in notes 3, 5, and 6. For another angle, see G.R. Gillett, "Medical Ethics in a Multicultural Context," *Journal of Internal Medicine* 238, no. 6 (1995): 531–37; L. Hipshman, "Attitudes towards Informed Consent, Confidentiality, and Substitute Treatment Decisions in Southern African Medical Students: A Case Study in Zimbabwe," *Social Science and Medicine* 49, no. 3 (1999): 313–28.

3 The dynamics of Hispanic cultures in the United States are of critical importance. Documented and undocumented peoples from these regions constitute a substantial minority of people residing in the country. For a brief discussion of these cultural issues as they relate to health-care, see C.A. Howard, S.J. Andrade, and T. Byrd, "The Ethical Dimensions of Cultural Competence in Border Health Care Settings," *Family and Community Health* 23, no. 4 (2001): 36–49.

4 I will use the words Latina/Latino interchangeably with Hispanic. However, there is some dispute about the use of these terms. According to a poll of 1200 readers of *Hispanic Magazine*, 65 percent preferred the term *Hispanic* to the term *Latino*. C. Granados, "'Latino' versus 'Hispanic'," Hispanic Magazine (December 2000), http://www.hispanicmagazine.com/2000/dec, accessed 6 August 2004. However, one must note that the name of the magazine as a possible caveat.

Kathie Neff Ragsdale suggested the term is rather one of social consciousness: the younger, more avant-garde prefer *Latino*; the more mature mainstream term is *Hispanic*. A second ground for demarcation is geographic versus linguistic. Neff Ragsdale suggests that *Latino* refers to the countries of Latin America, while *Hispanic* refers to speaking Spanish. K. Neff Ragsdale, "'Hispanic' vs. 'Latino'," *Eagle Tribune* (Andover, Mass.), 23 May 1999.

Others, such as the Hispanic Genealogy Forum, emphasize two different linguistic origins: one from Latin Italy and one from España (aka the latinized Hispania). See the forum's website: http://home.att.net/~Alsosa/whoarewe.htm.

All three of these positions (social consciousness, geography versus linguistics, and linguistic origins) as well as further implications for social policy are explored in a collection of essays edited by M.C. Gutman, *Perspectives on Las Américas: A Reader in Culture, History, and Representations* (Malden, MA: Blackwell, 2003). Since there is no standard usage at the writing of this essay, I will try to remain neutral by using the terms interchangeably.

5 The question on where to draw cultural boundaries is a difficult one. Guatemala may be an overly restrictive window to access by itself. One contemporary study by Edward F. Fischer suggests that the Central American region, including all of the ancient Mayan empire, really creates the most identifiable unit for examination, see E.F. Fischer, *Cultural Logics and Global Economics* (Austin, TX: University of Texas Press, 2002). For a recent overview of Guatemalan culture in its particularity, see M.E. Shea, *Culture and Customs of Guatemala* (Westport, CT: Greenwood, 2000).

6 L.R. Chavez et al., "Understanding Knowledge and Attitudes about Breast Cancer: A Cultural Analysis" *Archives of Family Medicine* 4 (1995): 145–52; C. Morgan, E. Park, and D.E. Cortes, "Beliefs, Knowledge, and Behavior about Cancer among Urban Hispanic Women," *Journal of the National Cancer Institute Monographs* 18 (1995): 57–63. Part of the problem may also be related to minority women's health. Recent studies of note that discuss cultural problems in treating Hispanic women who have had medical problems are discussed in P. McCartney, "Internet Resources on Minority Women's Health," *American Journal of Maternal Child Nursing* 27, no. 6 (Nov/Dec 2002): 355 and R. Riegel et al., "Standardized Telephonic Case Management in a Hispanic Heart Failure Population: An Effective Intervention," *Disease Management and Health Outcomes* 10, no. 4 (2002): 241–9.

7 Obviously, money is often an issue in hospitals that deal with indigent patients. However, too many variables can make any case more difficult. In the case of money, it is either the dominant factor or it isn't. Since ability to pay personally or with insurance or through a government program constitutes another sort of issue, I will leave this variable for a future essay.

8 Among some urban Hispanic communities in the United States, there is the belief that surgery is not an effective treatment for breast cancer. See Morgan, Park, and Cortes, note 6 above.

9   This is a rather controversial issue. What is at stake here (and in case two) is a sense of a universally recognized set of biomedical ethical principles. This sort of position has been advocated by G. Neitzke, "Global Aspects of Medical Ethics: Conditions and Possibilities," *Wiemer Medizinische Wochenschrift* 151, no. 9–10 (2002): 208–12; F.A. Chervenak and L.B. McCullough, "The Moral Foundation of Medical Leadership: The Professional Virtues of the Physician as Fiduciary of the Patient," *American Journal of Obstetrics and Gynecology* 184, no. 5 (2001): 875–9, discussion 879–89; E.D. Pellegrino, "Intersections of Western Biomedical Ethics and World Culture: Problematic and Possibility," *Cambridge Quarterly of Healthcare Ethics* 1, no. 3 (1992): 191–6.

10 Some might demur, saying that counter example 1 really supports the absolute value of human life, except that in this case it quantifies it such that if x is valuable, then 2x is twice as valuable. In this case we are involved merely in a calculation concerning saving one life or many. Utilitarians will take this tack, but I am aiming to focus on whether there are ever any good reasons for one to question whether the spy should continue to live. If there are, then my point is made.

11 For a discussion on this, see J. Savulescu and R.W. Momeyer, "Should Informed Consent be Based on Rational Beliefs?" *Journal of Medical Ethics* 23 (1997): 282–8.

12 See my discussion of the fact-value distinction (co-written with J.A. Donahue) in *Ethics Across the Curriculum: A Practice-Based Approach* (Lanham, MD: Lexington Books, 2003), chap. 2.

13 The role of coherentism in modern epistemology is discussed by K. Lehrer, *Theory of Knowledge* (Boulder, CO: Westview, 1990); W. Sellars, *Science, Perception and Reality* (London: Routledge & Kegan Paul, 1963); N. Rescher, *The Coherence Theory of Truth* (Oxford: Clarendon Press, 1973); A. Plantinga, *Warrant: The Current Debate* (Oxford: Oxford University Press, 1993). It is the position of this author that, in the particular situation described in the text, a pragmatic coherentism would constitute the most workable solution to the problem of the "rationality of the patient." Thus, if the patient presents a series of propositions that are internally coherent and are grounded in an established cultural milieu, the physician should accept them as rational.

14 I make this argument in my book, *Basic Ethics* (Upper Saddle River, NJ: Prentice Hall, 2000), introduction.

15 I am thinking of cases such as lying: telling that which is untrue with intent to deceive another. Some cultural traditions assume that all speech acts are veridical; others put a higher value on compassion in cases where the truth will hurt someone. All parties in the latter culture know this so that it mitigates the condition of deceiving another because the social convention exists to promote human caring. Thus in culture #1 if a terminally ill family member asks, "Will I die?" one must always say, "yes." This is because the relevant subsumption is under the moral institution of lying. In culture #2 the answer to "Will I die?" is "no," because the loved one knows the pain of the opposite answer and wishes to make the last days of life more joyful. In this second culture, the proper subsumption is under the moral convention of loving compassion. Most moral principles (save for exploitation and murder) are subject to such social interpretation in their application.

16 I should note that some schools of legal positivism hold to this doctrine. For a discussion of these issues, see *Basic Ethics*, see note 14 above, chap. 8.

17 Hegel writes influentially on the master/slave paradigm in *Phenomenology of Spirit*, trans. A.V. Miller (Oxford: Oxford University Press, 1977), 111–8.

18 The Stockholm syndrome in a domestic situation has been recently addressed by K. O'leary and R.D. Roland, ed., *Psychological Abuse in Violent Domestic Relations* (New York: Springer, 2001). For a view into the difficulties of detecting and measuring this syndrome, see S.M. Auerbach *et al.*, "Interpersonal Impacts and Adjustments to the Stress of Simulated Captivity: An Empirical Test of Stockholm Syndrome," *Journal of Social and Clinical Psychology* 13, no. 2 (1994): 207–11.

19 Part of the problem with the issue of "what is the physician to do" is that physician training in medical ethics is still not where it needs to be–especially concerning cultural literacy. Medical schools need to engage far more in cultural literacy to train and nurture budding physicians to be sensitive to these ethical issues. This training needs to extend not only for the four years of medical school, but in residency as well. For a discussion of this, see J. Coulehan and P.C. Williams, "Vanquishing Virtue: The impact of Medical Education," *Academic Medicine* 76, no. 6 (2001): 598–605.

20 I have made a stab at describing this process in chapter 8 of *Basic Ethics*, see note 14 above.

21 The Argument for the Moral Status of Basic Goods:

1. Before anything else, all people desire to act.—Fact
2. Whatever all people desire before anything else is natural to that species.—Fact
3. Desiring to act is natural to *Homo sapiens*.—1,2
4. People value what is natural to them.—Assertion
5. What people value they wish to protect.—Assertion
6. All people wish to protect their ability to act beyond all else.—1,3,4,5
7. The strongest interpersonal "oughts" are expressed via our highest value systems: religion, morality, and aesthetics.—Assertion
8. All people must agree, on pain of logical contradiction, that what is natural and desirable to them individually is natural and desirable to everyone collectively and individually.—Assertion
9. Everyone must seek personal protection for her own ability to act via religion, morality, and/or aesthetics.—6,7
10. Everyone, on pain of logical contradiction, must admit that all other humans will seek personal protection of their ability to act via religion, morality, and/or aesthetics.—8,9
11. All people must agree, on pain of logical contradiction, that since the attribution of the basic goods of agency are predicated generally, that it is inconsistent to assert idiosyncratic preferences.—Fact
12. Goods that are claimed through generic predication apply equally to each agent and everyone has a stake in their protection.—10,11
13. *Rights and duties are correlative.—Assertion*
14. Everyone has at least a moral right to the basic goods of agency and others in the society have a duty to provide those goods to all.—12,13

A slightly modified version of this argument in my book, *A Just Society* (Lanham, MD: Oxford: Rowman and Littlefield, 2004), chap. 3.

22 The discussion of the communitarian-individualism dynamics in traditional Chinese cultures has been a subject of interest of late. Some of the social institutions are complex and are by no means uniform. For a taste of this discussion, see J.B. Nie, "The Plurality of Chinese and American Moralities: Toward an Interpretive Cross-Cultural Bioethics," *Kennedy Institute of Ethics Journal* 10, no. 3 (2000): 239–60; M.C. Pang, "Protective Truthfulness: the Chinese way of Safeguarding Patients in Informed Treatment Decisions," *Journal of Medical Ethics* 25, no. 3 (1999): 247–53; on the medical ethos of China and Japan, J.R. McConnell, III, "The Ambiguity about Death in Japan: An Ethical Implication for Organ Procurement," *Journal of Medical Ethics* 25, no. 4 (1999): 315–21; D.F. Tsai, "Ancient Chinese Medical Ethics and the Four Principles of Biomedical Ethics," *Journal of Medical Ethics* 25, no. 4 (1999): 315–21; Z. Guo, "Chinese Confucian Culture and the Medical Ethical Tradition," *Journal of Medical Ethics* 21, no. 4 (1995): 239–46; R. Ishiwata and A. Sakai, "The Physician-Patient Relationship and Medical Ethics in Japan," *Cambridge Quarterly of Healthcare Ethics* 3, no. 1 (1994): 60–6.

23 Obviously these risk assessments are rather subjective and will vary with the advances in medical practice. However, for our purposes it is enough to admit that treatments have various risks and rewards that in some way must be discussed with the patient.

24 Resultant risk here means the risk of death after one of the paths (A D) is followed.

25 For a wide-ranging discussion of some of the causal relationships among the individual family-society in contemporary America, see D.S. Browning and G.B. Rodriguez, *Reweaving the Social Tapestry: Toward a Public Philosophy and Policy for Families* (New York: Norton, 2002).

26 W.D. Hamilton is one of the earliest proponents of kin selection as an alternative to Sewall Wright's group selection model, see "The Evolution of Altruistic Behavior," *American Naturalist* 97 (1963): 354–356 and "The Genetical Evolution of Social Behavior I," *Journal of Theoretical Biology* 7 (1964): 1–16; "The Genetical Evolution of Social Behavior II," *Journal of Theoretical Biology* 7 (1964): 17–52. Two other scholars of note in this tradition are John Maynard Smith and George Price. See J.M. Smith, "How to Model Evolution," in *The Latest on the Best: Essays on Evolution and Optimality*, ed. J. Dupré (Cambridge: Cambridge University Press, 1987), pp. 119–31 and G. Price, "Selection and Covariance," *Nature* 277 (1970): 520–1.

27 My depiction of a normative standard for world-views is set out in the Personal Worldview Imperative: "All people must develop a single comprehensive and internally coherent world-view that is good and that we strive to act out in our daily lives." This imperative is described in chapter 8 of *Basic Ethics*, see note 14 above, and, in the biomedical realm, in M. Boylan and K.E. Brown, *Genetic Engineering: Science and Ethics on the New Frontier* (Upper Saddle River, NJ: Prentice Hall, 2002), 6–8, 121–122, 132, 141, 146, 150–151, 154–155, 167.

Healthcare Disparity and Changing the Complexion of Orthopedic Surgeons

RICHARD E. GRANT AND MICHAEL BOYLAN

Introduction

If any country on earth seeks fairness in the delivery of essential goods of life, such as access to basic healthcare, then there should be equal access to all (Boylan, 2014). This is because all people count as one, and the right to healthcare is on par with the right to clean water, food, shelter, and protection from unwarranted bodily harm.[1] The best healthcare in the United States goes to white, straight, males who have health insurance and are middle-class or above (White, 1999; White and Chanoff, 2011). A good general measure of this assertion is to look at mortality rates. The assumption is that significant differences between various group mortality rates indicate healthcare disparity (including public health issues; Boylan, 2008). African-Americans, for example, have significantly higher mortality rates as measured against Americans of European descent. Nationally, for example, the difference in life expectancy between African-Americans and European-descent Americans is 4.8 years (in 2007); infant mortality is 2.3 times higher, and maternal mortality is 2.7 times higher (Xu *et al.*, 2010). In addition, when access to healthcare is raised in artificial test situations there is an increase in the patient population's sense of well-being (Tovar-Murray, 2010). These studies are statistically significant (Smedley *et al.*, 2003). They correlate with a low percentage of ethnic minority physicians in the United States, of only 4% (Rao and Flores, 2007). They point to a macro assessment of healthcare disparity in the United States. Healthcare disparity ignores the basic right to healthcare noted above. Since all legitimate moral rights imply correlative moral duties, the documented existence of healthcare disparity represents a societal duty unfulfilled. Something needs to be done about this.

Healthcare Disparity

The face of America is changing. The Pew Research Center estimates that by 2050 the majority of Americans will be a combination of minority groups – the so-called majority minority trend.[2] What this means is that if there is a problem in healthcare disparity between recognized minority groups and the European descent population, then this outcome will only get progressively worse.

One example of healthcare disparity comes from research done by Schulman *et al.* (1999). In this well-controlled study it was found that there was a statistically significant difference in the way European-descent Americans and African-Americans were treated when they presented with identical heart symptoms that called for cardiac catheterization. African-Americans were far less likely to be offered the standard treatment option. The authors hypothesized several reasons why the attending physicians offered this different level of care:

1. The procedure was judged to be too expensive (when African-American patients were involved).
2. The physicians made differential judgments about the value of the patient's life (without any other corroboration).
3. They cited anticipated complications that might occur in African-Americans (that were not evidenced-based).

These judgments are not made with the explicit intent of conscious animus against African-Americans. However, it has that effect. Individuals can possess attitudes that they do not feel are racist in origin, but can result in racist outcomes. When these outcomes are deleterious to a recognized racial, gender, ethnic, or sexual orientation group, then they reinforce healthcare disparity. For simplicity, let us refer to this sort of medical bias as suppressed worldview disorder (SWD). Those physicians who have SWD are not fully aware of their own personal worldview and how it affects their practice as a physician. Michael Boylan has advocated that all people undergo a structural process of personal analysis called the Personal Worldview Imperative: "All people must develop a single, comprehensive and internally coherent worldview that is good and that we strive to act out in our daily lives."[3] This imperative calls on everyone to lead a life that is self-reflective according to the criteria found in the imperative. The Personal Worldview Imperative may be the best cure for SWD. However, how we stimulate physicians to undergo this sort of critical self-reflection will require further exploration.

There are other instances of SWD that are demonstrated via statistically significant forms of healthcare disparity, such as foot disorders among Mexican Americans and European-descent Americans. Mexican Americans were offered far fewer joint-sustaining options as compared to European-descent Americans (White and Chanoff, 2011). This led to far more amputations among Mexican Americans.

A final example in this section is total joint arthroplasty. This is a procedure that can greatly relieve pain from arthritis, a painful condition that has no cure and is present in many middle-aged and elderly people. Despite its effectiveness and relative cost-effectiveness on the long run, this procedure is only available to 3.82 African-Americans per 1000 over 65 as opposed to 9.71 European-descent Americans per 1000 (White and Chanoff, 2011). This is even worse when we learn that 40% of African-Americans aged over 65 suffer from arthritis while only 25% of European-descent whites do. This means that the disparity in arthritis treatment by total joint arthroplasty favors European-descent Americans by more than 50%.

These examples point to a contemporary picture of healthcare in America: it fails the test of equality. One reason may be SWD but there may be other causes as well. Before we get there, let us examine how these disparities might affect a typical patient's perspective.

The Problem from the Patient's Perspective

One study by Ibrahim *et al.* (2002) suggests that Veterans Administration patients are less likely than European-descent Americans to be employed, married, or high school grads. African-Americans are more likely to live below the poverty line than European-descent Americans. This creates a class distinction. As White and Chanoff (2011) point out, this can create a worldview perspective of separate societies living together in a hierarchy. Those at the top feel that they *have achieved* whatever they have based *solely* upon their own merit, and that those *without* deserve their lesser state. This follows from a logically flawed understanding of *desert*. What does it mean to *deserve* something? The authors of this essay believe that desert refers to hard work by the agent involved without regard to birth preference regarding race, wealth, religion, or other factors that simply fall into some people's lap upon birth as a preferential gift (Boylan and Grant, 2004).

So what do you do if you are poor and the *other*? There are various possible perspectives: (a) the idealistic perspective, (b) the despondent perspective, and (c) the protester perspective. Let's examine each of these in order. In the idealistic perspective the patient *trusts* in his or her physician to be a fair and objective healthcare provider who is color blind and blind to social class. This sort of patient assumes that all patients admitted with a given condition will receive the same sort of care including all appropriate medical options (where "appropriate" means the general standard of care shown throughout the entire United States without regard to race, gender, sexual orientation, or social class). This idealistic worldview perspective is often more present in young people who have not been knocked around too much in their lives. Most people begin here – though for many the length of residency is very short.

Many would scoff at the idealistic perspective. We do not. It is the *way things are supposed to be*. If reality does not meet the ethical and professional demands of the profession and the society that supports the institution of medicine, then something is severely wrong. It is the idealists who continue to exhibit *outrage* when real conditions in Newark, NJ; Washington, DC; Selma, AL; Gary, IN; Fargo, ND; Colorado Springs, CO; and Los Angeles, CA (just to mention a cross-section) do not meet minimum standards measured upon the justified basic rights expectations of all people for healthcare delivered fairly.

Let's be clear about what is meant by "fairly." We intend an egalitarian meaning. This entails equal consideration of all. It does not necessitate identical treatments since patients are all different and their conditions present in unique ways. But what egalitarianism does is require that the physician seriously engage with each patient to the extent necessary to obtain the proper personalized prognosis in order to determine a course of treatment. This course of treatment will have only one objective: to be the very best accepted medical treatment given all the situational facts about the case. It will be an evidence-based assessment that has nothing to do with the patient being from a majority or from a minority group.

As we have seen in the last section this is not always the case. This leads to the second sort of response to perceived healthcare disparity: despondency. This reaction is very common among oppressed groups—especially as one ages. The fight flows out of the soul and the personal worldview strategy is one of endurance. The strong turn their fortitude toward putting up with an unfair structure that they believe is beyond their ability to change. They accept point blank that life is unfair and they are prepared to live with that reality.

Of course the macro result of many turning to despondency is that the inertia of the unequal system becomes that of stasis. The status quo becomes entrenched and solutions become that much harder to effect.

The third reaction is that of the protester. The protester often began as an idealist but became fed up with the difference between what *should be* and *things as they are*. A feeling of moral outrage is born. Most protesters begin within the system and try to reform it from within. But when the system is unresponsive patients turn to the court system for redress. The end result is further distance between patient and physician. As the battle lines form through this process power is the only operating principle. But medicine is about care and not about wielding legal and political power. Thus, reform from this angle is generally not productive.

The patient's perspective is always that of someone who is at a disadvantage. In the power scheme, patients (even if they were not diminished by their sickness or injury) are at the bottom of a very robust institutional power structure (unless they enlist the help of outside forces). That is why all three of the above patient responses will not be adequate to create positive change. The onus for change must pass to the medical community itself.

Creating Real Diversity in the Physician Population

In the last section it was argued that healthcare disparity based upon a patient's membership in various minority groups is a fact and that the three common responses (idealist, despondent, or protester) are generally not effective to bring about real change. Rather, the call was for physicians to heal themselves.

The first step in this process is to return to the suppressed worldview disorder (SWD) mentioned above. If this is a major source of the problem, then what is the solution? We said earlier that getting physicians to undergo a critical self-reflection process called the personal worldview imperative must be the end result. The problem is getting physicians to this point. Let's begin by returning to the patient. It is hard to assess how all three sorts of patient reaction view the SWD of the offending physician or hospital staff. When one confronts another whose personal worldview difference is so great that it almost becomes a difference in *kind* rather than just one of *degree*, then the patient is at a loss. The avenue of authentic communication is impassable. Another route must be chosen: the road of charade. This path is one of theater and performance. But because it is all make-believe, there is no lasting positive result.

The best antidote for SWD is for the hospital or regional medical community to diversify. Diversity is the proper medication for SWD. The reason for this is simple: most failures of personal worldview occur because people do not know any better. They do not know any better because they only see one model around them. Most people are rather lazy at self-worldview criticism and renewal. Therefore, they need an environmental change such that their own personal worldview is challenged by its existence among other, different worldview perspectives. Either a new accommodation has to be reached or the majority worldview retreats into a secure enclave. This latter strategy will not be prudentially effective over the long run. Therefore, diversity is the best public health strategy to cure SWD: it will force physicians to undergo critical worldview reflection. If they don't then they will not survive in the new community order.

Next, is to address strategies to make this happen. The goal is to reduce SWD in the medical community. The means is to increase diversity. But how do we increase diversity? One strategy is affirmative action. Affirmative action is understood in various ways.[4] The least controversial of its various guises is to appeal to desert theory (mentioned above). In desert theory those applying in higher education, professional schools, government contracts, and other desirable community roles should be able to present a portfolio of themselves that represents the *road traveled* by the applicant. Those who have had to achieve more in their lives because they have no access to family or social preferment should be given credit for this (Boylan and Grant, 2004). Our society does recognize the road traveled when it comes to giving preference in hiring to veterans. Why not extend this to those who have had to overcome considerable obstacles to get to where they are, for example, first-generation college graduate, lower socioeconomic background, membership in a minority population, among others? We think that this is essential in order to achieve the diversity necessary to cure SWD. But how do we get there? One approach initiated by Richard E. Grant is to create a context in which minority candidates for residency who wanted to compete for the very competitive subspecialty of orthopedic surgery might be given a value-added experience that might help them imagine themselves within the subspecialty as well as giving them additional functional qualifications so that they could move into residency programs based upon this enhanced understanding of deserts. Enter the Stephens Fellowship Program (as one prototype for the future).

The Timothy L. Stephens Orthopedic Fellowship Program for Minority Medical Students: Its Goals and Its Progress

In order to take a first step toward addressing healthcare disparity among orthopedic surgeons, the Stephens Orthopedic Fellowship Program was started. It was supported by a $916 000 grant from the St Luke's Foundation, University Hospitals Case Medical

Center in Cleveland, Ohio. The fellowship has launched an innovative educational program supervised by the Department of Orthopedic Surgery University Hospitals Case Medical Center. This fellowship program is the first of its kind in the nation and is designed to strengthen and expand the participation of minority medical students in the profession of orthopedic surgery. Named in honor of the first African-American orthopedic surgeon in the State of Ohio, Timothy L. Stephens, the orthopedic fellowship for minority medical students will afford a select group of minority medical students the opportunity to take a one-year break from their medical school studies. The program will last approximately 10 years and one fellow will be selected each year for participation. During the fellowship year, the student will be embedded in the activity of University Hospitals Case Medical Center Orthopedic Residency program, which is chaired by Randall Marcus.

The Stephen's fellow medical student will spend a full academic year at Case Medical Center where, under the supervision of a distinguished orthopedic faculty, he/she will participate along with current Case orthopedic residents in subspecialty lectures, weekly grand rounds, daily clinics, orthopedic surgical procedures, and basic science research. The Stephens fellow will also attend and present at national and regional orthopedic conferences, annual Orthopedic Research Society meetings, the American Academy of Orthopedic Surgeons conventions, and the J. Robert Gladden Society luncheon, which occurs during the American Academy of Orthopedic Surgery, where the fellow will have the opportunity to network with other minority medical students attending the Annual American Academy of Orthopedic Surgery Convention.

By the completion of their fellowship year, participating minority medical students will have been exposed to a highly competitive orthopedic residency program and will have been fully immersed in the culture of the postgraduate study of orthopedic surgery at University Hospitals Case Medical Center. They will have gained familiarity with musculoskeletal research scientists as well as orthopedic clinicians, and will have had extensive exposure to orthopedic surgical techniques through direct observation within the operating room theater. Experiences gained during the fellowship year will enable participants to become strong contenders for positions in orthopedic residency programs nationwide upon graduation from their respective medical schools.

By providing opportunities for minority medical students to pursue careers in orthopedic medicine, this new and unique initiative is seeking to overcome the racial, ethnic, and gender disparities that exist both within the academic realm in orthopedics as well as among practitioners in other surgical subspecialties. These chronic disparities, in turn, have a strong impact on minority access to quality orthopedic care. The issue is critical.

The St Luke's educational grant was designed to help minority medical students overcome the barriers to diversity in pursuit of specialized orthopedic study, research, and clinical practice. There are several challenges with respect to pipeline issues prior to the application process for minority medical students. Orthopedics reports an underwhelming acceptance of women and minorities within its ranks. Orthopedics currently stands at the bottom of an inverse pyramid of all surgical subspecialties with respect to the participation of women and minority candidates. There are at least 152 to 156 orthopedic residency educational programs in the United States. Many of these programs have never admitted female or minority applicants.

According to the American Academy of Orthopedic Surgery's self-reported survey on race, completed in 2006, only 1.5% of all American Academy of Orthopedic Surgery fellows practicing as board-certified orthopedic surgeons were African-American. This number should be contrasted to the presence of 1.6% Hispanic or Latinos, 4.2% Asian Americans, 2.2% other, and 90.5% Caucasians. There was a new census developed in 2008. At that time, women constituted only 3% of the total of the orthopedic workforce. Ten percent of practicing orthopedic surgeons were members of minority groups; and Asian Americans remain the largest minority group represented in the rank of the orthopedic surgical workforce.

Over the past two decades, the traditional African-American orthopedic residencies included Harlem and Columbia in New York City; Cook County in Chicago, Illinois; Morehouse in Atlanta, Georgia; Meharry and Vanderbilt in Nashville; King Drew UCLA in Los Angeles, California; and Howard University Hospital in Washington, DC. Dr Charles H. Epps Jr presented a review of the statistics at the meeting of the American Orthopedic Association in Asheville, North Carolina, in 2005 and indicated that Howard University Hospital usually graduated four residents from its Orthopedic Residency Program. At the time of his report, the King Drew Medical School Residency Program also produced another two residents from its Orthopedic Residency Program, providing a total of six graduates representing at that time 25% of the annual increase in diversity within the United States.

In order to effect change through education and leadership opportunities, the Timothy Stephens Fellowship Program is targeting candidates who have completed the first two years of their basic science education and are about to enter into their third year or their clinical year. These students would have to apply for a one-year hiatus from the normal course of their medical studies. This would allow them to participate in a 365-day course of total embedding into the educational, surgical, and research activities of Case University Hospitals Orthopedic Residency Program, which has been in existence for approximately 142 years. The current Chair of that program is Dr Randall Marcus, who has noted that the program averages over 500 applications per year for six residency slots. The program at University Hospitals (UH) Case Medical Center is considered in the top 10% of preferred residency programs in the United States and has remained at that level for well over 140 years.

As far as the fellowship nuts and bolts are concerned, fellows are allowed to review the basic science research activities within the Department of Orthopedic Surgery under the direction of Dr Edward Greenfield and Dr Claire Rimnac. This will allow them to select the research projects of their choice that expose them to bench research and intensive musculoskeletal basic science research projects. On the clinical side, research is also available under the auspices and direction of UH Orthopedic Department faculty members. Additionally, the Stephens fellow will be allowed exposure to all aspects of the didactic subspecialty activities, including multispecialty lectures occurring in the early morning, afternoon conferences, and weekly grand rounds and journal clubs.

Stephens fellows would be expected to attend and present at national and regional conferences, and to attend the annual Orthopedic Research Society meetings, and the American Academy of Orthopedic Surgery (already mentioned before). In addition, they will accompany Dr Richard E. Grant, Dr Randall Marcus, and other members of the full-time orthopedic staff and attend their clinics at the University Hospitals. Residents will also be exposed to the Otis Moss Jr Health Center biweekly and will shadow Dr Carla Harwell, who is the Medical Director of the Otis Moss Jr Health Center. The 360-degree exposure will cover a period of July 1 through June 30 of the following year and emphasizes the translational aspects of the program from basic science bench work to clinical bedside.

Outcomes and expectations include an enhanced exposure to a highly competitive academic Orthopedic Residency Program and the culture thereof, with complete immersion in the culture of the University Hospitals Case Medical Center Orthopedic Residency and observation of the demands of a typical resident day within the Department of Orthopedic Residency. It is our expectation that such intimate exposure will provide the fellow with a quantum leap in their musculoskeletal database with respect to basic science and to clinical applications. The other expectations include the production of peer-reviewed clinical and basic science publications. The one-year exposure to basic science lectures and grand rounds and their publications should markedly enhance the fellow's curriculum vitae. Ostensibly, this should afford the Stephens fellow great familiarity with Case research scientists and clinical attending physicians, and help him or her to develop career-long relationships with various attending physicians. The fellows will also be exposed to surgical techniques in the operating room and will learn some of the nuances of surgical discipline and surgical decision-making.

The anticipated outcome will affect the pipeline of competent and highly competitive medical students who hopefully in the future will apply for residency positions within the Department of Orthopedic Surgery at the University Hospitals Case Medical Center. The goal is to create competitive applicants who have the potential for becoming AOA (American Osteopathic Association) graduates from their medical school. Most applications should reflect high USMLE (the national medical testing agency) scores. The fellows are expected to become familiar with the level of competition and expectations of the majority culture currently being accepted into the University Hospitals Case Medical Center Orthopedic Program. In view of their increased exposure to basic science and basic science research, we are anticipating the development of clinician scientists who might become future faculty members at University Hospitals Case Medical Center Department of Orthopedic Surgery.

To date, we have had three participants in the program, all of whom completed the activities as outlined above. For the purpose of this essay we wish to share a summary of the activities of the first graduate participant of the Timothy L. Stephens Orthopedic Fellowship Program from August 2009 through June 2010, namely the medical student Havalee Henry from the University of Rochester. Ms Henry lauded the program and its founders for their foresight with regards to the needs of healthcare service and the importance of diversity in the providers of orthopedic services. She also expressed gratitude and appreciation for the tremendous opportunity to enhance her skill and knowledge and to interact with distinguished faculty in the field.

- Her primary research experience centered on the expansion of human chondrocytes. Dr Henry and her mentor (Dr Jim Dennis) used a bioreactor system to investigate what growth factors and conditions would be optimal for the development of cartilage sheets from human articular chondrocytes.

- Dr Henry and her mentor used a bioreactor system to investigate what growth factors and conditions would be optimal for the development of cartilage sheets from human articular chondrocytes. Her role with respect to the research project included responsibility for conducting a literature search and developing the experimental design. She conducted every aspect of the experiment, which included mastering tissue culture techniques (thawing cells, culturing cells, using expansion medium, developing aggregate cultures, counting cells, subculturing cells). She also conducted phase microscopy; tissue staining for histological purposes (collagen type II and type X immunohistochemical staining); quantitative analysis of DNA; glycosaminoglycan assays; and all data analysis on the results of the experiment.
- The result of these studies indicated that fibroblast growth factor-18 (FGF-18) held potential to increase chondrocyte proliferation during expansion. This project culminated in an article reviewing growth factors impacting growth of human articular chondrocytes, which was published in the Case Western Reserve Orthopedic Journal.
- Dr Henry's second project involved production and implantation of tissue-engineered neotrachea from rabbit auricular chondrocytes. These chondrocytes were cultured to produce a mechanically stable trachea-like tissue. The project investigated whether the tissue-engineered trachea could function as an effective substitute when implanted into a segmental tracheal defect. This project was successful in developing sheets of cartilage but was unable to maintain the patency of the neotrachea due to fibrosis.
- Her third project was aimed at developing a straightforward and time-efficient method of calculating femoral anteversion intraoperatively by combining measurements of the apparent femoral neck shaft angle, the true femoral neck shaft angle, and femoral inclination with measurements obtained from lateral X-rays of the femoral neck. It was felt that this information would allow the surgeon to quickly and easily calculate femoral version, which is considered vital to the performance of rotational osteotomies. She undertook this project under the direction of Dr Daniel Cooperman. Seventy-two femora from the Cleveland Museum of Natural History were photographed and relevant measurements obtained and combined with previously obtained data to determine the accuracy of calculating femoral version intraoperatively. It was concluded that these were precise measurements and correlated nicely with anteversion measured using the method of Kingsley and Olmsted.
- With respect to her surgical exposure, medical student Henry was exposed to and participated in a total of 76 surgeries encompassing the orthopedic subspecialties of foot and ankle, total joint reconstruction, tumor, sports, hand and upper extremity, and trauma. Ms Henry also participated in multiple lectures that were either subspecialty lectures or lectures related to our weekly Grand Rounds conferences.

With respect to the future changes in the program, we are working on identification and leveraging of stakeholder expertise and resources, both within the Department of Orthopedic Surgery at University Hospitals Case Medical Center, and externally such as medical schools, societies, and professional organizations, that will allow us to create a pipeline bridge through which the number and percentage of under-represented minor medical students who transition into orthopedic residencies in this competitive specialty can be increased.

To date, our initiative is consistent with the theory of change as evidenced by the engagement of fellows in the immersion process over the past 1.75 cycles of the grant from St Luke's Foundation. Over the past 12 months, two of our fellows will be seeking residency slots in Orthopedic Residency Programs and have submitted manuscripts and abstracts that should have received responses. Our strategy continues to be that of a 12-month exposure to a highly competitive academic Orthopedic Residency Program allowing familiarity with Case basic science research. The desired outcome is to markedly enhance the fellow's curriculum vitae to create a so-called "super candidate." We want to provide each candidate with a quantum leap in their musculoskeletal database, encourage the development and submission of peer-reviewed clinical and basic science manuscripts for publication, podium presentations, surgical and clinical shadowing, and clinical shadowing and community health fair exposure at the Otis Moss Jr University Case Medical Health Center.

As far as the basic science mentoring is concerned, on average for quarter three, the program spent over $5287 on each fellow; with respect to the Department of Orthopedic Surgery the cost of mentoring and shadowing was $98 000; and at the Otis Moss Jr Medical Center the mentoring program cost $4415.

With respect to the challenges and lessons learned, based on the performance of each fellow, there have been modifications to the strategy for moving fellows to the program. We now have joint objectives, have re-evaluated our support, and have instituted innovations and adopted new challenges with respect to the program.

In the process of recruiting for the 2011–12 academic year, we are still seeking candidates who do not require remediation with respect to their academic achievements prior to the time that they were accepted into the program. We hope to increase the portfolio of highly competitive candidates who are interested in securing an orthopedic residency slot in their fourth year match process. We will be retooling the program's outreach and recruitment so that interested second- and third-year medical students who fit the profile for the program can be aggressively recruited for the 2012–13 academic year. In order to achieve these goals, we will have to leverage social capital of the entire professional academic orthopedic community and create a national advisory board of orthopedic surgical academic colleagues and organizations and utilize social media to highlight the program and to spread the word with respect to the program.

Conclusion

This essay began by demonstrating that there are healthcare disparities in the United States. These disparities affect minority populations the hardest. One of the causes of these disparities comes from the healthcare community's suppressed worldview disorder (SWD). A SWD keeps people from adequate personal worldview introspection that would allow them to see how they are part of the problem of healthcare disparity. The cure for SWD is to increase diversity in the healthcare community – particularly in power positions such as physicians. The essay then described one program that is operating with that goal in mind: the Timothy L. Stephens Orthopedic Fellowship

Program. Though this program is still in its early stages, it promises to stand as a model for other residency programs as a positive way to offer opportunity for a more diversified academy of practitioners. It is hoped that the success of this program will demonstrate a pattern for other outstanding residency programs to follow – not just in orthopedic surgery but in all under-represented medical subspecialties. Programs such as the Stephens Program (and others that have the same objectives) will go a long way to improving healthcare diversity, which, in turn, will help cure the healthcare community of its SWD. The end result will be to improve healthcare delivery to all people – regardless of race, sexual orientation, or economic class. And this is a goal that we all should support.

Notes

1 Boylan (2004, 2011), cf. "The Moral Right to Healthcare: Part Two" (see p. 157 of this volume).
2 www.pewresearch.org (April 10, 2010).
3 Boylan (2004), p. 21.
4 For a brief sample of these views see: Beauchamp (1998), Bell (2003), Boylan (2002), and Pojman (1998).

References

Beauchamp, T.L. (1998) In defense of affirmative action. *Journal of Ethics* 2: 143–58.

Bell, D. (2003) Diversity's distraction. *Columbia Law Review* 103: 1622–33.

Boylan, M. (2002) Affirmative action: strategies for the future. *Journal of Social Philosophy* 33: 117–30.

Boylan, M. (2004) *A Just Society*. Lanham, MD, and Oxford: Rowman & Littlefield Publishers.

Boylan, M. (2008) Clean water. In: M. Boylan (ed.), *International Public Health Policy and Ethics*. Dordrecht: Springer; pp. 273–88.

Boylan, M. (2011) *Morality and Global Justice: Justifications and Applications*. Boulder, CO: Westview.

Boylan, M. (2014) The moral right to healthcare – part two. In: M. Boylan (ed.), *Medical Ethics*, 2nd edn. Malden, MA: Wiley-Blackwell, pp. 283–97.

Boylan, M. and Grant, R.E. (2004) Diversity and professional ethics. *Journal of the National Medical Association* 96(10): 188–200.

Ibrahim, S.A., Siminoff, L.A., Burant, C.J., and Kwoh, C.K. (2002) Understanding ethnic differences in the utilization of joint replacement for osteoarthritis: The role of patient level factors. *Medical Care* 40(1) (suppl.): 144–51.

Pojman, L. (1998) The case against affirmative action. *Public Affairs Quarterly* 6: 181–206.

Rao, V. and Flores, G. (2007) Why aren't there more African-American physicians? *Journal of the National Medical Association* 99(9) (September): 986–93.

Schulman, K.A., Berlin, J.A., Harless, W., *et al.* (1999) The effect of race and sex on physician's recommendations for cardiac catheterization. *New England Journal of Medicine* 340(14): 1130.

Smedley, B., Stith, A., and Nelson, A. (eds) (2003) *Unequal Treatment: Confronting Racial and Ethnic Disparities in Health Care*. Washington, DC: Institute of Medicine, The National Academies Press.

Tovar-Murray, D. (2010) Social health and environmental quality of life: their relationship to positive physical health and subjective well-being in a population of urban African Americans. *Western Journal of Black Studies* 34(3): 358–66.

White, A.A. III (1999) Guest editor. *Clinical Orthopaedics and Related Research*. 363.

White, A.A. III and Chanoff, D. (2011) *Seeing Patients*. Cambridge, MA: Harvard University Press.

Xu, J., Kochanek, K.D., Murphy, S.L., and Tejada-Vera, B. (2010) Deaths: final data for 2007. *National Vital Statistics Reports* 58(19); available at: http://www.cdc.gov/nchs/data/nvsr/nvsr58/nvsr58_19.pdf [accessed February 20, 2013].

Evaluating a Case Study
Finding the Conflicts

After establishing an ethical point of view (including a segue to application), we are ready to approach cases. The first stage in handling cases effectively is to analyze the situation according to normal practice and potential ethical issues. Obviously, sometimes ethical issues are involved in what one will do, and at other times they are not. It is your job to determine when ethical issues are involved. Let us consider specific cases.

Case 1

You are a nurse who has an obnoxious patient in room 28. He claims that his medication dosage is wrong and should be reevaluated immediately. This patient has made this complaint many times before. Each time the dosage was checked and was found to be correct. The normal practice with problem complainers is to be slow in responding to their demands. After all, other patients who do not create such a fracas need your time.

Does this case involve any ethical issues? If so, what are they? How do they affect normal practice?

Case 2

You run a medical research facility at a major university and are testing a drug for one form of cancer. The preliminary results of your research after two years are not promising; in fact, the drug seems to have a deleterious effect in some instances. Your project has been funded for four years. The drug's results could change, but meanwhile people who might have had several more years of life under conventional treatments are dying. If you stop the experiment now, however, you may put people out of work, jeopardize future funding, and affect your entire university's science program.

Does this case involve any ethical issues? If so, what are they? How do they affect prudential (self-interested) concerns?

Checklist for Detecting Ethical Issues

Directions. Read your case carefully. Determine your ethical viewpoint (see "Developing a Practical Ethical Viewpoint," p. 58ff.). Decide which individual's perspective you will develop in your comments. Create one or more detection questions that will identify ethical issues. These detection questions will follow from your own ethical perspective. For example, from my practical ethical perspective, I have chosen the following two detection questions to bring moral issues to my attention. These questions follow from a deontological viewpoint.

1. *Is any party being exploited solely for the advantage of another?* (Exploitation can include instances of lying, injuring, deliberately falsifying, creating an unequal competitive environment, and so forth.)
2. *Is every effort being made to assist and affirm the human dignity of all parties involved?* (Affirming human dignity can include instances of encouraging the fulfillment of legal and human rights as well as taking personal responsibility for results that are consonant with these principles. Thus, you cannot hide behind nonfunctioning rules.)

By asking these questions within the context of the case, I am able better to understand the moral dimensions that exist with other professional concerns.

A few other comments may be useful concerning my detection questions. Question 1 concerns "prohibitions" (i.e., actions that you must refrain from doing). Question 2 concerns "obligations" (i.e., actions that you are required to do). Anything that is not an ethical obligation or a prohibition is a "permission" (i.e., an action that you may do if you choose). Thus, if the case you present does not invoke a prohibition or an obligation, then you may act solely according to the dictates of your professional practice. It is often useful to group your detection questions as prohibitions and obligations, which emphasizes different types of moral duty.

Try creating detection questions and apply them to the earlier two cases. What do they reveal about the moral issues involved in the cases? How do different detection questions emphasize different moral issues? How different are these perspectives? How similar are they?

Once you have completed this preliminary ethical assessment, you can return to the ethical theory you have adopted and determine *how* and *why* the prohibitions and obligations are applicable to this theory.

Read the following macro and micro cases and follow the steps outlined:

A. Identify your practical ethical viewpoint including any linking principles.
B. Determine which character's perspective you will adopt.
C. Identify two or more detection questions that define obligation and prohibition within the ethical theory you have chosen.
D. Apply the detection questions to the cases to bring attention to the ethical issues.
E. Discuss the interrelationships between the dictates of the ethical issues and those of the professional practice. How might they work together? How might they be opposed?

Macro and Micro Cases[1]

Macro Case 1. You are the head of a research lab at a for-profit genetic engineering company. The National Institutes of Health (NIH) has just put online (open source) its latest work on the operation of various key proteins that turn off at a certain time in a male's life. This discovery came from clinical research conducted at the NIH. It is also common knowledge that this activity is connected to phenotypic hair loss. Now, for the first time, it seems that the genetic understanding of male baldness is understood. You bring this fact up at a high-level staff meeting. Your supervisor, the president of the company, says that the company should submit a patent for the genetic process. You say that patents can only be granted when the idea is novel. The fact that it was already published on the Web by NII I makes it unoriginal. Your boss says, "But applications are patentable. I want you to submit the patent showing that we have solved the way to cure male baldness." "But we *haven't* discovered that yet." "Be creative. Be ambiguous. But put it in the ball park. If we don't have the real solution by the time they rule on this, then you are out of a job." What do you do?

Macro Case 2. There is a new genetic screening test called "Let it All Hang Out" (LIAHO). This test can screen for 50 common genetic tendencies such as alcoholism, diabetes, Huntington's disease (fatal), melanoma of the eye (fatal), etc. It also says whether you are gay.

You are the Human Resources Director for the ABC Corporation (a Fortune 100 company). A salesperson is trying to sell you LIAHO to use on all new hires. The salesman shows you how these genetic diseases can cost the company money so that you should use this information in your hiring decisions. It is also true that your main plants are located in states in which there is a virulent anti-gay sentiment. This could also hurt sales if it turned out you were hiring gays. The question is: should you recommend that the company use the LIAHO test on all new employment applicants? What are the pros and cons? Your boss has asked you to write a memo assessing the test and whether ABC should get on board and use it. Write the memo.

Macro Case 3. The U.S. Senate is about to consider a new patients' bill of rights. The parts of the bill that concern you are three policy directives aimed at paternalism versus patient autonomy. In this case, identify three issues you believe would be controversial regarding federal legislation covering patient autonomy and paternalism (these will be the three policy directives contained within the Senate bill).

After you identify three issues, describe the two sides of each issue. Then write a mock Senate debate in the form of a dialogue between two or more senators discussing your three points from the floor of the Senate. Structure the debate so that it involves moral arguments. Identify a winner of the debate from your own viewpoint.

Macro Case 4. Metropolitan Gotham City (any major U.S. city) needs to share medical information as the result of the creation of a consortium among local hospitals allowing certain ones to specialize in particular areas of treatment that require very expensive medical equipment. Thus, many inter-hospital referrals are made.

The regional consortium has a request for proposals for a new information system that will facilitate this information exchange. Various vendors will submit proposals to a committee appointed by the consortium to evaluate them. Because there is a conflict between privacy protections and efficiency, each vendor must write a proposal that addresses each but supports one side over the other.

You must take the persona of either (a) the vendors (at least two opposing positions) or (b) the selection committee evaluating at least two opposing proposals (which you will create). If you choose the vendor point of view, argue the case for a proefficiency system and a proprivacy system (one vendor will argue one position and another will take the other position). In each instance, be sure to use major ethical theories to make your point.

If you choose the selection committee perspective, you must justify your choice of a system that either emphasizes (a) efficiency or (b) privacy. Again, you must use a major ethical theory to support your eventual conclusion.

Macro Case 5. You are an upper-level male administrator at a large teaching hospital. You have just been to a conference in which a speaker described the female voice within the hospital. The speaker indicated how much better the hospital would function if it listened to that female voice and incorporated it into the institution's operations in fulfilling its mission.

You wonder what would happen if you tried to do this in your hospital. All the senior officers at the hospital are men, and only one female is on the governing board. Making such changes could cause you to be viewed as a trouble maker and could hurt your career. On the other hand, you went into hospital administration to do some good in the world. You agree in theory with what the speaker said, but doing something about it is rather different.

List three areas in which a hospital might benefit by giving more expression to the female voice. Then list all the negative repercussions that might occur if you make incorporating the female voice into the hospital's mission a top-level priority. Finally, if you are in favor of doing this, write a memo to the appropriate person arguing that position. If you are against doing this, write a memo to yourself that you will put into your files detailing why you do not think that you should support this position at this time. In either case, refer to a majority ethical theory.

Macro Case 6. You have been appointed chairperson of the governor's task force on health care allocations for the next decade. The state is divided into four large health care regions, but at this moment you are thinking about Region 2, which encompasses a major city.

One of the findings that has interested you is that allocation requests from inner city poverty areas differ from those from affluent suburban areas. Requests from the inner cities are for basic medical supplies for low-tech medical services delivery. This group needs more physicians, subsidized pharmaceuticals (such as medicine for hypertension), and extensive prenatal and pediatric care, along with basic health care information so that patients in this area can make informed health care decisions that will affect their lives.

The suburbs request sophisticated diagnostic and surgical facilities to meet high-tech needs in sports medicine, cosmetic surgery, and less invasive operating procedures.

The committee's decisions must go through the normal political process. At the moment, many on the committee believe that the affluent areas should get the major share of this money. Their reasons are that the affluent people in the suburbs (a) support the society with their taxes and therefore should be cared for first; (b) vote in much higher numbers so that they are more important in political decisions; and (c) have lobbying groups that will support their interests. Because they "put their money where their mouths are," they should be rewarded with funding.

In contrast, the poor in the inner city (a) pay fewer taxes, (b) vote in small numbers and therefore have little influence in political decisions, and (c) are not the movers and shakers of society. They are disproportionately female, black, Hispanic, and native American, and many of them are children. These groups do not have a powerful constituency.

How can you balance the needs of these two groups? What moral principles should be used to guide the allocation of resources? You must write a preliminary report to the governor in three days. Use ethical principles to guide your recommendation of resource allocation.

Micro Case 1. You had an accident. You were taken to the emergency department of the hospital and required surgery. They had to remove part of your spleen. You signed an informed consent for your surgery that said discarded tissue could be used for medical research. However, after your recovery, you discover that Dr Janice Gold was a founding partner in *Genomic Futures*, a firm that seeks to patent genes for new future cures. In this case you discover (after hiring an investigative law firm) that Dr Gold used the tissue from your spleen to come up with a new understanding of how the spleen reacts to a common disease, mononucleosis. This, in turn, made the company stock go way up. Dr Gold is now 20 million dollars richer for those parts of your spleen. How should you think about this? Are you owed compensation? Can doctors simply use your tissue and enrich themselves? Pretend you are the judge hearing the case.

Micro Case 2. You are a job applicant. The company that you want to work for is asking you to take the LIAHO test (see above) as a precondition for employment. You don't really know all the conditions that they list on their disclosure sheet. You aren't even sure whether you want to know whether you have a fatal inherited condition. Besides, it seems to you a little creepy to have your genetic information in a possible employer's hands. The hang-up is that you've lost your job. You have a family and if you don't get a new job soon, you will have to sell your house. Moving somewhere else will mean relocating the family, and so forth. This job will pay more than your last job. But there is still the nagging sense of being violated by taking this test. You are going home to talk to your spouse about this. Set out your dialogue with him/her.

Micro Case 3. You are a physician in private practice. John Smith and Mary Jones have been your patients for years. During a physical exam, Mr. Smith informs you that he is engaged to be married to Ms. Jones. You ask whether Mr. Smith has disclosed his HIV condition to Ms. Jones. "We've always practiced safe sex," Mr. Smith answers. "She can't possibly be infected."

"But don't you think she has a right to know? *Before* you are married?"

"That's nobody's business but mine," Mr. Smith replies.

Mr. Smith leaves, and you begin to consider the situation. You swore an oath of confidentiality when you became a physician. But you also swore an oath to do no harm. Would you be doing harm by not preventing possible harm? Does Mary Jones have a right to know that her husband-to-be is HIV positive? And if he refuses to tell her, should you tell her?

Identify issues involved from the physician's point of view, using a major ethical theory to justify telling Ms. Jones. Be sure to refer to the practice of medicine according to the Hippocratic Oath. (As an optional assignment, list arguments that Mr. Smith and Ms. Jones might make about their own interests in this case. Do these considerations change what the physician should do? Why or why not?)

Micro Case 4. You are a nurse in the maternity section of a suburban hospital. One of your patients, Ms. Younger, has just had her first child. Her health insurance allows her a 48-hour stay, however, Ms. Younger's baby, Sally, is quite jaundiced. You know from your twelve years of experience that such severe cases can easily be treated in two or three days under a bilirubin light. You also know that Ms. Younger is due to be discharged in three hours. The physician in charge took the position of the hospital and the insurance company that patients should be discharged in 48 hours.

When you brought up the jaundice problem to the physician, he replied, "Well, she can put the baby in front of a window to get a similar effect, and if that doesn't work, the insurance company will send out a nurse with a portable bilirubin light. It will work out."

"But you don't know this woman like I do," you answered. But the physician would not change his position. You tried to explain that Ms. Younger is a first-time mother without a car and coming back to the hospital for blood checks would be impossible. In addition, Ms. Younger does not understand the seriousness of her baby's condition.

The physician replied that the hospital and the insurance company had well-conceived procedures for everything. It would all be fine.

You believe, however, that the baby's life is at stake. You believe that the only way to solve the problem is to bring more people into the dialogue so that they might understand the true extent of the situation. If a conversation were enjoined, then surely an effect that was good for all parties would result.

What are the possible options that are open to you? Provide at least three alternatives and then, using this list, outline an action plan based on principles of human relationship and ethical theory to guide your actions. How do principles of justice and care interact in the various options you set out?

Micro Case 5. You are a physician. Your patient, Sam, has heart problems caused by some venal blockage near the heart. You have presented the possible treatment options to Sam: (a) do nothing, (b) use drug therapy to thin his blood, (c) perform angioplasty, or (d) perform by-pass surgery. Sam is a very fearful person and is in favor of the drug therapy.

What Sam fails to account for, however, is that he is at high risk right now. Although drug therapy is the safest treatment (vis-à-vis its side effects alone), it still leaves him with the greatest risk. You try to explain this to Sam: risk of treatment (the risk inherent in the treatment itself) plus resultant risk (one's risk of death after undergoing treatment) = total risk. In a simplified model, you tell Sam that the risk of treatment for the four alternatives ranks as follows (based on an ascending risk scale of 1–10):

A. No therapy: = 0 / resultant risk = 9.5 / total risk = 9.5
B. Drug therapy: = 0.5 / resultant risk = 8 / total risk = 8.5

C. Angioplasty: $= 1.5$ / resultant risk $= 6$ / total risk $= 7.5$

D. By-pass surgery: $= 5$ / resultant risk $= 1$ / total risk $= 6.0$

Although Sam is not a risk taker, he is making a choice that is really riskier for him. This seems to you to be an irrational choice.

What should you do? Should you try to bully Sam into options C or D? Should you enlist others to help convince Sam that C or D is best? Should you enlist family members to help Sam make the decision? Or should you let Sam make his own decision? After all, it is his life. Write an essay justifying your decision.

Micro Case 6. You are an emergency room physician at an inner city hospital. Mrs. Lopez, a poor first-generation immigrant from Central America, comes to see you since she has no regular doctor. She has a bronchial infection that can be treated with antibiotics. In the course of your examination of Mrs. Lopez, you discover a lump on her right breast. This lump concerns you and you suggest some tests. Through the hospital's interpreter, you inform her of your plan.

Mrs. Lopez does not want tests. She just wants to get her medicine and leave, but you fear that her breast lump may be malignant and that only by prompt treatment can you save her life. Mrs. Lopez does not like talking about her breasts with strangers, and her husband would never allow anyone to cut her in that area of her body.

You feel certain that the reasons that Mrs. Lopez wants to leave and forgo any tests are that she does not fully appreciate the danger she is in and she comes from a cultural tradition in which the husband's likes or dislikes (concerning the appearance of his wife's breasts) are decisive.

Cite at least three alternatives for action. Then show why one of these alternatives is the best. Use a major ethical theory and linking principle to justify your action.

Note

1   For more on macro and micro cases, see the overview on p. 58ff.

Issues of Life and Death

General Overview: It is certainly no surprise that life and death are a daily part of the practice of medicine. In the United States, each individual state has exact instructions for testing whether or not a patient who has been admitted to the hospital is dead. In the old days, things were simpler. When a patient's heart stopped pumping, he or she was dead. This origin of life (in the Western tradition) goes back to Aristotle. However, this test became obsolete when medicine's ability to keep a heart beating artificially extends well past the failure of other organs—especially the brain. Though respirators can keep a body functioning, it is the functioning brain that is thought to be the essential element in determining whether someone is alive.

This does not mean that there is not some controversy. For example, the case of Terri Schiavo sparked a prolonged legal debate as her body was kept functioning for the seven years from 1998 to 2005 although she was shown to be in a persistent vegetative state, having suffered massive irreversible brain damage. Because patients in this state often display autonomic musculature responses, some non-medical family members mistake these for conscious actions. Nowhere is the gap between professional and layperson greater than in cases such as these.

In this chapter we will examine two perennially controversial issues surrounding life and death: euthanasia and abortion.

A. Euthanasia

Overview: *Euthanasia* means "good death" in classical Greek. It also has come to mean mercy killing, which involves taking an *action* that will end a life that is afflicted with a terminal disease and that is characterized by intense suffering. *Passive euthanasia* entails stopping the life-support system or other artificial life-sustaining support of a patient who is terminally ill. The patient or their family may seek this solution. Some due

Medical Ethics, Second Edition. Edited by Michael Boylan.
© 2014 John Wiley & Sons, Inc. Published 2014 by John Wiley & Sons, Inc.

process is generally required before the request can be granted. Although the doctor may be the agent who brings about the patient's death by discontinuing treatment, it is not considered active euthanasia because nothing is administered to *cause* the death—that would be the role of the illness or accident that brought the patient to the hospital in the first place. Among some philosophers there is a debate on whether there is a legitimate distinction between active and passive euthanasia.

An associated concept is assisted suicide, in which a physician or another person provides the means necessary for a patient to end his or her own life. The late Dr Jack Kevorkian created an apparatus that could be set up and then manipulated by the patient to effect his own death. Assisted suicide is a form of euthanasia because the patient requesting to die is not in the calm, dispassionate state necessary for free rational choice but likely is in pain, needing help. In such circumstances, it is not unusual for the patient to plead for death. When providing the patient the means to grant this wish, is the doctor or other person acting differently than if they themselves actually administered the death-causing substance to the patient?

Opinions concerning euthanasia and assisted suicide are strongly held. Some believe that they are the most compassionate responses to a person who will die anyway and is suffering greatly. Nonetheless, active euthanasia is illegal in most of the world. It is considered murder. Among the industrialized nations of the world, Holland has the most liberal laws relating to euthanasia. In 1985 the Royal Dutch Medical Association formed guidelines for a national Commission on Euthanasia. Under these guidelines, if a patient acts voluntarily, makes a well-considered request that is reviewed by the physician's colleagues, has a durable death wish, and suffers to an unacceptable degree, the physician will not be prosecuted for engaging in active euthanasia or assisted suicide.

Other issues involved in this debate are withholding or withdrawing nutrition to newborns with severe congenital abnormalities or a very low birthweight (and thus judged to be *premature*). This example brings the question of what constitutes euthanasia to a specific level. If active euthanasia were to be made legal, these are the sorts of questions that would arise.

One way that bioethicists think about problems such as this is by returning to the model of persistent vegetative state. As we saw in the case of Terri Schiavo, such individuals are thought to be already dead in the sense of brain death. But when we think about abnormal newborns is the situation analogous or different? If it were analogous, it means that newborns have neither a developed sense of self nor a rich sense of consciousness that modern definitions of life require. So, if the newborn baby has a severe physical defect or disease that will mean certain death in months or a few years (at most), then should the parents and physicians be able to make the life and death choice *for the child*? The opposing argument would say that the cases are very different. The persistent vegetative state person has no consciousness or sense of self because of disease or accident and *will never recover*. This is not the case with newborns. Their brain is just fine, but has not developed yet. Who is to say whether a life that lasts only 6 months to a few years is not worth living? The choice of one's moral theory (set out in Chapter 1) might steer you to one of the options.

In the first essay Daniel Callahan argues for a distinction between killing and letting die. He bases this argument upon two key premises: (a) the metaphysical premise that thinking that a person's own actions in removal of life support are the sole cause of another's death is arrogant; and (b) the moral premise that distinguishes between causing death and being morally responsible for that death. In passive euthanasia, Callahan asserts, one causes death without being ethically responsible for it.

In the second essay, Pieter V. Admiraal argues that human suffering is the greatest of evils. Therefore, when a patient is suffering without hope of recovery and meets various other criteria, then the physician may perform euthanasia. Dr Admiraal has performed euthanasia himself and thinks that the so-called distinction between active and passive euthanasia is specious.

Leon Kass forms his argument based upon an examination of the Hippocratic Oath and its injunction against administering a poison. If the Hippocratic Oath defines medical professionalism, and if the physician wishes to be a professional, then she or he should not administer a poison (i.e., perform active euthanasia or assisted suicide). However, Kass does allow for engaging in passive euthanasia along the lines outlined by Callahan.

B. Abortion

Overview: Another controversial question concerns abortion. In the United States, since the Supreme Court decision *Roe v. Wade* (1973),[1] abortion has been legal. However, unlike many High Court decisions, this one is continually revisited by dissenters. The decision declared unconstitutional a Texas law that restricted legal abortions in cases affecting the life of the mother. This decision had the effect of legalizing abortion. The ruling established three guidelines affecting abortion legislation: (a) until the end of the first trimester, the decision to have an abortion is completely up to the woman; (b) after the first trimester, the state may regulate abortion health; and (c) when the fetus is viable (in the third trimester), the state may regulate or prohibit abortion except when the mother's life is at stake.

Emotion on this issue runs so high that some extremist dissenters have resorted to violence—including murder, as in the case of Dr George Tiller who was killed while attending a church service.

The section on abortion presents two very influential essays in the history of this debate and an article of mine that seeks some sort of middle ground. In the first essay, John Noonan reviews various criteria concerning the recognition of biological personhood. For Noonan (and many foes of abortion), the definition of when an organism becomes human is crucial to the abortion debate (since to kill an innocent human at will is generally thought to be a definition of murder). He looks for biological events that might be taken as significant in the creation and development of a fetus. He chooses a model that describes chances of survival. Before conception, the potential fetus (as viewed from the probability of conception) is less than 1 in 200 million. After conception, the odds drastically change to 4 in 5. Noonan takes the change in probability to indicate a change in the biological status of the fetus that is so significant that he believes confers personhood.

Judith Jarvis Thomson accepts the premise that the fetus may be a person (for the purpose of discussion). Her argument is that the killing of an innocent is sometimes permissible. In other words, it is not tantamount to murder (killing in self-defense is an example of this). She suggests that there is no absolute right to life for any innocent. This is especially true in pregnancy, when the fetus depends on the pregnant woman's body for its well-being. If a person has absolute control over her body and is not obliged to put her life or well-being at risk, then the woman who allows a pregnancy to develop makes a choice that is entirely a moral permission—not an obligation. She may or may not allow the pregnancy to develop since her body will be used in the process.

Thomson argues that those who go beyond their moral duties to help others are called good Samaritans. Being a good Samaritan may be the decent thing to do, but it is not obligatory. In the same way, bringing a pregnancy to term (especially one that began voluntarily) may be the decent thing to do, but it is not obligatory.

My own essay proposes a middle ground by recognizing the truth and falsehood of both positions. I believe that by using the methodology of the Personal Worldview Imperative, we can enter into the worldviews of both sides and understand what compels them to hold their various positions. From there the anti-abortion foes are shown to be wrong because the status of the fetus and even the post-birth infant does not confer dialectically necessary rights. I create proportional respect owed to the fetus beginning at the end of the first trimester. I then integrate this position with the Aristotelian sense of potentiality that also relates to the moment of conception until the end of the first trimester. The sense of respect due to the embryo at this basic level is proportionally diminished but not absent entirely. I also show the omni-pro-abortion position to be wrong because it does not differentiate levels of threat that motivate a pregnant woman to seek an abortion. Not all levels are equal. It is important to differentiate these levels and compare them to the levels of respect due to the embryo and to identify when in pregnancy to act.

The model of the Personal Worldview Imperative seeks to create a new context through which advocates of both sides can justify their positions and gain an understanding of the opposing side. This is not a position of relativism, but it does open the door for dialogue.

Note

1   *Roe v. Wade* 410 US 113, 93 S, Ct. 705, 1/22/73.

A. Euthanasia

Killing and Allowing to Die

Daniel Callahan

… No valid distinction, many now argue, can be made between killing and allowing to die, or between an act of commission and one of omission. The standard distinction

"Killing and Allowing to Die," by Daniel Callahan, was originally published in the *Hastings Center Report* 1989; 19 (Special Suppl.): 5–6. Reprinted by permission. © The Hastings Center.

being challenged rests on the commonplace observation that lives can come to an end as the result of: (a) the direct action of another who becomes the cause of death (as in shooting a person), and (b) the result of impersonal forces where no human agent has acted (death by lightning, or by disease). The purpose of the distinction has been to separate those deaths caused by human action, and those caused by nonhuman events. It is, as a distinction, meant to say something about human beings and their relationship to the world. It is a way of articulating the difference between those actions for which human beings can be held rightly responsible, or blamed, and those of which they are innocent. At issue is the difference between physical causality, the realm of impersonal events, and moral culpability, the realm of human responsibility.

The challenges encompass two points. The first is that people can become equally dead by our omissions as well as our commissions. We can refrain from saving them when it is possible to do so, and they will be just as dead as if we shot them. It is our decision itself that is the reason for their death, not necessarily how we effectuate that decision. That fact establishes the basis of the second point: if we *intend* their death, it can be brought about as well by omitted acts as by those we commit. The crucial moral point is not how they die, but our intention about their death. We can, then, be responsible for the death of another by intending that they die and accomplish that end by standing aside and allowing them to die.

Despite these criticisms—resting upon ambiguities that can readily be acknowledged—the distinction between killing and allowing to die remains, I contend, perfectly valid. It not only has a logical validity but, no less importantly, a social validity whose place must be central in moral judgments. As a way of putting the distinction into perspective, I want to suggest that it is best understood as expressing three different, though overlapping, perspectives on nature and human action. I will call them the metaphysical, the moral, and the medical perspectives.

Metaphysical

The first and most fundamental premise of the distinction between killing and allowing to die is that there is a sharp difference between the self and the external world. Unlike the childish fantasy that the world is nothing more than a projection of the self, or the neurotic person's fear that he or she is responsible for everything that goes wrong, the distinction is meant to uphold a simple notion: there is a world external to the self that has its own, and independent, causal dynamism. The mistake behind a conflation of killing and allowing to die is to assume that the self has become master of everything within and outside of the self. It is as if the conceit that modern man might ultimately control nature has been internalized: that, if the self might be able to influence nature by its actions, then the self and nature must be one.

Of course that is a fantasy. The fact that we can intervene in nature, and cure or control many diseases, does not erase the difference between the self and the external world. It is as "out there" as ever, even if more under our sway. That sway, however great, is always limited. We can cure disease, but not always the chronic illness that comes with the cure. We can forestall death with modern medicine, but death always wins in the long run because of the innate limitations of the body, inherently and stubbornly beyond final human control. And we can distinguish between a diseased body and an aging body, but in the end if we wait long enough they always become one and the same body. To attempt to deny the distinction between killing and allowing to die is, then, mistakenly to impute more power to human action than it actually has and to accept the conceit that nature has now fallen wholly within the realm of human control. Not so.

Moral

At the center of the distinction between killing and allowing to die is the difference between physical causality and moral culpability. To bring the life of another to an end by an injection kills the other directly; our action is the physical cause of the death. To allow someone to die from a disease we cannot cure (and that we did not cause) is to permit the disease to act as the cause of death. The notion of physical causality in both cases rests on the difference between human agency and the action of external nature. The ambiguity arises precisely because we can be morally culpable for killing someone (if we have no moral right to do so, as we would in self-defense) and no less culpable for allowing someone to die (if we have both the possibility and the obligation of keeping that person alive). Thus there are cases where, morally speaking, it makes no difference whether we killed or allowed to die; we are equally responsible. In those instances, the lines of physical causality and moral culpability happen to cross. Yet the fact that they can cross in some cases in no way shows that they are always, or even usually, one and the same. We can normally find the difference in all but the most obscure cases. We should not, then, use the ambiguity of such cases to do away altogether with the distinction between killing and allowing to die. The ambiguity may obscure, but does not erase, the line between the two.

There is one group of ambiguous cases that is especially troublesome. Even if we grant the ordinary validity between killing and allowing to die, what about those cases that combine (a) an illness that renders a patient unable to carry out an ordinary biological function (to breathe or eat on his own, for example), and (b) our turning off a respirator or removing an artificial feeding tube? On the level of physical causality, have we killed the patient or allowed him to die? In one sense, it is our action that shortens his life, and yet in another sense his underlying disease brings his life to an end. I believe it reasonable to say that, since his life was being sustained by artificial means (respirator or feeding tube) made necessary because of the fact that he had an incapacitating disease, his disease is the ultimate reality behind his death. But for its reality, there would be no need for artificial sustenance in the first place and no moral issue at all. To lose sight of the paramount reality of the disease is to lose sight of the difference between our selves and the outer world.

I quickly add, and underscore, a moral point: the person who, without good moral reason, turns off a respirator or pulls a feeding tube, can be morally culpable; that the patient has been allowed to die of his underlying condition does not morally excuse him. The moral question is whether we are obliged to continue treating a life that is being artificially sustained. To cease treatment may or may not be morally acceptable; but it should be understood, in either case, that the physical cause of death was the underlying disease.

Medical

An important social purpose of the distinction between killing and allowing to die has been that of protecting the historical role of the physician as one who tries to cure or comfort patients rather than to kill patients. Physicians have been given special knowledge about the body, knowledge that can be used to kill or to cure. They are also given great privileges in making use of that knowledge. It is thus all the more important that physicians' social role and power be, and be seen to be, a limited power. It may be used only to cure or comfort, never to kill. They have not been given, nor should they be given, the power to use their knowledge and skills to bring life to an end. It would open the way for powerful misuse and, no less importantly, represent an intrinsic violation of what it has meant to be a physician.

Yet if it is possible for physicians to misuse their knowledge and power to kill people directly, are they thereby required to use that same knowledge always to keep people alive, always to resist a disease that can itself kill the patient? The traditional answer has been: not necessarily. For the physician's ultimate obligation is to the welfare of the patient, and excessive treatment can be as detrimental to that welfare as inadequate treatment. Put another way, the obligation to resist the lethal power of disease is limited—it ceases when the patient is unwilling to have it resisted, or where the resistance no longer serves the patient's welfare. Behind this moral premise is the recognition that disease (of some kind) ultimately triumphs and that death is both inevitable sooner or later and not, in any case, always the greatest human evil. To demand of the physician that he always struggle against disease, as if it was in his power always to conquer it, would be to fall into the same metaphysical trap mentioned above: that of assuming that no distinction can be drawn between natural and human agency.

A final word. I suggested [in an earlier discussion] that the most potent motive for active euthanasia and assisted suicide stems from a dread of the power of medicine. That power then seems to take on a drive of its own regardless of the welfare or wishes of patients. No one can easily say no—not physicians, not patients, not families. My guess is that happens because too many have already come to believe that it is their choice, and their choice alone, which brings about death; and they do not want to exercise that kind of authority. The solution is not to erase the distinction between killing and allowing to die, but to underscore its validity and importance. We can bring disease as a cause of death back into the care of the dying.

Euthanasia in The Netherlands
Justifiable Euthanasia

Pieter V. Admiraal

In recent years I have spoken on numerous occasions about various aspects of euthanasia practice in general hospitals. I always limit myself to that group of patients who are in the terminal phase of an incurable, usually malignant disease, and I have always placed emphasis upon the desirability of good terminal supportive care by a team of doctors, nurses, and pastors. At the same time I have repeatedly pointed out that the practice of euthanasia occurs only as a last resort and that the majority of patients die without recourse to euthanasia.

I shall limit myself to just two aspects of euthanasia. First, I wish to discuss what causes a patient to make a request for euthanasia to the doctor who is treating him; and secondly, to address the question of what we are to understand by "passive euthanasia".

What Makes a Patient Request Euthanasia

A patient in the terminal phase will only request euthanasia if he considers his suffering to be unbearable and chooses to die rather than to live under these circumstances. I assume that the request is the result of a lengthy decision process by a patient who is fully conscious of the consequences of his request to himself, to his relatives, and to the doctor to whom he directs his request. At the same time I assume that all persons involved are agreed that the suffering of the patient cannot be relieved in any way and that the performance of euthanasia is only and exclusively in the interest of the patient. Euthanasia then becomes the ultimate act of care for the dying.

What brings the patient to the point of requesting euthanasia from his doctor? Which factors cause the suffering of the patient to become unbearable? Objective considerations lead us to distinguish physical and psychological causes which are closely related to each other.

Physical causes of requests for euthanasia

Loss of strength
Especially in cachectic patients, a serious loss of strength occurs as a result of greatly increased protein breakdown and poor peripheral circulation. As a result, the patient

"Euthanasia in The Netherlands: Justifiable Euthanasia," by Pieter V. Admiraal, is reprinted by permission of the publisher, *Issues in Law and Medicine* 1988; 3(4, Spring). Copyright © 1988 by the National Legal Center for the Medically Dependent & Disabled, Inc. pp. 361–70.

in a terminal phase no longer is capable of any physical exertion. The patient then becomes totally dependent on nursing care both day and night.

Fatigue
The loss of strength practically always is accompanied by extreme fatigue even without any physical effort at all. This fatigue cannot be influenced in any way at all and is experienced as exhausting by the patient.

Pain
Until recently pain was the most important cause of physical and psychological suffering. Nowadays, in most cases, pain can be adequately controlled without the normal psychological functions of the patient being adversely affected.

As examples of pain treatment one can mention pharmacotherapy with the administering of analgesics and psychopharmaceuticals, the continuous epidural application of morphine-like analgesics, and the fixed blocking of the sensitive nerve-paths of the sympathetic nervous system.

Unfortunately, the above methods of controlling pain are not yet known or applicable everywhere. Pain can then become unbearable. In a small number of instances pain cannot be subjected to acceptable control even with the most advanced techniques. One may be compelled to administer morphine and/or psychopharmaceuticals intravenously on a continuous basis in such high doses that it has serious harmful effects on the psychic functioning of the patient.

Shortness of breath
An increasing shortness of breath and belabored breathing often occurs in the terminal phase. Some of the causes can be:

- Specific lung aberrations such as inflammations of tumors, which increasingly diminish lung capacity, resulting in the development of dyspnea. But also the growth of small tumors in the lungs, for example in the trachea or in the bronchi, can result in a serious stridor.
- Growth of tumors in the mouth cavity can cause a serious obstruction to breathing and even result in suffocation.
- A large quantity of liquid in the lungs as a result of insufficient coughing up due to loss of strength or in consequence of a cardial decompensation.
- A diminished tissue oxygenation will by reflex action lead to faster breathing which can be experienced as shortness of breath by the patient.

Sleeplessness
Although sleeplessness may occur as a complaint all by itself, it is especially patients who suffer fatigue, shortness of breath, and pain who sleep badly, and this can result in exhaustion. When pain is the cause, one will have to administer an analgesic late in the evening or increase the dosage.

Persistent sleeplessness in patients without pain often necessitates the administering of barbiturates as a result of which the patient may be dull and drowsy during the daytime. Just as in the case of healthy people, waking periods appear to be longer at night than they actually are. Conversely, after a short period of sleep the patient can get the false impression that he has slept a long time, and that can be very disappointing and make the waking period seem even longer.

Nausea and vomiting

Nausea can be a side effect of analgesics or of cytotoxics. The administering of anti-emetics is then indicated, but the effect is often disappointing. In the case of a total blockage of the stomach intestine, vomiting will be continuous, sometimes even when there is continuous suctioning by means of a stomach siphon. Vomiting is exhausting and disorients the patient.

Flow of saliva

When there is a total blockage of the esophagus or the throat cavity, the saliva produced must be spit out constantly and that is psychically burdensome.

Thirst

Thirst occurs when there is a disturbance of the electrolyte content of the blood and with dehydration. Especially when the patient is being treated at home it can be difficult to administer sufficient liquids by means of an infusion or a stomach siphon. The routine (almost ritual) moistening of the lips does not then offer relief.

Incontinence

There are several causes which can lead to the patient being incontinent with respect to urine or to feces for a shorter or longer period during an illness. Incontinence requires constant intensive nursing care and is experienced by the patient as humanly degrading.

Decubitis

Bedsores will easily develop in patients as a result of bad blood circulation in the skin, and definitely so in the case of cachectic patients who can no longer move themselves because of the loss of strength and the increase of fatigue. If the patient in addition is incontinent, then bedsores can scarcely be averted in intensive nursing. Through tissue deterioration and secondary infections the bedsores are often accompanied by a very penetrating, unpleasant odor.

Miscellany

Some miscellaneous causes are:

- Constipation, especially with the administering of morphine-like analgesics.
- Perspiration
- Hunger
- Itching, especially with jaundice
- Coughing
- Ascites [Dropsy of the abdomen]

- Cystitis with an [implanted] catheter
- Fungi infections of the mouth cavity
- Hiccupping with [organic] processes in the upper abdomen

Side effects of therapeutic treatments
Finally, our therapeutic actions can cause the patient minor or serious side effects for a shorter or longer period of time. Thus, there is the general malaise after major surgical operations or extended X-ray therapy. Repeated cytotoxic treatments cause not only a general feeling of malaise but usually also the loss of body hair which is experienced as something extremely unpleasant, especially by women. As pointed out earlier, patients suffer from nausea for a long time when analgesics and cytotoxics are administered, while painful muscle indurations can occur with the extended administering of intramuscular injections.

The above summation is not intended to suggest the order of frequency in which these problems occur. Fatigue, shortness of breath, nausea, pain, incontinence, and decubitis are in general the biggest problems. But an isolated symptom, like an itch or hiccups can also in the long run be experienced as unbearable by a patient.

Psychological causes of requests for euthanasia

The most important psychic causes are as follows:

Somatic deviations
This includes psychic suffering as a result of the above described somatic problems. All of the somatic deviations mentioned above can become a serious psychic burden to the patient.

Many of the above deviations last during an extended period of the illness, and almost all of them get increasingly worse, often to the very time of death, which in the long run leads to the psychical exhaustion of the patient, despite all nursing and spiritual care. It is especially incontinence, decubitis, and the loss of all strength which the patient in the end experiences as humanly degrading. Under these circumstances many patients consider this last phase as an affront to human dignity, as suffering without any use or purpose, as undeserved and as the disintegration of their humanness.

Anxieties
Practically every patient is plagued by anxiety during the course of his illness. From the very beginning, from the moment that an unfavorable diagnosis has been made and death is inevitable, many patients develop a fear of pain and grievous suffering. This anxiety is based on hearsay or on one's own experience, and even today is seemingly confirmed by the texts of some obituary announcements. [For example: after long and painful suffering, patiently endured, the Lord called home to his eternal rest, our dearly beloved....] But information provided by lay-persons is often not very encouraging. Whereas, many doctors betray their task as physicians by providing poor information or by falling short in the doctor-patient relationship. Regrettably, many doctors still talk and publish about "the pain of cancer" as something that is worse than any other pain.

Much more difficult to combat or to refute is the anxiety about spiritual and physical decay and deformation. After all, we cannot guard the patient against these. The only help we can give here is the promise to alleviate suffering when possible or if necessary to end it. The same thing holds for the anxiety about needing total nursing care and becoming totally dependent. Loneliness and isolation are also anxious threats and indeed many patients are lonely in long nights of waking, alone with their thoughts and fearful expectations. Isolated nursing in the end phase, however much needed from a nursing perspective, encourages this loneliness at home or in the hospital. Only the experience of a warm shared humanity can afford relief in this situation.

Anxiety about dying itself can have various causes. In dying there comes, of course, the inevitable parting from this life, the world in which one has lived and worked, and from beloved relatives. But there can also be anxiety about the moment of dying, the anxiety that then "something" will happen that is unpleasant and threatening without your having any definite idea of what that might be. It is certain that the theatrical portrayal of dying on the stage, or on the screen, usually is far removed from reality. The death scene in an opera is a flagrant example of this.

Anxiety about what comes after death is culturally and religiously determined and can vary from a vague anxiety about the unknown to a literal deathly fear of punishment, which may or may not be eternal. Fortunately, many persons also die in the firm conviction of another, blessed life, united with those who went before. There are also more and more people who, in consequence of the present Western cultural pattern, no longer believe in a hereafter and consequently do not have any anxiety about the hereafter. Fears about dying can be discussed with both the spiritual counselor and the doctor.

As a result of intoxications from one's own body or from various pharmaceuticals, anxious hallucinations or confusions can occur. It requires competent medical and professional knowledge to prevent or to combat these anxieties.

Grief

However much we all realize that death is inevitable and unbreakably linked to life, the certainty of the approaching end of our lives makes us sorrowful. Grief can be about the loss of family and friends or about the loss of earthly things, the possession of which has now become so useless.

Grief will become worse in the measure that less expression can be given to it. Especially in the beginning of the illness process, when the diagnosis is just received, it often happens that the patient, his family and his friends, conceal their grief from each other; and sometimes, out of fear to show their own grief, they are not open to the grief of the other. Grief is then crowded out and bottled up. Grief then becomes sorrow and it would be better to listen to each other's grief and to give each other the opportunity to cry out one's feelings. Mutual understanding is after all the basis of the saying: "Company in distress, makes sorrow less." Grief becomes unbearable when it is not recognized, and the patient is left alone with it, and not understood [by others].

Grief becomes bitter when the patient poses the question of why this happens to him who does not deserve it, and not to another who does seem to deserve it; also when he asks why this should happen to him now, at this point in his life. We see this especially in young people who see their future cut off and by older persons who, after a life of hard work, anticipated enjoying a well earned rest, or who finally wanted to get at fulfilling their long cherished and long postponed ideals.

Such a grief can easily turn into rancor, revolt, and aggression. There can also be grief about the grief of those left behind or about the uncertain, perhaps even precarious future which confronts those left behind. Cares, for example, about less income when the provider dies, or cares about the further nurturing of children when the mother dies young. Such grief depresses the patient and can easily turn into a serious depression.

Some strict believers can experience their grief as wrong in the sight of God who "proposes and disposes," and they may feel guilty about the fact that they do not accept and cheerfully bear their grief.

Rancor, resistance, aggression, and denial but also acceptance
and acquiesence play an important role in the terminal phase
They were clearly described for the first time by Kubler-Ross and it is to her great merit that she prepared the way for meaningful terminal care of the dying. Without in any way minimizing her work, I must point out that her observations are for the most part based on observations of American patients with a different life style and a different cultural pattern from that of the European. The above physical and psychological problems can become unbearable suffering for the patient and create the occasion for a request for euthanasia.

Suffering is specific for each human being: an animal does not suffer in the sense that we mean here. An animal feels pain, a human being suffers pain. Only that person can suffer who is capable of deliberate comparative retrospective and prospective contemplation in which one compares, weighs, and evaluates. Suffering therefore includes grief, depression, concern, and anxiety. But fortunately, there is also hope, acquiescence, and acceptance. These too are specifically human.

The suffering of a human being is strictly individual and is determined by the psychological tension and inner resources of that person in enduring dire distress. The suffering of the other is largely withdrawn from our objective observation and consequently it is difficult to weigh and to judge.

It is therefore just as wrong to admiringly attribute to one heroism or martyrdom and to reproach the other for a cowardly attitude toward life. We must seriously ask ourselves where some among us derive the right to judge the suffering of another to be bearable when that person tells us that his suffering is unbearable.

In my honest opinion, it is the inalienable right of each person to make the judgment that his individual suffering is no longer bearable and to request euthanasia from the doctor who is treating him. But then that doctor may not and cannot refrain from making a judgment about the suffering of the person who requests euthanasia. After all, a request for euthanasia, by itself, does not legalize its application. The doctor must then attempt, on the basis of observable facts and on the basis of feeling his way into the situation of the patient, apart from his own emotions, arrive at a judgment which is as honest as possible. He shall have to try to realize in his own mind why the patient under these circumstances prefers death to life. Above all he will have to ask himself whether the circumstances can be improved. His judgment will become more mature and more balanced as his experience in providing terminal care to the dying increases.

He must always remain aware that he continues to bear the final responsibility for his decision. It is therefore desirable and necessary that the doctor seek the counsel and assistance of others so that he may in this way constantly test his opinion against that of others.

It is my opinion that every doctor has the right and the duty after prolonged and thorough deliberation to carry out euthanasia; at the request of the other person and in his interest, knowing that he is responsible to himself, to the other, and to the law. Similarly, every doctor has the unassailable right under any circumstances to refuse to carry out euthanasia, knowing that he is responsible to himself and to the other.

The carrying out of euthanasia can only be based on the acknowledgment of unbearable suffering. Here I wish consciously to pass over the Christian view that suffering purifies or, in a broader sense, that suffering is part of life and therefore must be accepted. Many do not subscribe to these views and I think it absolutely wrong to impose such a value judgment on another person or to make him dependent on it. A doctor can refuse to carry out euthanasia on those grounds, provided he does not block the way for a doctor who is prepared to act on the request of the patient.

It would be wrong to give the impression that the request of a patient who is terminally ill with cancer must always and only be based on the above examples of unbearable suffering. Thus, a patient who has arrived at the point of acceptance and acquiescence may no longer attach any value to his life, his relatives, or to his environs. We then speak of a total detachment, one that is especially difficult for relatives to understand and accept. Such a patient only longs for the end. We see this with some frequency in patients of advanced age who have lost all their relatives and friends. As indicated earlier, the desire for reunion can play a role in believing patients.

Carrying Out "Passive Euthanasia"

In the Netherlands the political discussion about the legalization of euthanasia is to a large extent controlled by the confessional parties which find themselves confronted with a dilemma: on the one hand the practice of euthanasia is considered acceptable by a large majority of the population, including the confessional part, but on the other hand, the Roman Catholic Church and some Protestant churches forbid the practice of active euthanasia.

In order to get out of this impasse, the term "passive euthanasia" has been introduced in recent years. In general, it is defined as "the discontinuance of life sustaining means or treatment as a result of which the patient dies after a shorter or longer period." This can be clarified by means of two examples:

1. Stopping existing [life support] medications such as antibiotics, cytotoxins, anti-arrythmia's [heart regulating medications], medications for increasing blood pressure, diuretics, cortico-steroids, or insulin.
2. Stopping existing nonmedication treatments such as kidney dialysis, blood transfusions, intravenous or tube feeding, reanimation, physiotherapy, or antidecubitis treatment.

Under passive euthanasia one could also place the carefully considered decision not to begin one of the above treatments or an agreement not to reanimate when breathing is arrested or the heart stops beating.

In passive euthanasia there is therefore a conscious decision by the doctor either to discontinue an existing treatment or not to initiate a possible treatment. Only fifty years ago the problems were not so great. The number of possible treatments was small and just about all were exclusively symptomatic so that the treating physician, already in an early stage of the illness, was compelled and justified in saying to the patient that he, as a doctor, could do no more.

Today it is quite different. Our therapeutic arsenal is very extensive, every year new medicines and methods are discovered so that the number of patients to whom the doctor must say, "I can do nothing more for you," is becoming smaller and smaller.

As we have discussed earlier, a number of these therapies cause so many unpleasant side effects that the continuance of the treatment becomes unacceptable to the patient and he asks his doctor to discontinue the treatment. Obviously in reaching this decision, other factors, for example, the hopeless prospect of symptomatic treatment without any chance of a definite cure, also plays an important role. Whereas in the past, it was a matter of necessity that the doctor himself had to discontinue a treatment, it now will be difficult for many doctors to discontinue a treatment at the patient's request. Indeed, there has been a case where the patient had to sign a declaration demanding the discontinuance of further treatment.

One thing is clear: if the doctor discontinues treatment and does no more the patient will die from the direct consequences of his disease. Using the example cited above, death will be the result of a serious sepsis, cardiac arrest, diabetic or uremic coma, anemia, malnutrition, breathing insufficiency, etc. This means that with passive euthanasia most patients will die only after a long pathway of suffering.

Under these circumstances the word euthanasia is completely mistaken and misleading. This is not at all the "gentle death" which is desired by the patient. The word "passive" here refers altogether to the attitude of the doctor.

Passive euthanasia is nothing but abstention. And abstention, doing nothing, is surely the very last thing a patient making a request [for euthanasia] is entitled to.

Of course, after abstention [nontreatment] it is possible to make dying easier in various ways. But if this occurs with analgesics and psychopharmaceuticals in high doses, then I see no difference at all with active euthanasia. The concept "passive euthanasia" then becomes a cover for the active euthanasia which is not allowed.

Even more dangerous, in my judgment, is the standpoint taken by some church people in the Netherlands who say that there is no euthanasia when a patient dies sooner than normal as a result of high doses of morphine-like analgesics. That opens the door to abuses!

First of all, the number of patients whose pain is untreatable is getting smaller and smaller; and secondly, to carry out euthanasia with morphine in patients who have been treated with morphine for a considerable period of time already, just will not work, because of the swiftly developing tolerance to the breath depressant effect. What must be prevented is that under the guise of controlling pain the lives of patients can be terminated in a wrong and uncontrolled manner without even calling this euthanasia.

In summary, I wish to posit that passive euthanasia is a hypocritical euphemism and not in the interest of the patient who is in a terminal phase.

Why Doctors Must Not Kill

Leon R. Kass

Do you want your doctor licensed to kill? Should he or she be permitted or encouraged to inject or prescribe poison? Shall the mantle of privacy that protects the doctor-patient relationship, in the service of life and wholeness, now also cloak decisions for death? Do you want *your* doctor deciding, on the basis of his own private views, when you still deserve to live and when you now deserve to die? And what about the other fellow's doctor—that shallow technician, that insensitive boor who neither asks nor listens, that unprincipled money-grubber, that doctor you used to go to until you got up the nerve to switch: do you want *him* licensed to kill? Speaking generally, shall the healing profession become also the euthanizing profession?

Common sense has always answered, "No." For more than two millennia, the reigning medical ethic, mindful that the power to cure is also the power to kill, has held as an inviolable rule, "Doctors must not kill." Yet this venerable taboo is now under attack. Proponents of euthanasia and physician-assisted suicide would have us believe that it is but an irrational vestige of religious prejudice, alien to a true ethic of medicine, which stands in the way of a rational and humane approach to suffering at the end of life. Nothing could be further from the truth. The taboo against doctors killing patients (even on request) is the very embodiment of reason and wisdom. Without it, medicine will have trouble doing its proper work; without it, medicine will have lost its claim to be an ethical and trustworthy profession; without it, all of us will suffer—yes, more than we now suffer because some of us are not soon enough released from life.

Consider first the damaging consequences for the doctor-patient relationship. The patient's trust in the doctor's wholehearted devotion to the patient's best interests will be hard to sustain once doctors are licensed to kill. Imagine the scene: you are old, poor, in failing health, and alone in the world; you are brought to the city hospital with fractured ribs and pneumonia. The nurse or intern enters late at night with a syringe full of yellow stuff for your intravenous drip. How soundly will you sleep? It will not matter that your doctor has never yet put anyone to death; that he is legally entitled to do so will make a world of difference.

And it will make a world of psychic difference too for conscientious physicians. How easily will they be able to care wholeheartedly for patients when it is always possible to think of killing them as a "therapeutic option"? Shall it be penicillin and a respirator one more time, or, perhaps, this time just an overdose of morphine? Physicians get tired of treating patients who are hard to cure, who resist their best efforts, who are on their way down—"gorks," "gomers," and "vegetables" are only

"Why Doctors Must Not Kill," by Leon Kass, was originally published in *Commonweal*, Aug. 9, 1991. Reprinted with permission of the Commonweal Foundation. For subscriptions, call 1-999-495-6755.

some of the less than affectionate names they receive from the house officers. Won't it be tempting to think that death is the best "treatment" for the little old lady "dumped" again on the emergency room by the nearby nursing home?

It is naive and foolish to take comfort from the fact that the currently proposed change in the law provides "aid-in-dying" only to those who request it. For we know from long experience how difficult it is to discover what we truly want when we are suffering. Verbal "requests" made under duress rarely reveal the whole story. Often a demand for euthanasia is, in fact, an angry or anxious plea for help, born of fear of rejection or abandonment, or made in ignorance of available alternatives that could alleviate pain and suffering. Everyone knows how easy it is for those who control the information to engineer requests and to manipulate choices, especially in the vulnerable. Paint vividly a horrible prognosis, and contrast it with that "gentle, quick release": which will the depressed or frightened patient choose, especially in the face of a spiraling hospital bill or children who visit grudgingly? Yale Kamisar asks the right questions: "Is this the kind of choice, assuming that it can be made in a fixed and rational manner, that we want to offer a gravely ill person? Will we not sweep up, in the process, some who are not really tired of life, but think others are tired of them; some who do not really want to die, but who feel that they should not live on, because to do so when there looms the legal alternative of euthanasia is to do a selfish or cowardly act? Will not some feel an obligation to have themselves 'eliminated' in order that funds allocated for their terminal care might be better used by their families or, financial worries aside, in order to relieve their families of the emotional strain involved?"

Euthanasia, once legalized, will not remain confined to those who freely and knowingly elect it—and the most energetic backers of euthanasia do not really want it thus restricted. Why? Because the vast majority of candidates who merit mercy-killing cannot request it for themselves: adults with persistent vegetative state or severe depression or senility or aphasia or mental illness or Alzheimer's disease; infants who are deformed; and children who are retarded or dying. All incapable of requesting death. They will thus be denied our new humane "assistance-in-dying." But not to worry. The lawyers and the doctors (and the cost-containers) will soon rectify this injustice. The enactment of a law legalizing mercy killing (or assisted suicide) on voluntary request will certainly be challenged in the courts under the equal-protection clause of the Fourteenth Amendment. Why, it will be argued, should the comatose or the demented be denied the right to such a "dignified death" or such a "treatment" just because they cannot claim it for themselves? With the aid of court-appointed proxy consenters, we will quickly erase the distinction between the right to choose one's own death and the right to request someone else's—as we have already done in the termination-of-treatment cases.

Clever doctors and relatives will not need to wait for such changes in the law. Who will be around to notice when the elderly, poor, crippled, weak, powerless, retarded, uneducated, demented, or gullible are mercifully released from the lives their doctors, nurses, and next of kin deem no longer worth living? In Holland, for example, a recent survey of 300 physicians (conducted by an author who supports euthanasia) disclosed that over 40 percent had performed euthanasia *without the patient's request*, and over 10 percent had done so in more than five cases. Is there any reason to believe that the average American physician is, in his private heart, more committed than his Dutch counterpart to the equal worth and dignity of every life under his care? Do we really want to find out what he is like, once the taboo is broken?

Even the most humane and conscientious physician psychologically needs protection against himself and his weaknesses, if he is to care fully for those who entrust themselves to him. A physician-friend who worked many years in a hospice caring for dying patients explained it to me most convincingly: "Only because I knew that I could not and would not kill my patients was I able to enter most fully and intimately into caring for them as they lay dying." The psychological burden of the license to kill (not to speak of the brutalization of the physician-killers) could very well be an intolerably high price to pay for the physician-assisted euthanasia.

The point, however, is not merely psychological: it is also moral and essential. My friend's horror at the thought that he might be tempted to kill his patients, were he not enjoined from doing so, embodies a deep understanding of the medical ethic and its intrinsic limits. We move from assessing consequences to looking at medicine itself.

The beginning of ethics regarding the use of power generally lies in nay-saying. The wise setting of limits on the use of power is based on discerning the excesses to which the power, unrestrained, is prone. Applied to the professions, this principle would establish strict outer boundaries—indeed, inviolable taboos—against those "occupational hazards" to which each profession is especially prone. *Within* these outer limits, no fixed rules of conduct apply; instead, prudence—the wise judgment of the man-on-the-spot—finds and adopts the best course of action in the light of the circumstances. But the outer limits themselves are fixed, firm, and non-negotiable.

What are those limits for medicine? At least three are set forth in the venerable Hippocratic Oath: no breach of confidentiality; no sexual relations with patients; no dispensing of deadly drugs. These unqualified, self-imposed restrictions are readily understood in terms of the temptations to which the physician is most vulnerable, temptations in each case regarding an area of vulnerability and exposure that the practice of medicine requires of patients. Patients necessarily divulge and reveal private and intimate details of their personal lives; patients necessarily expose their naked bodies to the physician's objectifying gaze and investigating hands; patients necessarily expose and entrust the care of their very lives to the physician's skill, technique, and judgment. The exposure is, in all cases, one-sided and asymmetric: the doctor does not reveal his intimacies, display his nakedness, offer up his embodied life to the patient. Mindful of the meaning of such nonmutual exposure, the physician voluntarily sets limits on his own conduct, pledging not to take advantage of or to violate the patient's intimacies, naked sexuality, or life itself.

The prohibition against killing patients, the first negative promise of self-restraint sworn to in the Hippocratic Oath, stands as medicine's first and most abiding taboo: "I will neither give a deadly drug to anybody if asked for it, nor will I make a suggestion to this effect. … In purity and holiness I will guard my life and my art." In forswearing the giving of poison, the physician recognizes and restrains a god-like power he wields over patients, mindful that his drugs can both cure and kill. But in forswearing the giving of poison, *when asked for it*, the Hippocratic physician rejects the view that the patient's choice for death can make killing him—or assisting his suicide—right. For the physician, at least, human life in living bodies commands respect and reverence—*by its very nature*. As its respectability does not depend upon human agreement or patient consent, revocation of one's consent to live does not deprive one's living body of respectability. The deepest ethical principle restraining the physician's power is not the autonomy or freedom of the patient; neither is it his own compassion or good intention. Rather, it is the dignity and mysterious power of human life itself, and, therefore, also what the oath calls the purity and holiness of the life and art to which he has sworn devotion. A person can choose to be a physician, but he cannot simply choose what physicianship means.

The central meaning of physicianship derives not from medicine's powers but from its goal, not from its means but from its end: to benefit the sick by the activity of healing. The physician as physician serves only the sick. He does not serve the relatives or the hospital or the national debt inflated due to Medicare costs. Thus he will never sacrifice the well-being of the sick to the convenience or pocketbook or feelings of the relatives or society. Moreover, the physician serves the sick not because they have rights or wants or claims, but because they are sick. The healer works with and for those who need to be healed, in order to help make them whole. Despite enormous changes in medical technique and institutional practice, despite enormous changes in nosology and therapeutics, the center of medicine has not changed: it is as true today as it was in the days of Hippocrates that the ill desire to be whole; that wholeness means a certain well-working of the enlivened body and its unimpaired powers to sense, think, feel, desire, move, and maintain itself; and that the relationship between the healer and the ill is constituted, essentially even if only tacitly, around the desire of both to promote the wholeness of the one who is ailing.

Can wholeness and healing ever be compatible with intentionally killing the patient? Can one benefit the patient as a whole by making him dead? There is, of course, a logical difficulty: how can any good exist for a being that is not? But the error is more than logical: to intend and to act for someone's good requires his continued existence to receive the benefit.

To be sure, certain attempts to benefit may in fact turn out, unintentionally, to be lethal. Giving adequate morphine to control pain might induce respiratory depression leading to death. But the intent to relieve the pain of the living presupposes that the living still live to be relieved. This must be the starting point in discussing all medical benefits: no benefit without a beneficiary.

Against this view, someone will surely bring forth the hard cases: patients so ill-served by their bodies that they can no longer bear to live, bodies riddled with cancer and racked with pain, against which their "owners" protest in horror and from which they insist on being released. Cannot the person "in the body" speak up against the rest, and request death for "personal" reasons?

However sympathetically we listen to such requests, we must see them as incoherent. Such person-body dualism cannot be sustained. "Personhood" is manifest on earth only in living bodies; our highest mental functions are held up by, and are inseparable from, lowly metabolism, respiration, circulation, excretion. There may be blood without consciousness, but there is never consciousness without blood. Thus one who calls for death in the service of personhood is like a tree seeking to cut its roots for the sake of growing its highest fruit. No physician, devoted to the benefit of the sick, can serve the patient as person by denying and thwarting his personal embodiment.

To say it plainly, to bring nothingness is incompatible with serving wholeness: one cannot heal—or comfort—by making nil. The healer cannot annihilate if he is truly to heal. The physician-euthanizer is a deadly self-contradiction.

But we must acknowledge a difficulty. The central goal of medicine—health—is, in each case, a perishable good: inevitably, patients get irreversibly sick, patients degenerate, patients die. Healing the sick is *in principle* a project that must at some point fail. And here is where all the trouble begins: How does one deal with "medical failure"? What does one seek when restoration of wholeness—or "much" wholeness—is by and large out of the question?

Contrary to the propaganda of the euthanasia movement, there is, in fact, much that can be done. Indeed, by recognizing finitude yet knowing that we will not kill, we are empowered to focus on easing and enhancing the *lives* of those who are dying. First of all, medicine can follow the lead of the hospice movement and—abandoning decades of shameful mismanagement—provide truly adequate (and now technically feasible) relief of pain and discomfort. Second, physicians (and patients and families) can continue to learn how to with-hold or withdraw those technical interventions that are, in truth, merely burdensome or degrading medical additions to the unhappy end of a life—including, frequently, hospitalization itself. Ceasing treatment and allowing death to occur when (and if) it will seem to be quite compatible with the respect life itself commands for itself. Doctors may and must allow to die, even if they must not intentionally kill.

Ceasing medical intervention, allowing nature to take its course, differs fundamentally from mercy killing. For one thing, death does not necessarily follow the discontinuance of treatment; Karen Ann Quinlan lived more than ten years after the court allowed the "life-sustaining" respirator to be removed. Not the physician, but the underlying fatal illness becomes the true cause of death. More important morally, in ceasing treatment the physician need not *intend* the death of the patient, even when the death follows as a result of his omission. His intention should be to avoid useless and degrading medical *additions* to the already sad end of a life. In contrast, in active, direct mercy killing the physician must, necessarily and indubitably, intend *primarily* that the patient be made dead. And he must knowingly and indubitably cast himself in the role of the agent of death. This remains true even if he is merely an assistant in suicide. A physician who provides the pills or lets the patient plunge the syringe after he leaves the room is *morally* no different from one who does the deed himself. "I will neither give a deadly drug to anybody if asked for it, nor will I make a suggestion to this effect."

Once we refuse the technical fix, physicians and the rest of us can also rise to the occasion: we can learn to act humanly in the presence of finitude. Far more than adequate morphine and the removal of burdensome machinery, the dying need our presence and our encouragement. Dying people are all too easily reduced ahead of time to "thinghood" by those who cannot bear to deal with the suffering or disability of those they love. Withdrawal of contact, affection, and care is the greatest single cause of the dehumanization of dying. Not the alleged humaneness of an elixir of death, but the humanness of connected living-while-dying is what medicine—and the rest of us—most owe the dying. The treatment of choice is company and care.

The euthanasia movement would have us believe that the physician's refusal to assist in suicide or perform euthanasia constitutes an affront to human dignity. Yet one of their favorite arguments seems to me rather to prove the reverse. Why, it is argued, do we put animals out of their misery but insist on compelling fellow human beings to suffer to the bitter end? Why, if it is not a contradiction for the veterinarian, does the medical ethic absolutely rule out mercy killing? Is this not simply inhumane?

Perhaps *inhumane*, but not thereby *inhuman*. On the contrary it is precisely because animals are not human that we must treat them (merely) humanely. We put dumb animals to sleep because they do not know that they are dying, because they can make nothing of their misery or mortality, and, therefore, because they cannot live deliberately—i.e., humanly—in the face of their own suffering and dying. They cannot live out a fitting end. Compassion for their weakness and dumbness is our only appropriate emotion, and given our responsibility for their care and well-being, we do the only humane thing we can. But when a conscious human being asks us for death, by that very action he displays the presence of something that precludes our regarding him as a dumb animal. Humanity is owed humanity, not humaneness. Humanity is owed the bolstering of the human, even/or especially in its dying moments, in resistance to the temptation to ignore its presence in the sight of suffering.

B. Abortion

An Almost Absolute Value in History

JOHN T. NOONAN JR.

The most fundamental question involved in the long history of thought on abortion is: How do you determine the humanity of a being? To phrase the question that way is to put in comprehensive humanistic terms what the theologians either dealt with as an explicitly theological question under the heading of "ensoulment" or dealt with implicitly in their treatment of abortion. The Christian position as it originated did not depend on a narrow theological or philosophical concept. It had no relation to theories of infant baptism.[1] It appealed to no special theory of instantaneous ensoulment.

"An Almost Absolute Value in History" is from John T. Noonan (ed.), *The Morality of Abortion: Legal and Historical Perspectives*. Cambridge, MA: Harvard University Press; pp. 267–272. Copyright © 1970 by the President and Fellows of Harvard College. Reprinted by permission of the publisher.

It took the world's view on ensoulment as that view changed from Aristotle to Zacchia. There was, indeed, theological influence affecting the theory of ensoulment finally adopted, and, of course, ensoulment itself was a theological concept, so that the position was always explained in theological terms. But the theological notion of ensoulment could easily be translated into humanistic language by substituting "human" for "rational soul"; the problem of knowing when a man is a man is common to theology and humanism.

If one steps outside the specific categories used by the theologians, the answer they gave can be analyzed as a refusal to discriminate among human beings on the basis of their varying potentialities. Once conceived, the being was recognized as man because he had man's potential. The criterion for humanity, thus, was simple and all-embracing: if you are conceived by human parents, you are human.

The strength of this position may be tested by a review of some of the other distinctions offered in the contemporary controversy over legalizing abortion. Perhaps the most popular distinction is in terms of viability. Before an age of so many months, the fetus is not viable, that is, it cannot be removed from the mother's womb and live apart from her. To that extent, the life of the fetus is absolutely dependent on the life of the mother. This dependence is made the basis of denying recognition to its humanity.

There are difficulties with this distinction. One is that the perfection of artificial incubation may make the fetus viable at any time: it may be removed and artificially sustained. Experiments with animals already show that such a procedure is possible. This hypothetical extreme case relates to an actual difficulty: there is considerable elasticity to the idea of viability. Mere length of life is not an exact measure. The viability of the fetus depends on the extent of its anatomical and functional development. The weight and length of the fetus are better guides to the state of its development than age, but weight and length vary. Moreover, different racial groups have different ages at which their fetuses are viable. Some evidence, for example, suggests that Negro fetuses mature more quickly than white fetuses. If viability is the norm, the standard would vary with race and with many individual circumstances.

The most important objection to this approach is that dependence is not ended by viability. The fetus is still absolutely dependent on someone's care in order to continue existence; indeed a child of one or three or even five years of age is absolutely dependent on another's care for existence; uncared for, the older fetus or the younger child will die as surely as the early fetus detached from the mother. The unsubstantial lessening in dependence at viability does not seem to signify any special acquisition of humanity.

A second distinction has been attempted in terms of experience. A being who has had experience, has lived and suffered, who possesses memories, is more human than one who has not. Humanity depends on formation by experience. The fetus is thus "unformed" in the most basic human sense.

This distinction is not serviceable for the embryo which is already experiencing and reacting. The embryo is responsive to touch after eight weeks and at least at that point is experiencing. At an earlier stage the zygote is certainly alive and responding to its environment. The distinction may also be challenged by the rare case where aphasia has erased adult memory: has it erased humanity? More fundamentally, this distinction leaves even the older fetus or the younger child to be treated as an unformed inhuman thing. Finally, it is not clear why experience as such confers humanity. It could be argued that certain central experiences such as loving or learning are necessary to make a man human. But then human beings who have failed to love or to learn might be excluded from the class called man.

A third distinction is made by appeal to the sentiments of adults. If a fetus dies, the grief of the parents is not the grief they would have for a living child. The fetus is an unnamed "it" till birth, and is not perceived as personality until at least the fourth month of existence when movements in the womb manifest a vigorous presence demanding joyful recognition by the parents.

Yet feeling is notoriously an unsure guide to the humanity of others. Many groups of humans have had difficulty in feeling that persons of another tongue, color, religion, sex, are as human as they. Apart from reactions to alien groups, we mourn the loss of a ten-year-old boy more than the loss of his one-day-old brother or his 90-year-old grandfather. The difference felt and the grief expressed vary with the potentialities extinguished, or the experience wiped out; they do not seem to point to any substantial difference in the humanity of baby, boy, or grandfather.

Distinctions are also made in terms of sensation by the parents. The embryo is felt within the womb only after about the fourth month. The embryo is seen only at birth. What can be neither seen nor felt is different from what is tangible. If the fetus cannot be seen or touched at all, it cannot be perceived as man.

Yet experience shows that sight is even more untrustworthy than feeling in determining humanity. By sight, color became an appropriate index for saying who was a man, and the evil of racial discrimination was given foundation. Nor can touch provide the test; a being confined by sickness, "out of touch" with others, does not thereby seem to lose his humanity. To the extent that touch still has appeal as a criterion, it appears to be a survival of the old English idea of "quickening"—a possible mistranslation of the Latin *animatus* used in the canon law. To that extent touch as a criterion seems to be dependent on the Aristotelian notion of ensoulment, and to fall when this notion is discarded.

Finally, a distinction is sought in social visibility. The fetus is not socially perceived as human. It cannot communicate with others. Thus, both subjectively and objectively, it is not a member of society. As moral rules are rules for the behavior of members of society to each other, they cannot be made for behavior toward what is not yet a member. Excluded from the society of men, the fetus is excluded from the humanity of men.[2]

By force of the argument from the consequences, this distinction is to be rejected. It is more subtle than that founded on an appeal to physical sensation, but it is equally dangerous in its implications. If humanity depends on social recognition, individuals or whole groups may be dehumanized by being denied any status in their society. Such a fate is fictionally portrayed in 1984 and has actually been the lot of many men in many societies. In the Roman empire, for example, condemnation to slavery meant the practical denial of most human rights; in the Chinese Communist world, landlords have been classified as enemies of the people and so treated as nonpersons by the state. Humanity does not depend on social recognition, though often the failure of society to recognize the prisoner, the alien, the heterodox as human has led to the destruction of human beings. Anyone conceived by a man and a woman is human. Recognition of this condition by society follows a real event in the objective order, however imperfect and halting the recognition. Any attempt to limit humanity to exclude some group runs the risk of furnishing authority and precedent for excluding other groups in the name of the consciousness or perception of the controlling group in the society.

A philosopher may reject the appeal to the humanity of the fetus because he views "humanity" as a secular view of the soul and because he doubts the existence of anything real and objective which can be identified as humanity. One answer to such a philosopher is to ask how he reasons about moral questions without supposing that there is a sense in which he and the others of whom he speaks are human. Whatever group is taken as the society which determines who may be killed is thereby taken as human. A second answer is to ask if he does not believe that there is a right and wrong way of deciding moral questions. If there is such a difference, experience may be appealed to: to decide who is human on the basis of the sentiment of a given society has led to consequences which rational men would characterize as monstrous.

The rejection of the attempted distinctions based on viability and visibility, experience and feeling, may be buttressed by the following considerations: Moral judgments often rest on distinctions, but if the distinctions are not to appear arbitrary *fiat*, they should relate to some real difference in probabilities. There is a kind of continuity in all life, but the earlier stages of the elements of human life possess tiny probabilities of development. Consider for example, the spermatozoa in any normal ejaculate: There are about 200,000,000 in any single ejaculate, of which one has a chance of developing into a zygote. Consider the oocytes which may become ova: there are 100,000 to 1,000,000 oocytes in a female infant, of which a maximum of 390 are ovulated. But once spermatozoon and ovum meet and the conceptus is formed, such studies as have been made show that roughly in only 20 percent of the cases will spontaneous abortion occur. In other words, the chances are about 4 out of 5 that this new being will develop. At this stage in the life of the being there is a sharp shift in probabilities, an immense jump in potentialities. To make a distinction between the rights of spermatozoa and the rights of the fertilized ovum is to respond to an enormous shift in possibilities. For about twenty days after conception the egg may split to form twins or combine with another egg to form a chimera, but the probability of either event happening is very small.

It may be asked, What does a change in biological probabilities have to do with establishing humanity? The argument from probabilities is not aimed at establishing humanity but at establishing an objective discontinuity which may be taken into account in moral discourse. As life itself is a matter of probabilities, as most moral reasoning is an estimate of probabilities, so it seems in accord with the structure of reality and the nature of moral thought to found a moral judgment on the change in probabilities at conception. The appeal to probabilities is the most commonsensical of arguments, to a greater or smaller degree all of us base our actions on probabilities, and in morals, as in law, prudence and negligence are often measured by the account one has taken of the probabilities. If the chance is 200,000,000 to 1 that the movement in the bushes into which you shoot is a man's, I doubt if many persons would hold you careless in shooting; but if the chances are 4 out of 5 that the movement is a human being's, few would acquit you of blame. Would the argument be different if only one out of ten children conceived came to term? Of course this argument would be different. This argument is an appeal to probabilities that actually exist, not to any and all state of affairs which may be imagined.

The probabilities as they do exist do not show the humanity of the embryo in the sense of a demonstration in logic any more than the probabilities of the movement in the bush being a man demonstrate beyond all doubt that the being is a man. The appeal is a "buttressing" consideration, showing the plausibility of the standard adopted. The argument focuses on the decisional factor in any moral judgment and assumes that part of the business of a moralist is drawing lines. One evidence of the nonarbitrary character of the line drawn is the difference of probabilities on either side of it. If a spermatozoon is destroyed, one destroys a being which had a chance of far less than 1 in 200 million of developing into a reasoning being, possessed of the genetic code, a heart and other organs, and capable of pain. If a fetus is destroyed, one destroys a being already possessed of the genetic code, organs, and sensitivity to pain, and one which had an 80 percent chance of developing further into a baby outside the womb who, in time, would reason.

The positive argument for conception as the decisive moment of humanization is that at conception the new being receives the genetic code. It is this genetic information which determines his characteristics, which is the biological carrier of the possibility of human wisdom, which makes him a self-evolving being. A being with a human genetic code is man.

This review of current controversy over the humanity of the fetus emphasizes what a fundamental question the theologians resolved in asserting the inviolability of the fetus. To regard the fetus as possessed of equal rights with other humans was not, however, to decide every case where abortion might be employed. It did decide the case where the argument was that the fetus should be aborted for its own good. To say a being was human was to say it had a destiny to decide for itself which could not be taken from it by another man's decision. But human beings with equal rights often come in conflict with each other, and some decision must be made as whose claims are to prevail. Cases of conflict involving the fetus are different only in two respects: the total inability of the fetus to speak for itself and the fact that the right of the fetus regularly at stake is the right to life itself.

The approach taken by the theologians to these conflicts was articulated in terms of "direct" and "indirect." Again, to look at what they were doing from outside their categories, they may be said to have been drawing lines or "balancing values." "Direct" and "indirect" are spatial metaphors; "line-drawing" is another. "To weigh" or "to balance" values is a metaphor of a more complicated mathematical sort hinting at the process which goes on in moral judgments. All the metaphors suggest that, in the moral judgments made, comparisons were necessary, that no value completely controlled. The principle of double effect was no doctrine fallen from heaven, but a method of analysis appropriate where two relative values were being compared. In Catholic moral theology, as it developed, life even of the innocent was not taken as an absolute. Judgments of acts affecting life issued from a process of weighing. In the weighing, the fetus was always given a value greater than zero, always a value separate and independent from its parents. This valuation was crucial and fundamental in all Christian thought on the subject and marked it off from any approach which considered that only the parents' interests needed to be considered.

Even with the fetus weighed as human, one interest could be weighed as equal or superior: that of the mother in her own life. The casuists between 1450 and 1895 were willing to weigh this interest as superior. Since 1895, that interest was given decisive weight only in the two special cases of the cancerous uterus and the ectopic pregnancy. In both of these cases the fetus itself had little chance of survival even if the abortion were not performed. As the balance was once struck in favor of the mother whenever her life was endangered, it could be so struck again. The balance reached between 1895 and 1930 attempted prudentially and pastorally to forestall a multitude of exceptions for interests less than life.

The perception of the humanity of the fetus and the weighing of fetal rights against other human rights constituted the work of the moral analysts. But what spirit animated their abstract judgments? For the Christian community it was the injunction of Scripture to love your neighbor as yourself. The fetus as human was a neighbor; his life had parity with one's own. The commandment gave life to what otherwise would have been only rational calculation.

The commandment could be put in humanistic as well as theological terms: Do not injure your fellow man without reason. In these terms, once the humanity of the fetus is perceived, abortion is never right except in self-defense. When life must be taken to save life, reason alone cannot say that a mother must prefer a child's life to her own. With this exception, now of great rarity, abortion violates the rational humanist tenet of the equality of human lives.

For Christians the commandment to love had received a special imprint in that the exemplar proposed of love was the love of the Lord for his disciples. In the light given by this example, self-sacrifice carried to the point of death seemed in the extreme situations not without meaning. In the less extreme cases, preference for one's own interests to the life of another seemed to express cruelty or selfishness irreconcilable with the demands of love.

Notes

1 According to Granville Williams (*The Sanctity of Human Life*, p. 193), "The historical reason for the Catholic objection to abortion is the same as for the Christian Church's historical opposition to infanticide: the horror of bringing about the death of an unbaptized child." This statement is made without any citation of evidence. [As previously argued], desire to administer baptism could, in the Middle Ages, even be urged as a reason for procuring an abortion. It is highly regrettable that the American Law Institute was apparently misled by Williams' account and repeated after him the same baseless statement. See American Law Institute, *Model Penal Code: Tentative Draft No. 9* (1959), p. 148, n. 12.

2 Thomas Aquinas gave an analogous reason against baptizing a fetus in the womb: "As long as it exists in the womb of the mother, it cannot be subject to the operation of the ministers of the Church as it is not known to men" (*In sententias Petri Lombardi* 4.6 1.1.2).

A Defense of Abortion[1]

Judith Jarvis Thomson

Most opposition to abortion relies on the premise that the fetus is a human being, a person, from the moment of conception. The premise is argued for, but, as I think, not well. Take, for example, the most common argument. We are asked to notice that the development of a human being from conception through birth into childhood is continuous; then it is said that to draw a line, to choose a point in this development and say "before this point the thing is not a person, after this point it is a person" is to make an arbitrary choice, a choice for which in the nature of things no good reason can be given. It is concluded that the fetus is, or anyway that we had better say it is, a person from the moment of conception. But this conclusion does not follow. Similar things might be said about the development of an acorn into an oak tree, and it does not follow that acorns are oak trees, or that we had better say they are. Arguments of this form are sometimes called "slippery slope arguments"—the phrase is perhaps self-explanatory—and it is dismaying that opponents of abortion rely on them so heavily and uncritically.

I am inclined to agree, however, that the prospects for "drawing a line" in the development of the fetus look dim. I am inclined to think also that we shall probably have to agree that the fetus has already become a human person well before birth. Indeed, it comes as a surprise when one first learns how early in its life it begins to acquire human characteristics. By the tenth week, for example, it already has a face, arms and legs, fingers and toes; it has internal organs, and brain activity is detectable.[2] On the other hand, I think that the premise is false, that the fetus is not a person from the moment of conception. A newly fertilized ovum, a newly implanted clump of cells, is no more a person than an acorn is an oak tree. But I shall not discuss any of this. For it seems to me to be of great interest to ask what happens if, for the sake of argument, we allow the premise. How, precisely, are we supposed to get from there to the conclusion that abortion is morally impermissible? Opponents of abortion commonly spend most of their time establishing that the fetus is a person, and hardly any time explaining the step from there to the impermissibility of abortion. Perhaps they think the step too simple and obvious to require much comment. Or perhaps instead they are simply being economical in argument. Many of those who defend abortion rely on the premise that the fetus is not a person, but only a bit of tissue that will become a person at birth; and why pay out more arguments than you have to? Whatever the explanation, I suggest that the step they take is neither easy nor obvious, that it calls for closer examination than it is commonly given, and that when we do give it this closer examination we shall feel inclined to reject it.

I propose, then, that we grant that the fetus is a person from the moment of conception. How does the argument go from here? Something like this, I take it. Every person has a right to life. So the fetus has a right to life. No doubt the mother has a right to decide what shall happen in and to her body; everyone would grant that. But surely a person's right to life is stronger and more stringent than the mother's right to decide what happens in and to her body, and so outweighs it. So the fetus may not be killed; an abortion may not be performed.

It sounds plausible. But now let me ask you to imagine this. You wake up in the morning and find yourself back to back in bed with an unconscious violinist. A famous unconscious violinist. He has been found to have a fatal kidney ailment, and the Society of Music Lovers has canvassed all the available medical records and found that you alone have the right blood type to help. They have therefore kidnapped you, and last night the violinist's circulatory system was plugged into yours, so that your kidneys can be used to extract poisons from his blood as well as your own. The director of the hospital now tells you, "Look, we're sorry the Society of Music Lovers did this to you—we would never have permitted it if we had known. But still, they did it, and the violinist now is plugged into you. To unplug you would be to kill him. But never mind, it's only for nine months. By then he will have recovered from his ailment, and can safely be unplugged from you." Is it morally incumbent on you to accede to this situation? No doubt it would be very nice of you if you did, a great kindness. But do you *have* to accede to it? What if it were not nine months, but nine years? Or longer still? What if the director of the hospital says, "Tough luck, I agree, but you've now got to stay in bed, with the violinist plugged into you, for the rest of your life. Because remember this. All persons have a right to life, and violinists are persons. Granted you have a right to decide what happens in and to your body, but a person's right to life outweighs your right to decide what happens in and to your body. So you cannot ever be unplugged from him." I imagine you would regard this as outrageous, which suggests that something really is wrong with that plausible-sounding argument I mentioned a moment ago.

In this case, of course, you were kidnapped; you didn't volunteer for the operation that plugged the violinist into your kidneys. Can those who oppose abortion on the ground I mentioned make an exception for a pregnancy due to rape? Certainly. They can say that persons have a right to life only if they didn't come into existence because of rape; or they can say that all persons have a right to life, but that some have less of a right to life than others, in particular, that those who came into existence because of rape have less. But these statements have a rather unpleasant sound. Surely the question of whether you have a right to life at all, or how much of it you have, shouldn't turn on the question of whether or not you are a product of a rape. And in fact the people who oppose abortion on the ground I mentioned do not make this distinction, and hence do not make an exception in case of rape.

Nor do they make an exception for a case in which the mother has to spend the nine months of her pregnancy in bed. They would agree that would be a great pity, and hard on the mother; but all the same, all persons have a right to life, the fetus is a person, and so on. I suspect, in fact, that they would not make an exception for a case in which, miraculously enough, the pregnancy went on for nine years, or even the rest of the mother's life.

Some won't even make an exception for a case in which continuation of the pregnancy is likely to shorten the mother's life; they regard abortion as impermissible even to save the mother's life. Such cases are nowadays very rare, and many opponents of abortion do not accept this extreme view. All the same, it is a good place to begin: a number of points of interest come out in respect to it.

1

Let us call the view that abortion is impermissible even to save the mother's life "the extreme view." I want to suggest first that it does not issue from the argument I mentioned earlier without the addition of some fairly powerful premises. Suppose a woman has become pregnant, and now learns that she has a cardiac condition such that she will die if she carries the baby to term. What may be done for her? The fetus, being a person, has a right to life, but as the mother is a person too, so has she a right to life. Presumably they have an equal right to life. How is it supposed to come out that an abortion may not be performed? If mother and child have an equal right to life, shouldn't we perhaps flip a coin? Or should we add to the mother's right to life her right to decide what happens in and to her body, which everybody seems to be ready to grant—the sum of her rights now outweighing the fetus's right to life?

The most familiar argument here is the following. We are told that performing the abortion would be directly killing[3] the child, whereas doing nothing would not be killing the mother, but only letting her die. Moreover, in killing the child, one would be killing an innocent person, for the child has committed no crime, and is not aiming at his mother's death. And then there are a variety of ways in which this might be continued. (1) But as directly killing an innocent person is always and absolutely impermissible, an abortion may not be performed. Or, (2) as directly killing an innocent person is murder, and murder is always and absolutely impermissible, an abortion may not be performed.[4] Or, (3) as one's duty to refrain from directly killing an innocent person is more stringent than one's duty to keep a person from dying, an abortion may not be performed. Or, (4) if one's only options are directly killing an innocent person or letting a person die, one must prefer letting the person die, and thus an abortion may not be performed.[5]

Some people seem to have thought that these are not further premises which must be added if the conclusion is to be reached, but that they follow from the very fact that an innocent person has a right to life.[6] But this seems to me to be a mistake, and perhaps the simplest way to show this is to bring out that while we must certainly grant that innocent persons have a right to life, the theses in (1) through (4) are all false. Take (2), for example. If directly killing an innocent person is murder, and thus is impermissible, then the mother's directly killing the innocent person inside her is murder, and thus is impermissible. But it cannot seriously be thought to be murder if the mother performs an abortion on herself to save her life. It cannot seriously be said that she *must* refrain, that she *must* sit passively by and wait for her death. Let us look again at the case of you and the violinist. There you are, in bed with the violinist, and the director of the hospital says to you, "It's all most distressing, and I deeply sympathize, but you see this is putting an additional strain on your kidneys, and you'll be dead within the month. But you *have* to stay where you are all the same. Because unplugging you would be directly killing an innocent violinist, and that's murder, and that's impermissible." If anything in the world is true, it is that you do not commit murder, you do not do what is impermissible, if you reach around to your back and unplug yourself from that violinist to save your life.

The main focus of attention in writings on abortion has been on what a third party may or may not do in answer to a request from a woman for an abortion. This is in a way understandable. Things being as they are, there isn't much a woman can safely do to abort herself. So the question asked is what a third party may do, and what the mother may do, if it is mentioned at all, is deduced, almost as an afterthought, from what it is concluded that third parties may do. But it seems to me that to treat the matter in this way is to refuse to grant to the mother that very status of person which is so firmly insisted on for the fetus. For we cannot simply read off what a person may do from what a third party may do. Suppose you find yourself trapped in a tiny house with a growing child. I mean a very tiny house, and a rapidly growing child—you are already up against the wall of the house and in a few minutes you'll be crushed to death. The child on the other hand won't be crushed to death; if nothing is done to stop him from growing he'll be hurt, but in the end he'll simply burst open the house and walk out a free man. Now I could well understand it if a bystander were to say, "There's nothing we can do for you. We cannot choose between your life and his, we cannot be the ones to decide who is to live, we cannot intervene." But it cannot be concluded that you too can do nothing, that you cannot attack it to save your life. However innocent the child may be, you do not have to wait passively while it crushes you to death. Perhaps a pregnant woman is vaguely felt to have the status of house, to which we don't allow the right of self-defense. But if the woman houses the child, it should be remembered that she is a person who houses it.

I should perhaps stop to say explicitly that I am not claiming that people have a right to do anything whatever to save their lives. I think, rather, that there are drastic limits to the right of self-defense. If someone threatens you with death unless you torture someone else to death, I think you have not the right, even to save your life, to do so. But the case under consideration here is very different. In our case there are only two people involved, one whose life is threatened, and one who threatens it. Both are innocent: the one who is threatened is not threatened because of any fault, the one who threatens does not threaten because of any fault. For this reason we may feel that we bystanders cannot intervene. But the person threatened can.

In sum, a woman surely can defend her life against the threat to it posed by the unborn child, even if doing so involves its death. And this shows not merely that the theses in (1) through (4) are false; it shows also that the extreme view of abortion is false, and so we need not canvass any other possible ways of arriving at it from the argument I mentioned at the outset.

2

The extreme view could of course be weakened to say that while abortion is permissible to save the mother's life, it may not be performed by a third party, but only by the mother herself. But this cannot be right either. For what we have to keep in mind is that the mother and the unborn child are not like two tenants in a small house which has, by an unfortunate mistake, been rented to both: the mother *owns* the house. The fact that she does adds to the offensiveness of deducing that the mother can do nothing from the supposition that third parties can do nothing. But it does more than this: it casts a bright light on the supposition that third parties can do nothing. Certainly it lets us see that a third party who says "I cannot choose between you" is fooling himself if he thinks this is impartiality. If Jones has found and fastened on a certain coat, which he needs to keep him from freezing, but which Smith also needs to keep him from freezing, then it is not impartiality that says "I cannot choose between you" when Smith owns the coat. Women have said again and again "This body is *my* body!" and they have reason to feel angry, reason to feel that it has been like shouting into the wind. Smith, after all, is hardly likely to bless us if we say to him, "Of course it's your coat, anybody would grant that it is. But no one may choose between you and Jones who is to have it."

We should really ask what it is that says "no one may choose" in the face of the fact that the body that houses the child is the mother's body. It may be simply a failure to appreciate this fact. But it may be something more interesting, namely the sense that one has a right to refuse to lay hands on people, even where it would be just and fair to do so, even where justice seems to require that somebody do so. Thus justice might call for somebody to get Smith's coat back from Jones, and yet you have a right to refuse to be the one to lay hands on Jones, a right to refuse to do physical violence to him. This, I think, must be granted. But then what should be said is not "no one may choose," but only "*I* cannot choose," and indeed not even this, but *I* will not *act*" leaving it open that somebody else can or should, and in particular that anyone in a position of authority, with the job of securing people's rights, both can and should. So this is no difficulty. I have not been arguing that any given third party must accede to the mother's request that he perform an abortion to save her life, but only that he may.

I suppose that in some views of human life the mother's body is only on loan to her, the loan not being one which gives her any prior claim to it. One who held this view might well think it impartiality to say "I cannot choose." But I shall simply ignore this possibility. My own view is that if a human being has any just, prior claim to anything at all, he has a just, prior claim to his own body. And perhaps this needn't be argued for here anyway, since, as I mentioned, the arguments against abortion we are looking at do grant that the woman has a right to decide what happens in and to her body.

But although they do grant it, I have tried to show that they do not take seriously what is done in granting it. I suggest the same thing will reappear even more clearly when we turn away from cases in which the mother's life is at stake, and attend, as I propose we now do, to the vastly more common cases in which a woman wants an abortion for some less weighty reason than preserving her own life.

3

Where the mother's life is not at stake, the argument I mentioned at the outset seems to have a much stronger pull. "Everyone has a right to life, so the unborn person has a right to life." And isn't the child's right to life weightier than anything other than the mother's own right to life, which she might put forward as ground for an abortion?

This argument treats the right to life as if it were unproblematic. It is not, and this seems to me to be precisely the source of the mistake.

For we should now, at long last, ask what it comes to, to have a right to life. In some views having a right to life includes having a right to be given at least the bare minimum one needs for continued life. But suppose that what in fact *is* the bare minimum a man needs for continued life is something he has no right at all to be given? If I am sick unto death, and the only thing that will save my life is the touch of Henry Fonda's cool hand on my fevered brow, then all the same, I have no right to be given the touch of Henry Fonda's cool hand on my fevered brow. It would be frightfully nice of him to fly in from the West Coast to provide it. It would be less nice, though no doubt well meant, if my friends flew out to the West Coast and carried Henry Fonda back with them. But I have no right at all against anybody that he should do this for me. Or again, to return to the story I told earlier, the fact that for continued life that violinist needs the continued use of your kidneys does not establish that he has a right to be given the continued use of your kidneys. He certainly has no right against you that *you* should give him continued use of your kidneys. For nobody has any right to use your kidneys unless you give him this right—if you do allow him to go on using your kidneys, this is a kindness on your part, and not something he can claim from you as his due. Nor has he any right against anybody else that *they* should give him continued use of your kidneys. Certainly he had no right against the Society of Music Lovers that they should plug him into you in the first place. And if you now start to unplug yourself, having learned that you will otherwise have to spend nine years in bed with him, there is nobody in the world who must try to prevent you, in order to see to it that he is given something he has a right to be given.

Some people are rather stricter about the right to life. In their view, it does not include the right to be given anything, but amounts to, and only to, the right not to be killed by anybody. But here a related difficulty arises. If everybody is to refrain from killing that violinist, then everybody must refrain from doing a great many different sorts of things. Everybody must refrain from slitting his throat, everybody must refrain from shooting him—and everybody must refrain from unplugging you from him. But does he have a right against everybody that they shall refrain from unplugging you from him? To refrain from doing this is to allow him to continue to use your kidneys. It could be argued that he has a right against us that *we* should allow him to continue to use your kidneys. That is, while he had no right against us that we should give him the use of your kidneys, it might be argued that he anyway has a right against us that we shall not now intervene and deprive him of the use of your kidneys. I shall come back to third-party interventions later. But certainly the violinist has no right against you that *you* shall allow him to continue to use your kidneys. As I said, if you do allow him to use them, it is a kindness on your part, and not something you owe him.

The difficulty I point to here is not peculiar to the right of life. It reappears in connection with all the other natural rights, and it is something which an adequate account of rights must deal with. For present purposes it is enough just to draw attention to it. But I would stress that I am not arguing that people do not have a right to life—quite to the contrary, it seems to me that the primary control we must place on the acceptability of an account of rights is that it should turn out in that account to be a truth that all persons have a right to life. I am arguing only that having a right to life does not guarantee having either a right to be given the use of or a right to be allowed continued use of another person's body—even if one needs it for life itself. So the right to life will not serve the opponents of abortion in the very simple and clear way in which they seem to have thought it would.

4

There is another way to bring out the difficulty. In the most ordinary sort of case, to deprive someone of what he has a right to is to treat him unjustly. Suppose a boy and his small brother are jointly given a box of chocolates for Christmas. If the older boy takes the box and refuses to give his brother any of the chocolates, he is unjust to him, for the brother has been given a right to half of them. But suppose that, having learned that otherwise it means nine years in bed with that violinist, you unplug yourself from him. You surely are not being unjust to him, for you gave him no right to use your kidneys, and no one else can have given him any such right. But we have to notice that in unplugging yourself, you are killing him; and violinists, like everybody else, have a right to life, and thus in the view we were considering just now, the right not to be killed. So here you do what he supposedly has a right you shall not do, but you do not act unjustly to him in doing it.

The emendation which may be made at this point is this: the right to life consists not in the right not to be killed, but rather in the right not to be killed unjustly. This runs a risk of circularity, but never mind: it would enable us to square the fact that the violinist has a right to life with the fact that you do not act unjustly toward him in unplugging yourself, thereby killing him. For if you do not kill him unjustly, you do not violate his right to life, and so it is no wonder you do him no injustice.

But if this emendation is accepted, the gap in the argument against abortion stares us plainly in the face: it is by no means enough to show that the fetus is a person, and to remind us that all persons have a right to life—we need to be shown also that killing the fetus violates its right to life, i.e., that abortion is unjust killing. And is it?

I suppose we may take it as a datum that in a case of pregnancy due to rape the mother has not given the unborn person a right to the use of her body for food and shelter. Indeed, in what pregnancy could it be supposed that the mother has given the unborn person such a right? It is not as if there were unborn persons drifting about the world, to whom a woman who wants a child says "I invite you in."

But it might be argued that there are other ways one can have acquired a right to the use of another person's body than by having been invited to use it by that person. Suppose a woman voluntarily indulges in intercourse, knowing of the chance it will issue in pregnancy, and then she does become pregnant; is she not in part responsible for the presence, in fact the very existence, of the unborn person inside? No doubt she did not invite it in. But doesn't her partial responsibility for its being there itself give it a right to the use of her body?[7] If so, then her aborting it would be more like the boys taking away the chocolates, and less like your unplugging yourself from the violinist—doing so would be depriving it of what it does have a right to, and thus would be doing it an injustice.

And then, too, it might be asked whether or not she can kill it even to save her own life: If she voluntarily called it into existence, how can she now kill it, even in self-defense?

The first thing to be said about this is that it is something new. Opponents of abortion have been so concerned to make out the independence of the fetus, in order to establish that it has a right to life, just as its mother does, that they have tended to overlook the possible support they might gain from making out that the fetus is *dependent* on the mother, in order to establish that she has a special kind of responsibility for it, a responsibility that gives it rights against her which are not possessed by any independent person—such as an ailing violinist who is a stranger to her.

On the other hand, this argument would give the unborn person a right to its mother's body only if her pregnancy resulted from a voluntary act, undertaken in full knowledge of the chance a pregnancy might result from it. It would leave out entirely the unborn person whose existence is due to rape. Pending the availability of some further argument, then, we would be left with the conclusion that unborn persons whose existence is due to rape have no right to the use of their mothers' bodies, and thus that aborting them is not depriving them of anything they have a right to and hence is not unjust killing.

And we should also notice that it is not at all plain that this argument really does go even as far as it purports to. For there are cases and cases, and the details make a difference. If the room is stuffy, and I therefore open a window to air it, and a burglar climbs in, it would be absurd to say, "Ah, now he can stay, she's given him a right to the use of her house—for she is partially responsible for his presence there, having voluntarily done what enabled him to get in, in full knowledge that there are such things as burglars, and that burglars burgle." It would be still more absurd to say this if I had had bars installed outside my windows, precisely to prevent burglars from getting in, and a burglar got in only because of a defect in the bars. It remains equally absurd if we imagine it is not a burglar who climbs in, but an innocent person who blunders or falls in. Again, suppose it were like this: people-seeds drift about in the air like pollen, and if you open your windows, one may drift in and take root in your carpets or upholstery. You don't want children, so you fix up your windows with fine mesh screens, the very best you can buy. As can happen, however, and on very, very rare occasions does happen, one of the screens is defective, and a seed drifts in and takes root. Does the person-plant who now develops have a right to the use of your house? Surely not—despite the fact that you voluntarily opened your windows, you knowingly kept carpets and upholstered furniture, and you knew that screens were sometimes defective. Someone may argue that you are responsible for its rooting, that it does have a right to your house, because after all you could have lived out your life with bare floors and furniture, or with sealed windows and doors. But this won't do—for by the same token anyone can avoid a pregnancy due to rape by having a hysterectomy, or anyway by never leaving home without a (reliable!) army.

It seems to me that the argument we are looking at can establish at most that there are *some* cases in which the unborn person has a right to the use of its mother's body, and therefore *some* cases in which abortion is unjust killing. There is room for much discussion and argument as to precisely which, if any. But I think we should sidestep this issue and leave it open, for at any rate the argument certainly does not establish that all abortion is unjust killing.

5

There is room for yet another argument here, however. We surely must all grant that there may be cases in which it would be morally indecent to detach a person from your body at the cost of his life. Suppose you learn that what the violinist needs is not nine years of your life, but only one hour: all you need do to save his life is to spend one hour in that bed with him. Suppose also that letting him use your kidneys for that one hour would not affect your health in the slightest. Admittedly you were kidnapped. Admittedly you did not give anyone permission to plug him into you. Nevertheless it seems plain to me you *ought* to allow him to use your kidneys for that hour—it would be indecent to refuse.

Again, suppose pregnancy lasted only an hour, and constituted no threat to life or health. And suppose that a woman becomes pregnant as a result of rape. Admittedly she did not voluntarily do anything to bring about the existence of a child. Admittedly she did nothing at all which would give the unborn person a right to the use of her body. All the same it might well be said, as in the newly amended violinist story, that she *ought* to allow it to remain for that hour—that it would be indecent of her to refuse.

Now some people are inclined to use the term "right" in such a way that it follows from the fact that you ought to allow a person to use your body for the hour he needs, that he has a right to use your body for the hour he needs, even though he has not been given that right by any person or act. They may say that it follows also that if you refuse, you act unjustly toward him. This use of the term is perhaps so common that it cannot be called wrong; nevertheless it seems to me to be an unfortunate loosening of what we would do better to keep a tight rein on. Suppose that box of chocolates I mentioned earlier had not been given to both boys jointly, but was given only to the older boy. There he sits, stolidly eating his way through the box, his small brother watching enviously. Here we are likely to say, "You ought not to be so mean. You ought to give your brother some of those chocolates." My own view is that it just does not follow from the truth of this that the brother has any right to any of the chocolates. If the boy refuses to give his brother any, he is greedy, stingy, callous—but not unjust. I suppose that the people I have in mind will say it does follow that the brother has a right to some of the chocolates, and thus that the boy does act unjustly if he refuses to give his brother any. But the effect of saying this is to obscure what we should keep distinct, namely the difference between the boy's refusal in this case and the boy's refusal in the earlier case, in which the box was given to both boys jointly, and in which the small brother thus had what was from any point of view clear title to half.

A further objection to so using the term "right" that from the fact that A ought to do a thing for B, it follows that B has a right against A that A do it for him, is that it is going to make the question of whether or not a man has a right to a thing turn on how easy it is to provide him with it; and this seems not merely unfortunate, but morally unacceptable. Take the case of Henry Fonda again. I said earlier that I had no right to the touch of his cool hand on my fevered brow, even though I needed it to save my life. I said it would be frightfully nice of him to fly in from the West Coast to provide me with it, but that I had no right against him that he should do so. But suppose he isn't on the West Coast. Suppose he has only to walk across the room, place a hand briefly on my brow—and lo, my life is saved. Then surely he ought to do it, it would be indecent to refuse. Is it to be said, "Ah, well, it follows that in this case she has a right to the touch of his hand on her brow, and so it would be an injustice in him to refuse"? So that I have a right to it when it is easy for him to provide it, though no right when it's hard? It's rather a shocking idea that anyone's rights should fade away and disappear as it gets harder and harder to accord them to him.

So my own view is that even though you ought to let the violinist use your kidneys for the one hour he needs, we should not conclude that he has a right to do so—we should say that if you refuse, you are, like the boy who owns all the chocolates and will give none away, self-centered and callous, indecent in fact, but not unjust. And similarly, that even supposing a case in which a woman pregnant due to rape ought to allow the unborn person to use her body for the hour he needs, we should not conclude that he has a right to do so; we should conclude that she is self-centered, callous, indecent, but not unjust, if she refuses. The complaints are no less grave; they are just different. However, there is no need to insist on this point. If anyone does wish to deduce "he has a right" from "you ought," then all the same he must surely grant that there are cases in which it is not morally required of you that you allow that violinist to use your kidneys, and in which he does not have a right to use them, and in which you do not do him an injustice if you refuse. And so also for mother and unborn child. Except in such cases as the unborn person has a right to demand it—and we were leaving open the possibility that there may be such cases—nobody is morally *required* to make large sacrifices, of health, of all other interests and concerns, of all other duties and commitments, for nine years, or even for nine months, in order to keep another person alive.

6

We have in fact to distinguish between two kinds of Samaritan: the Good Samaritan and what we might call the Minimally Decent Samaritan. The story of the Good Samaritan, you will remember, goes like this:

> A certain man went down from Jerusalem to Jericho, and fell among thieves, which stripped him of his raiment, and wounded him, and departed, leaving him half dead.
>
> And by chance there came down a certain priest that way: and when he saw him, he passed by on the other side.
>
> And likewise a Levite, when he was at the place, came and looked on him, and passed by on the other side.
>
> But a certain Samaritan, as he journeyed, came where he was; and when he saw him he had compassion on him.
>
> And went to him, and bound up his wounds, pouring in oil and wine, and set him on his own beast, and brought him to an inn, and took care of him.
>
> And on the morrow, when he departed, he took out two pence, and gave them to the host, and said unto him, "Take care of him; and whatsoever thou spendest more, when I come again, I will repay thee." (Luke 10:30–35)

The Good Samaritan went out of his way, at some cost to himself, to help one in need of it. We are not told what the options were, that is, whether or not the priest and the Levite could have helped by doing less than the Good Samaritan did, but assuming they could have, then the fact they did nothing at all shows they were not even Minimally Decent Samaritans, not because they were not Samaritans, but because they were not even minimally decent.

These things are a matter of degree, of course, but there is a difference, and it comes out perhaps most clearly in the story of Kitty Genovese, who, as you will remember, was murdered while thirty-eight people watched or listened, and did nothing at all to help her. A Good Samaritan would have rushed out to give direct assistance against the murderer. Or perhaps we had better allow that it would have been a Splendid Samaritan who did this, on the ground that it would have involved a risk of death for himself. But the thirty-eight not only did not do this, they did not even trouble to pick up a phone to call the police. Minimally Decent Samaritanism would call for doing at least that, and their not having done it was monstrous.

After telling the story of the Good Samaritan, Jesus said, "Go, and do thou like-wise." Perhaps he meant that we are morally required to act as the Good Samaritan did. Perhaps he was urging people to do more than is morally required of them. At all events it seems plain that it was not morally required of any of the thirty-eight that he rush out to give direct assistance at the risk of his own life, and that it is not morally required of anyone that he give long stretches of his life—nine years or nine months—to sustaining the life of a person who has no special right (we were leaving open the possibility of this) to demand it.

Indeed, with one rather striking class of exceptions, no one in any country in the world is *legally* required to do anywhere near as much as this for anyone else. The class of exceptions is obvious. My main concern here is not the state of the law in respect to abortion, but it is worth drawing attention to the fact that in no state in this country is any man compelled by law to be even a Minimally Decent Samaritan to any person; there is no law under which charges could be brought against the thirty-eight who stood by while Kitty Genovese died. By contrast, in most states in this country women are compelled by law to be not merely Minimally Decent Samaritans, but Good Samaritans to unborn persons inside them. This doesn't by itself settle anything one way or the other, because it may well be argued that there should be laws in this country—as there are in many European countries—compelling at least Minimally Decent Samaritanism.[8] But it does show that there is a gross injustice in the existing state of the law. And it shows also that the groups currently working against liberalization of abortion laws, in fact working toward having it declared unconstitutional for a state to permit abortion, had better start working for the adoption of Good Samaritan laws generally, or earn the charge that they are acting in bad faith.

I should think, myself, that Minimally Decent Samaritan laws would be one thing, Good Samaritan laws quite another, and in fact highly improper. But we are not here concerned with the law. What we should ask is not whether anybody should be compelled by law to be a Good Samaritan, but whether we must accede to a situation in which somebody is being compelled—by nature, perhaps—to be a Good Samaritan. We have, in other words, to look now at third-party interventions. I have been arguing that no person is morally required to make large sacrifices to sustain the life of another who has no right to demand them, and this even where the sacrifices do not include life itself; we are not morally required to be Good Samaritans or anyway Very Good Samaritans to one another. But what if a man cannot extricate himself from such a situation? What if he appeals to us to extricate him? It seems to me plain that there are cases in which we can, cases in which a good Samaritan would extricate him. There you are, you were kidnapped, and nine years in bed with that violinist lie ahead of you. You have your own life to lead. You are sorry, but you simply cannot see giving up so much of your life to the sustaining of his. You cannot extricate yourself, and ask us to do so. I should have thought that—in light of his having no right to the use of your body—it was obvious that we do not have to accede to your being forced to give up so much. We can do what you ask. There is no injustice to the violinist in our doing so.

7

Following the lead of the opponents of abortion, I have throughout been speaking of the fetus merely as a person, and what I have been asking is whether or not the argument we began with, which proceeds only from the fetus's being a person, really does establish its conclusion. I have argued that it does not.

But of course there are arguments and arguments, and it may be said that I have simply fastened on the wrong one. It may be said that what is important is not merely the fact that the fetus is a person, but that it is a person for whom the woman has a special kind of responsibility issuing from the fact that she is its mother. And it might be argued that all my analogies are therefore irrelevant—for you do not have that special kind of responsibility for that violinist, Henry Fonda does not have that special kind of responsibility for me. And our attention might be drawn to the fact that men and women both *are* compelled by law to provide support for their children.

I have in effect dealt (briefly) with this argument in section 4 above; but a (still briefer) recapitulation now may be in order. Surely we do not have any such "special responsibility" for a person unless we have assumed it, explicitly or implicitly. If a set of parents do not try to prevent pregnancy, do not obtain an abortion, but rather take it home with them, then they have assumed responsibility for it, they have given it rights, and they cannot *now* withdraw support from it at the cost of its life because they now find it difficult to go on providing for it. But if they have taken all reasonable precautions against having a child, they do not simply by virtue of their biological relationship to the child who comes into existence have a special responsibility for it. They may wish to assume responsibility for it, or they may not wish to. And I am suggesting that if assuming responsibility for it would require large sacrifices, then they may refuse. A Good Samaritan would not refuse—or anyway, a Splendid Samaritan, if the sacrifices that had to be made were enormous. But then so would a Good Samaritan assume responsibility for that violinist; so would Henry Fonda, if he is a Good Samaritan, fly in from the West Coast and assume responsibility for me.

8

My argument will be found unsatisfactory on two counts by many of those who want to regard abortion as morally permissible. First, while I do argue that abortion is not impermissible, I do not argue that it is always permissible. There may well be cases in which carrying the child to term requires only Minimally Decent Samaritanism of the mother, and this is a standard we must not fall below. I am inclined to think it a merit of my account precisely that it does *not* give a general yes or a general no. It allows for and supports our sense that, for example, a sick and desperately frightened fourteen-year-old schoolgirl, pregnant due to rape, may *of course* choose abortion, and that any law which rules this out is an insane law. And it also allows for and supports our sense that in other cases resort to abortion is even positively indecent. It would be indecent in the woman to request an abortion, and indecent in a doctor to perform it, if she is in her seventh month, and wants the abortion just to avoid the nuisance of postponing a trip abroad. The very fact that the arguments I have been drawing attention to treat all cases of abortion, or even all cases of abortion in which the mother's life is not at stake, as morally on a par ought to have made them suspect at the outset.

Second, while I am arguing for the permissibility of abortion in some cases, I am not arguing for the right to secure the death of the unborn child. It is easy to confuse these two things in that up to a certain point in the life of the fetus it is not able to survive outside the mother's body; hence removing it from her body guarantees its death. But they are importantly different. I have argued that you are not morally required to spend nine months in bed, sustaining the life of that violinist; but to say this is by no means to say that if, when you unplug yourself, there is a miracle and he survives, you then have a right to turn round and slit his throat. You may detach yourself even if this costs him his life; you have no right to be guaranteed his death, by some other means, if unplugging yourself does not kill him. There are some people who will feel dissatisfied by this feature of my argument. A woman may be utterly devastated by the thought of a child, a bit of herself, put out for adoption and never seen or heard of again. She may therefore want not merely that the child be detached from her, but more, that it die. Some opponents of abortion are inclined to regard this as beneath contempt—thereby showing insensitivity to what is surely a powerful source of despair. All the same, I agree that the desire for the child's death is not one which anybody may gratify, should it turn out to be possible to detach the child alive.

At this place, however, it should be remembered that we have only been pretending throughout that the fetus is a human being from the moment of conception. A very early abortion is surely not the killing of a person, and so is not dealt with by anything I have said here.

Notes

1 I am very much indebted to James Thomson for discussion, criticism, and many helpful suggestions.

2 Daniel Callahan, *Abortion: Law, Choice and Morality* (New York, 1970), p. 373. This book gives a fascinating survey of the available information on abortion. The

Jewish tradition is surveyed in David M. Feldman, *Birth Control in Jewish Law* (New York, 1968). Part 5, the Catholic tradition in John T. Noonan, Jr., "An Almost Absolute Value in History," in *The Morality of Abortion*, ed. John T. Noonan, Jr. (Cambridge, Mass., 1970).

3   The term "direct" in the arguments I refer to is a technical one. Roughly, what is meant by "direct killing" is either killing as an end in itself, or killing as a means to some end, for example, the end of saving someone else's life. See note 6, below, for an example of its use.

4   Cf. *Encyclical Letter of Pope Pius XI on Christian Marriage*, St. Paul Editions (Boston, n.d.), p. 32: "However much we may pity the mother whose health and even life is gravely imperiled in the performance of the duty allotted to her by nature, nevertheless what could ever be a sufficient reason for excusing in any way the direct murder of the innocent? This is precisely what we are dealing with here." Noonan *(The Morality of Abortion,* p. 43) reads this as follows: "What cause can ever avail to excuse in any way the direct killing of the innocent? For it is a question of that."

5   The thesis in (4) is in an interesting way weaker than those in (1), (2), and (3): they rule out abortion even in cases in which both mother *and* child will die if the abortion is not performed. By contrast, one who held the view expressed in (4) could consistently say that one needn't prefer letting two persons die to killing one.

6   Cf. the following passage from Pius XII, *Address to the Italian Catholic Society of Midwives*: "The baby in the maternal breast has the right to life immediately from God.—Hence there is no man, no human authority, no science, no medical, eugenic, social, economic or moral 'indication' which can establish or grant a valid juridical ground for a direct deliberate disposition of an innocent human life, that is a disposition which looks to its destruction either as an end or as a means to another end perhaps in itself not illicit.—The baby, still not born, is a man in the same degree and for the same reason as the mother" (quoted in Noonan, *The Morality of Abortion*, p. 45).

7   The need for a discussion of this argument was brought home to me by members of the Society for Ethical and Legal Philosophy, to whom this paper was originally presented.

8   For a discussion of the difficulties involved, and a survey of the European experience with such laws, see *The Good Samaritan and the Law*, ed. James M. Ratcliffe (New York, 1966).

The Abortion Debate in the Twenty-First Century

Michael Boylan

Very few conversations in the public arena have had such a long life with so little agreement to show for it as the abortion debate. This essay does not intend to settle the issue in a manner that everyone will accept but to outline a way to view the problem so that each person may develop a universal moral theory and a linking principle to resolve this problem.[1] I suggest that the means for doing so lies in the Personal Worldview Imperative: "All people must develop a single comprehensive and internally coherent worldview that is good and that we strive to act out in our daily lives."[2]

To this end, I present my argument in the following way. First, I review some of the history of the debate. Next, I critically examine the key premises in a version of the arguments from each side. Finally, I suggest a way to think about the problem that does not force a single solution on the reader but suggests a way to frame the problem so that each reader might determine his or her own universal maxim.

The History of the Debate

One can summarize the debate over abortion as being between two camps, proabortion and antiabortion.

The Proabortion Position[3]

1. A woman's body is her own—assertion.
2. Whatever is one's own is under her discretion to dispose of at will—fact.
3. A woman's body is under her discretion to dispose of at will—1, 2.
4. The fetus is wholly dependent on the woman's body (at least through most of the first two trimesters of pregnancy)—fact.
5. That which is wholly dependent on one's body is (baring any other intervening duties) wholly under one's discretion to dispose of at will—assertion.
6. The fetus inside a woman is hers to dispose of at will—3–5.
7. To abort a fetus is to remove it from one's body—fact.
8. Removing a fetus from a mother's body will, in most cases, cause it to be biologically nonfunctional—fact.
9. To abort a fetus is to cause it to be biologically nonfunctional—7, 8.
10. Removing something from one's body (which is at one's disposal, at will) is permissible—2, 3.
11. Removing the fetus from a woman's body is permissible even if such removal renders the fetus biologically nonfunctional—6, 9, 10.

The Antiabortion Position

1. From the moment of conception, there is a person—assertion.
2. All persons should be accorded full human rights—fact.
3. To kill an innocent human agent at will is impermissible—fact (generally accepted by most moral theories).
4. A fetus is an innocent human agent—assertion.
5. To kill a fetus is impermissible—1–4.
6. All morally impermissibly acts should be sanctioned by society as impermissible—fact.
7. Abortion kills the fetus—fact.
8. Abortion is impermissible and should be considered by society as impermissible—5–7.

Obviously, a tremendous gap exists between these two arguments. To properly review an ethical argument, I believe that we must assess the worldview(s) of those who make such arguments. Let us examine some aspects of the worldviews to which each side subscribes and then turn to key premises in the preceding arguments and other classic renditions of the argument. To make the worldview of each group understandable and sympathetic, I adopt the persona of an advocate of each as I encourage each of you to explore these worldviews to evaluate what positive and negative points they offer.

The worldviews of proabortionists

I believe that much of the power of proabortionists' argument is tied to (1) the unequal consequences that women face in sexual relations, (2) the issue of personal autonomy, and (3) the general societal repression of women. Let us examine these in order.

1. A consequence of a woman engaging in sexual intercourse is the possibility of a pregnancy. A man can engage in intercourse as often as he chooses, but he will never become pregnant. He can (if he is a purely egoistic sort of fellow) walk away when his sexual partner becomes pregnant. Although the consequence of their action is just as much his responsibility as it is hers, only she will have to bear the physical results of their joint behavior. This is unfair. If both the man and woman engaged in an action *jointly*, then they should have to bear the consequences jointly. History has shown, however, that has not always been the case. In fact, some have speculated that the entire institution of marriage evolved solely to protect women from this brute inequality.

   Why should men not have to suffer the consequences? The large number of single mothers around the world who must raise families is a testament to the brute inequality of the biological scenario that some sociobiologists have termed a battle of genetic strategies, which suggests that all organisms have a single biological imperative: to send their genes into future filial generations. The best strategy for a man is to inseminate as many women as possible, hoping that some of these actions will result in pregnancies and thus fulfill his biological imperative.

   The best strategy for a woman is to be very selective and to try to obtain a commitment from the biological father to assist her because a pregnant woman loses a proverbial step or two in competing for food and shelter. Also, when the child is born, the woman needs to nurse it for at least six months and needs some protection.

   If this scenario has any truth to it, the brute biological reproductive strategies of men and women clearly differ. For thousands of years, a mistake on the part of women in the execution of their strategy has had far more deleterious consequences than any failures on the part of men.

   Many women often see as a curiosity the fact that some of the most vocal critics of women and their reproductive decisions are men (who bear no biological consequences for their actions: "It is easy for *you* to say …").

   Thus, I believe that it is fairly clear why women would want the same *option* as men have to be able to walk away from an unfortunate sexual relationship.

Some critics say that men and women ought to face equal consequences. However, how are such consequences to be enforced? Even in the United States (which aspires to be a nation under law), we have not been able to make divorced fathers and men who abandon their reproductive partner pay legally sanctioned child support. How can we ever realistically aspire to make men pay the same price that women pay for the consequences of sexual intercourse?

2. The issue of autonomy relates to the ownership of one's own body. All things equal, it is difficult to know who would own your body except yourself.[4] This means that whatever you own is yours (unless some intervening duty can be proven). If you want to tattoo yourself, put piercing rings in various places, or cut off a limb, it is your privilege to do so because whatever is entirely yours is at your disposal. Thus, if you do not choose to use your body as a growth chamber for an embryo, you need not do it. It is your body to do with as you wish.

3. The general station of women in this society, as in most societies in history, has been as a repressed and enslaved group. This is a broad, sociological statement. This does not mean that there are not individual men who are sensitive and nurturing of their spouses, daughters, and women in general. One need only engage in some volunteer work with women's shelters and other facilities that deal with those in need, however, to recognize the truth of this generalization. Despite all our laws and aspirations as a society, women are treated differently from men. This difference is an added hurdle that women must overcome but that men do not face.

To make the point more clearly, women are the oppressed gender. For men to say to women that they must abide by laws enacted by men that constrict their reproductive freedom (so that they might not be as free as men) is an act of political enslavement. In this way, *freedom of choice* is essential, not the actual execution of an act of abortion. Most women would never want to have an abortion and will never have an abortion. Many women will even carry an impaired infant to term rather than abort it. Nonetheless, despite the fact that most women will never take advantage of the right of abortion (within the United States and a number of other countries), it is important to maintain the freedom of choice.

This freedom of choice is a cornerstone in the edifice that stands against gender enslavement. The struggle of oppressed women demands that they not be subjected to the will of men on something so essential to their biological nature as their reproductive equality. The ability to choose to terminate a pregnancy is merely one part of a very large structure. Not very long ago women who had to pay for the outcomes of their loving relationships were relegated to unlicensed physicians who used dirty tools and whose rates of sepsis was exceeded only by their blood-alcohol levels.[5]

The image of a woman alone, abandoned by her partner and by society, resonates with most women (even if they feel that such a situation will never happen to them). It is a there but for the grace of God, go I scenario. For this reason, most women feel solidarity for their sisters in need and strive to protect them from a solitary journey into hell.

The freedom of choice is an important symbol as a balance against gender oppression.

The worldviews of antiabortionists

The second group views reality much differently. To begin with, this group has a very strong belief in relatively unencumbered free will. Each person can act as she pleases without much real perturbation. This means all consequences are deserved. The idea that one gender is oppressed is viewed in several ways by different sides.

1. First, the group believes that this issue revolves around the female sex, which is already protected and is given more than ample opportunities in society. This group might say that a woman today has advantages in job searches over men because all she needs to have is a skill level that approaches a man's level and she will be automatically hired.
2. This group believes that sexual intercourse is an activity given by God for the creation of children. When people go against the laws of God, they must be prepared to accept the consequences. They consider abortion to be an easy way out. This group might say that living with a few more unfortunate consequences in life would be good for most of these unrelated young people.
3. The third perspective held by this group is more profound. It asserts that human life is precious and that everything should be done to preserve the life of the unborn, which cannot protect themselves.

When someone is impaired, s/he needs the protection and support of others. A fetus is in a similar position, but the impairment is not due to a defect in the genotype or in development but is a natural consequence of the current biological stage of this individual. All other things being equal, this embryo will become a human agent capable of reason and of action. This is an acceptance of the normal process of nature.

According to the doctrine of *novus actus interveniens*, the normal process of nature is taken to be the standard. This doctrine, which is well entrenched in the law,[6] states that a person who interferes with the normal operation of nature is responsible for all the ensuing consequences. For example, John is robbing a bank and says to the teller, "If you move, I'll shoot." The teller moves slightly as she presses the alarm button with her foot. The bank robber shoots, and his bullet ricochets off one of the iron bars of the teller's cage and lodges in the neck of a person standing in line behind the gunman.

Who caused the person to be shot? If one holds the inciting incident theory of causation (which is often considered definitive in the philosophy of science), then the teller is to blame. But this is ridiculous. The gunman put the teller into an abnormal situation. The gunman with his gun and his demands had changed the natural order. Thus, according to the doctrine of *novus actus interveniens*, the gunman, not the teller, is at fault for the bullet in the customer's neck because the gunman charged the natural order, and thus all ensuing events (in an appropriately fashioned action description) can be attributed to him.

How does this apply to abortion? The natural order would have the fetus grow and develop in the normal process. Any action that stops this process is considered to be causally responsible for the fetus's demise. If the fetus is a person, then the action is murder. Thus, abortion is murder.

If you were part of a society that institutionalized murder and did nothing to change the situation, then you would be considered an accessory to the murder. Thus, to live in a society that permits abortion and to do nothing to stop it is to be like someone who lived in the societies of Hitler, Stalin, or Pol Pot or in the world at large and could have reacted in some meaningful way to these dictators' actions but did not.

We in the United States have created a society that legalizes the continued killing of thousands of fetuses every year. If these fetuses are humans, are we not then guilty of mass murder? Is our society comparable to the murdering societies of history? Is this not cause enough to prohibit abortion now?

A Critical Examination of the Premises of Each Side

The preceding section presented a version of the pro and con arguments and explored in brief the worldviews of each side. Let us begin here by defining what I mean by *abortion*, which is the removal of a fetus from the female by natural or artificial means. The natural abortion is called *spontaneous abortion* and occurs in 20 to 25 percent of all pregnancies (depending on how one frames the data). Most spontaneous abortions, also called miscarriages, occur during the first trimester of pregnancy generally because the developing embryo is malformed. The miscarriage is nature's way of ensuring that potential children with no real chance of survival are given an exit at the beginning of life's journey.

Artificial abortion is the removal of a fetus from the female by medical means. The process of abortion does *not* kill that fetus. As a matter of fact, many embryos removed from the female do die. They do not die just because they are removed from the mother. If equipment such as an artificial womb were available, an embryo removed from a woman could continue to gestate, and would not necessarily die. All this is to say that if there is a right to abortion, it is a right to remove the fetus from a woman's body. But killing the fetus is not a right. If the fetus, for example, were able to be preserved, abortion would be a separate issue from that of what to do with that fetus.[7] One could remove the fetus and allow it to develop without any further contact with its biological mother. The right to abortion, *simpliciter*, is a right to remove a fetus from one's body. This follows from the sample argument and the worldview enhancement necessary to accept that argument. Therefore, the abortion issue changes drastically after the point of viability. In theory, one might be able to remove the fetus from the female and raise it separately. In this case, removing a fetus would not be tantamount to causing it to die.

Having clarified the definition of abortion, let us turn to a few key premises in the arguments on each side. First is the proabortion position as represented by the generic argument I presented. The argument given the world-view background is very persuasive. Detractors are likely to focus on premise 5: That which is wholly dependent on one's body is (baring any other intervening duties) wholly under one's discretion to dispose of at will—assertion.

The logical move is from autonomy over one's own body part to sovereignty over entities dependent on one's body. This is an argument that Judith Jarvis Thomson elaborates in her famous article.[8] Deontologists might object to a blanket endorsement of this position. It seems to violate the "duty to rescue," which is a moral obligation to aid another when the other person's basic goods of agency are threatened so long as doing so does not cause the rescuer to risk his or her own basic goods of agency.[9] The duty to rescue is supported by Kant, Gewirth, and Donagan.[10] For example, in the case of Kitty Genovese (which Thomson cites), the apartment dwellers watching her being attacked and killed could have screamed from their windows at the attacker or called the police or both. I can attest from personal experience that this is an effective way to thwart a criminal in the inner city. Thus, if a person can aid another whose basic goods of agency are being threatened without risking his own basic goods of agency, then he is obliged to do so. This is a little different from the depiction given by Thomson. She says that a person is not obliged to go out and confront the attacker but that a person who does is a Good Samaritan. This implies that there are only two responses to the Kitty Genovese case—either fight or flight. This is too simple, however. Surely everyone is obliged to aid another when doing so does not risk his or her own basic goods of agency. But what of abortion?

Is abortion properly analogous to one of these options in the Kitty Genovese example: (a) calling the police and yelling from their windows or (b) leaving the apartment complex to physically stop the assailant? Option (a), involves merely fulfilling a moral duty, which does not deserve praise but a mere statement of gratitude. Option (b) involves risking basic goods of agency, which could result in death. People choosing option (b) are heroes. Is the woman who chooses to carry a fetus to term more like the person doing her duty or the hero? The answer to this question can be an important component in evaluating this argument.

Returning to premise 5, we can also note that what one does to one's own body and what one does to entities that are not part of one's body are different. We pay no mind to eliminating bacteria, viruses, cysts, and growths. They are not of our body and have no intrinsic worth, nor would a reasonable interpretation of precautionary reasoning dictate that they have any worth.[11]

A fetus is certainly different, however; it will, all things being equal, develop into a moral agent who has absolute rights to freedom and well-being. Thus, the argument for potentiality is not wholly without merit. Although the fetus is not actually a person in the strong sense of the word, it is a *potential* person. This potentiality of personhood is not trivial and cannot be dismissed.

Next, let us examine the antiabortion position as represented by the generic argument as I presented it. Given its worldview background, the argument is very persuasive. Detractors are likely to focus on premise 3: To kill an innocent human agent at will is impermissible—fact (generally accepted by most ethical theories). Some would want to discuss the nature of "innocence." Is the word an absolute term (i.e., in no way deserves to die) or relative to the action description at hand (i.e, is in no way threatening the life of any other agent—knowingly or unknowingly).[12] The first sense is rather silly as depicted because it presupposes many unstated propositions that would need to be argued and defended. The second sense, on the other hand, has merit. *Innocent* in this reading implies that a person is not materially involved in the loss of fundamental rights of agency for another (intended or otherwise).

For example, consider the deer hunter who shoots another person thinking she was a deer. That person being shot at could justifiably kill the person who is shooting at her. (We assume that the only way to stop the shooting is to use lethal force.[13]) Under this reading, the unwitting hunter is not innocent but is materially guilty because he jeopardizes the life of another.

Under this definition, a person may be innocent only if she is not materially threatening the life of another.[14] Thus, killing a fetus that threatens the life of its mother is not a case of killing an innocent.

Let us explore the word *threatens*, which has many meanings. One meaning is a danger to the mother's life. A fetus (without motive) may be the cause of its mother's death. Another meaning refers to ripping apart the world-view in which the pregnant woman lives. This threatens her because it challenges everything that she holds as precious in her life plan (stated or only imagined). This is not trivial. People kill themselves for as much because threats to one's worldview are very serious. Contained within one's world-view is the very ground of personal well-being. A threat to worldview, in this fundamental interpretation, can be ranked after life itself as the most potent of threats. Thus, when an individual engages in protecting her fundamental worldview, she is entitled to use extreme measures. This can include harming materially innocent agents in order to protect this fundamental worldview.

The story is not so simple, however. One's worldview is comprised of various elements—not all of which are of equal importance and weight. This means that the level of threat is variable as is the appropriate response to the threat. Is this a question of balance?

It is always a question of balancing. The difference between theories that explicitly balance—Utilitarianism, Intuitionism, and Virtue Ethics—and those that are often depicted as nonbalancing (such as deontology) is that the former group balances at the back end, that is, at the moment of decision.

Deontological theories also balance, but they aspire to balance at the front end, that is, in the depiction of the act to be judged. An individual seeks balance in judging what type of action is involved. Forming an action description is not value neutral but involves balancing competing understandings of what is happening (i.e., what is relevant). Thus, there is always balancing. The issue is what drives the decision making. I suggest that what drives the decision making ought to be the Personal Worldview Imperative. The consistency portion of this imperative requires a person to treat all cases alike and create rules that do not contradict each other and fulfill the aspirations of that ethical theory.

Thus, one must define what "threatens" his worldview. For example, when I was a track runner, a very talented runner in our club had the potential to be an Olympic runner. He had joined the club because it had four other runners who were favorites to make the 1976 Olympic team. The only problem was that this runner never finished a race in the four years I ran with the club. Something would always get in the way. Either his splits were not exactly as he had wanted them to be, a black bird flew over the track (he hated black birds), he thought he heard someone yelling something at him, or the humidity suddenly changed, and so forth. Surely, although these distractions were real and important to him, the rest of us ultimately viewed them as trivial. The same is true for some meanings of *threaten*. What is a legitimate meaning of the word? To make this point more effectively, let me contrast seven reasons for an abortion that women might consider threats to themselves.[15]

A. Ms. A is pregnant. It has been determined that if she were to bring this fetus to term, she will die. She feels threatened because her life is in danger.

B. Ms. B is pregnant. She is a married mother of five children with very little financial means. If she carries this fetus to term, her other five children will be pushed over the edge of starvation. Ms. B feels threatened because the lives of her other children are at stake.

C. Ms. C is pregnant. She is married, and her obstetrician has told her that the baby she is carrying has a fatal disease that will kill the child by the age of six. The death will be painful. Medical science might find a cure for this disease, but probably not in time to save her child. Ms. C feels threatened on behalf of her unborn child.

D. Ms. D is pregnant. She is "thirty-something," single, and in a career that is just about to take off. Her profession is so competitive and limited that it is reasonable to assume that if she misses this opportunity, she will never have another one. Ms. D feels threatened because her career and personal life plan are at stake.

E. Ms. E is pregnant. She is a high school senior who has been admitted to a very selective college. Her college admission might not be renewable if she does not attend this fall. Her parents would be furious if they knew she is pregnant. Her whole future is at stake, her plans did not include a pregnancy. She could not be a good mother at this point in her life. Ms. E feels threatened because her future and her reputation are at stake.

F. Ms. F is pregnant. She is married and has decided that she would like to have a boy and a girl. She already has the girl and amniocentesis has indicated that this fetus is also a girl. She and her husband do not want to have more than two children because it is not part of their life plan. Ms. F feels threatened because she has a girl within her when she wanted a boy.

G. Ms. G is pregnant. She is married and has decided that she would like a male child who is intelligent and has the physical features that she believes represent the perfect child: blonde hair, blue eyes, 6 feet in height, and intelligence capable of scoring 1,500+ on the SATs. Assume that a battery of tests can predict a genotype that is most compatible with the desired phenotype/developmental end product. Ms. G's test results indicate that her fetus is deficient in several areas: several shades of brown hair seem likely, brown eyes, height of slightly less than 6 feet, and intelligence capability of scoring only 1200 on the SAT. Ms. G feels threatened because she has a fetus that will not meet her standard for the child she really wants.

Each of these scenarios illustrates a threat on a sliding scale. If a person is entitled to kill an otherwise innocent agent who is materially guilty because it threatens her, then it is important to create a line that separates acceptable threats from unacceptable threats.

Case A involves a pure sense of self-defense. Case B may be said to be an act of self-defense on behalf of another (the other children), although this case is somewhat more difficult because it has several contingencies. These contingencies include calculations on whether the family *will* starve or whether intervening events—such as better employment prospects or higher crop yields—might alter the situation. Other possible scenarios could also be constructed, but the point of this example is to illustrate self-defense on behalf of another. In Case C, the situation is similar to one addressed in active euthanasia. The decision maker is paternalistically acting on behalf of another's best interest. The mother may think that she knows that this child will not want to die so early and with so much suffering. She may also think that she cannot face the trial of caring for another knowing that the future is both fixed and fatal.

Cases D and E are similar except for the age of the women. The age issue can work both ways. One might give greater latitude to the younger woman because she is not fully mature and responsible for her actions. Or one might give greater latitude to the older woman because as one ages, doors of opportunity close. The consequences to the older woman are probably more severe than to the younger. Each case uses *threaten* in the context of "very disruptive to my life plan."

Cases F and G are similar because they indicate a sense of eugenics. In fact, a large number of abortions are performed in the world because of the sex of the fetus. Thousands of female fetuses have been aborted because the mother desired a son. Case G involves a science fiction scenario in which people desire to have "designer babies." This is a desirable future to some but a nightmare to others.

More will be said about these meanings of *threaten* in the next section of this essay.

The other aspect of premise 3 concerns the definition of an agent. This issue has been much discussed in the literature with few definitive results.[16] I would like to preface my remarks by referring to the essay on precautionary reasoning by Deryck Beyleveld and Shaun Pattinson.[17] Beyleveld makes the point that *full human rights*, that is, those that confer absolute respect for freedom and well-being, become operative only when there is an agent who clearly meets the criteria of being a prospective, purposive agent. His point would not be evident without objection until some time in a child's second year of life.[18] If we grant this, all infants less than 30 months of age have no dialectically necessary claim to agency. Q.E.D., these infants have no dialectically necessary claim to life (one of the aspects of well-being).

This standard is certainly very high. Surely it does not mean that we are entitled to kill at will all infants under the age of 30 months. Precautionary reasoning indicates that various actions such as walking and feeding oneself indicate that the infant may be more cognizant than we can scientifically document. Many other animals also are able to perform these actions,[19] yet we do not ascribe to them the rights we afford to human agents. To determine why this is so, we need to turn back to the Personal World Imperative.

The Personal Worldview and Abortion

According to the Personal Worldview Imperative, all people must develop a single comprehensive and internally coherent worldview that is good and that they strive to act out in their daily lives. It enjoins each of us to create both a comprehensive and internally coherent vision of life. One aspect of this is to be able to will ourselves to have actions performed on us without violating the laws of nature as we understand them.[20] This is similar to the Kantian notion of imperfect duties.[21]

A fetus cannot will its own demise (i.e., being aborted) without contradicting the natural law that says that ceteris paribus all humans act for their own preservation and happiness.

What if we could not will? Certainly, this situation may occur when we are at the beginning of life. The fetus does not act; and because *willing* is a precondition to action, the fetus does not will. This seems to be an exception to the Kantian interpretation of the Personal Worldview Imperative referred to earlier. However, some might claim that this situation should be judged as we would assess a person who is asleep (to use Aristotle's example—the fetus is not willing *now* but will be in the position to will in the near future).[22] This argument is a form of precautionary reasoning.

The essence of this doctrine (as I choose to use it) is to make precautionary reasoning a form of Aristotelian potentiality that holds open the possibility that the individual in question may be more empowered than we can scientifically determine. At some time, we must determine a point beyond which it is impossible (from the worldview perspective of the speaker) for the individual in question to be afforded the moral rights of agency—even using precautionary reasoning. Does this mean that past the point of affording the fetus proportional rights[23] through precautionary reasoning we are entitled to give the fetus no consideration at all and thus be entitled to kill it at will? The answer is no because I have linked "precaution" with a sense of Aristotelian potentiality. Under this interpretation of *precautionary* reasoning, we must give some level of respect to any fetus, no matter how immature. On the principle of proportionality that I have been espousing, we would give more respect to a 13-week fetus than to a 4-week fetus because the 13-week fetus is closer to enjoying precautionary reasoning than is a 4-week fetus. The pregnant woman must determine just how much respect, vis-à-vis various threats that face her.

In this process, a person must first establish the floor of precautionary reason; this requires judgment. Personally, I would put the floor at the end of the first trimester of pregnancy (13 weeks). Before this point, the brain and spinal cord are not connected; therefore, according to my own best understanding, it would be impossible for the fetus to deliberate, plan, and act. Others may disagree with me and put the floor in either direction (i.e., earlier or later in pregnancy).

Second, each individual must determine the limit of respect to accord a fetus who is neither (a) an actual agent nor (b) a possible agent (even under a liberal sense of precautionary reasoning). The agent in question is *potentially* a possible agent. As a *potentially* possible agent, the fetus is accorded some respect because, baring intervention, it will become a possible agent (protected by precautionary reason) and eventually a full-blown agent (protected by most theories of morality).

This interpretation invalidates the given form of the proabortion argument because it suggests that the at-will provision is incorrect. A person may eliminate some entity at will only when the entity receives no justifiable respect. Under the interpretation just outlined, some level of respect is always due to potentiality tied to precautionary reasoning; the agent involved must determine the *level of respect*. This is a personal assessment, but to say so does not imply relativism. Instead, this expression is the proper expression of the Personal Worldview Imperative in which a person legislates a universal interpretation of reality (which would include valuing this level of respect).

I do not believe that a woman may abort a fetus at will. I believe that the fetus must represent a threat that supersedes the level of respect the woman has assigned to the fetus. I would say that the threats represented by F and G in the preceding examples do not meet this standard. Thus, abortion on the basis of the baby's sex or some eugenic desire is impermissible at any stage of pregnancy. The level of respect due the fetus as a mere potential possible agent is greater than the level of maternal threat.

I assess cases A through E in the examples as meeting this standard of threat that supersedes the level of respect for the fetus during the first trimester of pregnancy. Others might demur because they would quarrel with me about balancing of threats. I view case A as meeting a sufficient standard of threat throughout the pregnancy.[24] In third-trimester abortions, however, the opportunity to remove the fetus without destroying it may exist. The right to an abortion is not a right to have the embryo destroyed but merely a right to have it removed from the mother's body.

Cases B, C, D, and E form two units that have similar themes (self-defense for the sake of another and severe disruption to one's personal life plan, respectively). Since averting death is more disastrous to agency than mere roadblocks (no matter how disruptive), I assess B and C as being higher-order threats than D and E. This differentiation must be considered in different stages of pregnancy in which an abortion may be permissible. For example, I lean toward D and E as being permissible only during the first trimester but B and C as being permissible during the first two trimesters.

The general principle in operation is how to weigh threat and response. In Cases D and E the nature of the response changes as the fetus develops. Thus, a response to a fetus in the first trimester is different from a response in the second trimester is different from a response in the third trimester. This is so because in the first trimester one has merely the principle of potentiality by which to refer.

After the first trimester, I believe that the principle of precautionary reason becomes operative and proportionally more relevant until the minimal stages of operationally verifiable agency are evidenced (30 months after birth—or less). After 30 months (or whatever time is chosen), killing the entity is absolutely impermissible unless it were materially threatening the life of the mother.[25]

Conclusion

In this essay, I have aspired to be suggestive rather than definitive on the question of abortion. To this end, I have suggested criteria that different people can use to set the universal limits of permissibility and impermissibility. This variation is due to the variation in personal worldviews in which one may weigh maternal threats and fetal respect differently. Instead of focusing on the definition of personhood or the expression of autonomy, I suggest that focusing on maternal threats versus fetal respect is more productive.

This approach suggests that three levels should be considered when evaluating how much respect anyone deserves: (a) full personhood (at some time in the first few years of development), (b) possible personhood (protected by precautionary reason from some base level to personhood; I put this moment at the end of the first trimester of pregnancy), and (c) potential possible personhood (from the moment of conception to possible personhood).

Full moral rights obtain necessarily to those enjoying full personhood (since they are actual deliberating agents). Something proportionally approaching full moral rights may be claimed for the possible agent, and some proportionally lower level of respect (with its associated rights) should be granted to those on the lowest level of personhood.

In contrast to the traditional antiabortion position that generally argues for full moral rights for the fetus from conception, my theory creates three levels of respect that move well past birth to be complete. In contrast to the traditional proabortionist position that generally argues for the right of abortion at will, my theory denies abortions at will. It requires the demonstration of a level of maternal threat that is greater than the level of respect we ought to give the developing (though not yet actual) person.

The levels that an individual sets for threats versus respect follow from his complex web of values that I call the *worldview*. Through a dialectical interaction between the abortion question and this person's values emerges personal ownership of a universal theory dealing with if, when, and under what conditions an embryo may be separated from its biological mother.

The question of abortion has been in the public forum so long because it addresses many key issues related to the rights of others versus our own individual expressions of autonomy. I believe that total consensus on this issue will never occur in the present framework because consensus is a derivative property of each person's worldview. And because worldviews differ, so will the imperatives they endorse. This is not a statement of relativism but a factual description of various people working on a common problem (each believing that she or he has *the* correct answer).

On the optimistic side, however, I believe that viewing the abortion question from the Personal Worldview Imperative will at least create increased understanding of (a) the other side's position and (b) a vocabulary that is structured so that it does not prejudge the issue (for example, the vocabulary of maternal threat versus fetal respect). This type of understanding will be essential if any real progress in the public debate on abortion is to be made.

Notes

1 I define a *linking principle* as one that follows from a moral theory but that is "action guiding" in its application. One example of a linking principle is precautionary reason.

2 An argument for the Personal Worldview Imperative is given in the Introduction of *Basic Ethics* and in an abbreviated form in Chapter 1 of this volume.

3 Obviously, no single argument represents either position entirely. There are, in fact, many distinct arguments for the conclusion that abortion is or is not permissible. My reconstructions here are meant to represent my opinion about the strongest version of each argument in a simple, generic form.

4 There are at least two objectors to this position. First, to say that one "owns" one's body splits the person in two. There is no proper distinction between one's self and one's body; they are one and the same. Thus, all metaphors of ownership are faulty and do not fit legal notions of ownership. For a statement of this position, see Hugh V. McLachlan, "Bodies Rights and Abortion," *Journal of Medical Ethics*, 23, no. 3 (1997): 176–80. Second, those who accept a theology that posits an all powerful creator God—such as Judaism, Christianity, and Islam (a sizable portion of the world's population)—will demur on this point since it is dogma that God created everything and therefore "owns" what she/he/it has created. In this case, one's body is not one's own but God's. This tenet can have an effect on the argument.

5   For a description of these times, see Leslie J. Reagan, *When Abortion Was a Crime: Women, Medicine, and Law in the United States, 1867–1973* (Berkeley CA: University of California Press, 1997).

6   H.L.A. Hart and A.M. Honoré, *Causation in the Law* (Oxford: Clarendon Press, 1959), pp. 129 ff.; compare with 127, 292–96.

7   In this case, the state would enter the equation as an interested party to govern the interests of the newly born, premature infant.

8   Judith Jarvis Thomson, "A Defense of Abortion," *Philosophy and Public Affairs* 1 (1971): 47–66. This article has had enormous response. Some of the most interesting of these include Robert N. Wennberg, *Life in the Balance: Exploring the Abortion Controversy* (Grand Rapids, MI: Eerdmans, 1985); John T. Wilcox, "Nature as Demonic in Thomson's Defense of Abortion," in *The Ethics of Abortion: Pro-Life vs. Pro-Choice*, ed. Robert M. Baird and Stuart E. Rosenbaum, rev. ed. (Buffalo, NY: Prometheus, 1993): 212–25; Mary Anne Warren, "On the Moral and Legal Status of Abortion," in *Arguing about Abortion*, ed. Lewis M. Schwartz (Belmont, MA: Wadsworth, 1993), pp. 227–34; Keith J. Pavlischek, "Abortion Logic and Paternal Responsibility: One More Look at Judith Thomson's 'A Defense of Abortion,'" *Public Affairs Quarterly* 7 (1993): 341–61; David Boonin-Vail, "A Defense of 'A Defense of Abortion': On the Responsibility Objection to Thomson's Argument," *Ethics* 107 (January 1997): 286–313.

9   The reason for this caveat is that a person is not *obliged* ever to risk his or her own basic goods of agency for the sake of another. To do so would be to admit that the other person has more of a right to the basic goods of agency than the rescuer. This would entail the other person being better *qua* an agent than the rescuer. There is no support for such an assertion under the deontological theories I am citing since all agents are equally entitled to the basic goods of agency simply by being human beings alive on this earth. Those who choose to risk their own basic goods of agency for the sake of others go "above and beyond" their moral duty (i.e., they are heroes). But one who fulfills only his or her duty to save another when his or her basic goods of agency are not at risk is only an ordinary person doing his or her duty.

10 Immanuel Kant, *Grundlegung zur Metaphysik der sitten*, vol. 4, Prussian Academy edition (Berlin: G. Reimer, 1903), p. 421; Alan Gewirth, "Replies to My Critics," in *Gewirth's Ethical Rationalism: Critical Essays with a Reply by Alan Gewirth*, ed. Edward Regis Jr. (Chicago: University of Chicago Press, 1984), pp. 228–29; Alan Donagan, *The Theory of Morality* (Chicago: University of Chicago Press, 1977), pp. 154 ff.

11 Derek Beyleveld and Shaun Pattinson, "Precautionary Reasoning as a Link to Moral Action," (first edition of this volume, p. 41 ff.).

12 I discuss what I mean by "action description" in the Introduction to *Basic Ethics*.

13 The proportionality of "threat" to "minimal response necessary to alleviate the threat" is very important in cases of self-defense. However, in the instance of abortion, the response (abortion) will have a fixed effect (the death of the fetus) until near the end of the second trimester. In this case, the only variable is the level of threat. After viability, of course, the situation changes if there is a policy to use an abortion procedure that seeks to preserve the fetus's life.

14 Alan Donagan makes a similar distinction; see *The Theory of Morality* (Chicago: University of Chicago Press, 1977), pp. 87 ff.

15 These cases are not meant to be comprehensive but merely suggestive of certain levels of threat. The cases assume only willing sexual intercourse. I would characterize all nonvoluntary acts of sexual intercourse (such as rape or incest) as creating a very high sense of threat for the woman, which might be characterized as being between "A" and "B." In this case, carrying the fetus (as innocent as it may be) constantly reinforces the horror and degradation of the initial act. This humiliation is a primary threat to human action and well-being so that the woman would be fully within her rights to remove the fetus from her body at any time.

16 For a discussion of this literature, see Bonnie Steinbock, *Life Before Birth: The Moral and Legal Status of Embryos and Fetuses* (Oxford: Oxford University Press, 1992).

17 Beyleveld, p. 39.

18 This is a troubling point because it invokes both methodologies and measurements. Some may want to push the point back a bit, but the ultimate

measure in this case is whether the child has shown that she or he has a sense of self and that the sense of self deliberates and carries out action. Thus, walking or beginning to speak might count. *Wherever* one wishes to set this point will be well past birth.

19 In most cases, human infants go through many developmental stages more slowly than do infants of other species. Thus, on this alone, one would afford more proportional status to puppies or to baby lizards than to humans. Obviously, we do not afford this status because we employ precautionary reasoning.

20 This interpretation of the Personal Worldview Imperative comes about through the sense of consistency. It would be inconsistent to view ourselves as being outside nature's laws. Therefore, to will exceptions for ourselves is irrational (because it is inconsistent).

21 The Kantian notion of imperfect duties is here taken to be positive duties requiring action on the part of the agent. One of these duties is the requirement that we aid others whenever we can do so without risking our basic goods of agency. For a discussion of my view of Kantian imperfect duties, see Michael Boylan, *Basic Ethics* (Upper Saddle River, NJ: Prentice Hall, 2000), Chapter 4.

22 Aristotle believes that a person may have the power of sight even when he is asleep and has his eyes shut. The idea is that when the person is awakened, he will be able to see. The fact that while asleep, this power is only potential does not diminish the claim that he will soon be able to see. Aristotle, *The Metaphysics: Text and Commentary*, W.D. Ross (Oxford: Clarendon University Press, 1924), 1048b 1–6.

23 The notion of proportional rights stems from the individual's best assessment of the possible degree of agency that *may* exist. This goes well beyond any demonstrated agency (which may be as late as 30 months after birth). This attribution of rights is given not because of demonstrated capacity on the part of the fetus but because it seems possible that an individual may possess attributes that confer agency, that is, a sense of inductive and deductive logic along with the capacity to deliberate about action (even in a very minimal way) *before* this is operationally evident to some observer. Therefore, out of precaution, we act as if the individual has these capacities (even though there is no demonstrable evidence for this). As a result, we confer precautionary rights of agency. These differ from full rights of agency only in the fact that they are not *dialectically necessary* (Gewirth) or *apodeitically necessary* (Kant). They are, in fact, contingently necessary (contingent because they are based on the assessment of the person making the attribution).

24 As well as those cases between A and B—as per footnote 15 (covering rape and incest—and all other cases of involuntary sex that has resulted in a pregnancy).

25 Such a situation would be bizarre and a person would have to stretch her imagination to identify a plausible case. Unfortunately my volunteer work experience has taught me that all too frequently adults feel threatened by children. They cry too much, they keep needing to have their diaper changed, or they drive me nuts with their fussiness are among adults' responses to children. Too often the threat threshold is far too low for these adults. Beating, abusing, and even killing infants is justified in the minds of these adults because the infants' needs interfered with the adults' life plans (as per F and G in the examples). Such a response to a perceived threat is far too great and is therefore morally impermissible.

Evaluating a Case Study
Assessing Embedded Levels

The goal in this series of exercises is for you to be able to write an essay that critically evaluates a biomedical problem involving ethical issues. Your essay should include an examination of aspects of medical practice as well as the ethical dimensions. In Chapter 3, we discussed how to bring the ethical dimensions to the fore through the use of detection questions. These were put side by side the principles of professional practice.

In this chapter, we compare these two types of issues. This comparison can be accomplished in multiple ways; the one offered here invokes a technique that rates professional practice as having three levels of complexity: surface, medium, and deep. The level of interaction allows you to see at a glance how professional practice issues and ethical issues conflict.

You need a model of some type to evaluate the professional practice issues and ethical issues that may conflict. When ethical issues and professional issues conflict, you do not *automatically* choose either. Some ethical problems can be solved easily and do not require forgoing the dictates of the professional practice. At other times, an ethical problem must be solved in such a way that professional practices must be overridden.

You need a methodology for comparison. The *embedded concept model* is one such methodology. I illustrate how this works with several examples that employ a chart to clarify the ways the concepts conflict. You may also want to use this technology if you have access to one of the popular computer spreadsheet programs, but the use of a spreadsheet is not necessary. A more conventional approach is to discuss these differences. The spreadsheet is no substitute for solid narrative description, but at the very least it simplifies and makes visual the model I propose.

Case 1

You are a senior hospital administrator and you have learned that dissatisfaction has been expressed concerning the manner in which staff members explain the consent forms patients must sign before their surgical procedures can be performed. Although your hospital's practice is within the law and the existing procedures used by other hospitals, your hospital serves an immigrant population with low education levels. To explain the medical procedure and its possible outcomes in more detail would require additional time and would involve additional hospital expenditures, and money is tight (as always). What should you do?

Professional Practice Issues

1. A professional is required only to follow the law and the guidelines of its professional association.
2. Implementing a new system could require additional costs.
3. Going beyond the law and the association's guidelines could be perceived as raising the standard that other hospitals would be required to follow. Meeting this additional standard could require the use of funds that had not been budgeted.

Ethical Issues

1. Physical health is crucial to every person because it is essential to purposive action. What is most important to a rational purposive agent should be within that agent's sphere of autonomy.
2. *Informed* consent is necessary for autonomous decision making.

In this simple case, the ethical guidelines override those of the professional practice guidelines. That means the ethical guidelines are "easier" to solve. When a great disparity exists between the imbeddedness of one alternative as opposed to the other (meaning deep as opposed to surface), that direction should drive the decision. One should implement the other side as it is possible. For example, in this case, the hospital administrator should implement a program to explain medical procedures and their outcomes to patients so that they can better understand the health care decisions they must make. Other professional practice considerations should be addressed in the context of the action to enhance patient understanding, which takes precedence.

Table 4.1 Analysis of consent practices at Mercy Hospital

	Surface	Medium	Deep
Professional Practice Issues			
A professional is required to follow only the law and the professional association's guidelines	x		
The hospital may be accused of raising the standard	x		
Implementation costs		x	
Ethical Issues			
One's personal health decisions should be within one's sphere of autonomy			x
Only a truly *informed* consent satisfies the conditions of autonomy			x

Case 2

This case is not so simple. You are a regional director at the World Health Organization. One of your duties is to supervise the distribution of birth control devices to women in less-developed countries. The product of choice has been the intrauterine device (IUD) that has proved to be effective and inexpensive. The problem is that in the United States, several hundred users of the IUD have contracted pelvic inflammatory infections that have been linked to use of the IUD. As regional director, you must decide whether to continue to supply IUDs to women in less-developed countries.

Professional Practice Issues

1. As a professional in the public health field, your responsibility is to choose public policy that maximizes the health and minimizes the health risks in the general population.
2. Sexual activity without birth control in less-developed countries will lead to an increasing population that, in turn, will lead to severe poverty and mass starvation.
3. Mass starvation kills millions; pelvic inflammatory infections kill hundreds. Thus, it is better to save the many (in the spirit of the profession's mission).

Ethical Issues

1. Each person's life is precious.
2. The end of saving more lives does not justify the means of sacrificing others.

This case differs from Case 1 because the ethical and professional guidelines are equal. In this case, the dictates of the ethical imperative must be followed because it is more deeply imbedded in a person's worldview than is the imperative of professional practice. The components of ethics enter the worldview generically as a feature of a

Table 4.2 Analysis of population control in the Third World

	Surface	Medium	Deep
Professional Practice Issues			
Public health mission to preserve the health of as many as possible			x
Sexual activity without birth control leads to mass starvation			x
The end justifies the means			x
Ethical Issues			
Human life is precious			x
The end does not justify the means			x

person's humanity. The imperatives of professionalism enter the worldview as one of many modes of personal fulfillment.

As with scientific theories, the dictates of a universally binding imperative founded on generic structures trump those of a particular person's individual interests. More details on this appear in the "Evaluating a Case Study" section in Chapter 5.

In this essay, the main concern is the ability to assess the levels of imbeddedness. Some common mistakes that my students have made in performing this assessment follow:

1. *Not giving the imperatives of professional practice their due.* Remember that whether you assess imbeddedness via a spreadsheet or through discursive paragraphs, you are working from your original analysis of the problem. A failure to uncover all the important facets will be reflected in your depiction of imbeddedness. You will notice gaps in the reasoning and will feel that something is missing. If this happens, go back over the issues lists. Rewrite the case in your own words; expand or recast the case in some way. By doing this, you become the author and are forced to recognize key elements in the case as presented.

2. *Seeing everything at the same level of imbeddedness.* You need to view imbeddedness as a way to describe the degree to which the professional practice or ethical issue is essential to the case. A less essential issue should be given less consideration. To better understand the essential structure of a professional practice, prepare short justifications of your choice of that element as an issue in the case. As you prepare your justifications, think about each element in its relation to the whole. If that relation could not be different without seriously altering the whole, then it is essential. If you can find substitutes that would work just as well, the relation is incidental.

3. *Listing too many professional and ethical issues.* This is the flip side to step 1. You have given too much detail that is not essential to the case at hand, or you are listing one issue in a number of different ways. In either event, preparing an essential description of your elements (as in step 2) can help you shorten your issue list to only those required for your evaluation.

Good solid work avoiding these mistakes will enable you to create a more satisfactory result in the argumentative stage, in which you may finally apply your ethical theory to your annotated imbeddedness charts.

Macro and Micro Cases[1]

Macro Case 1. You are the senior administrator of a national chain of nursing homes. At your recent annual meeting with the directors, a problem among the nursing staff was identified. A sizable number of inhabitants of your nursing homes are in great pain and voice a will to die. The nurses are seeking a policy that will allow them some discretion in dealing with these patients, vis-à-vis allowing nature to take its course. The nurses would like to know the company's position if they delay certain treatments or if they actually hasten death by administering overdose injections in severe cases.

Anecdotal evidence suggests that the relatives of these individuals would not pursue costly lawsuits if this "informal" policy were carried out (although that is always a possibility). In fact, the same evidence indicates that family members long for closure on what seems to be inevitable.

You know that state laws explicitly prohibit active euthanasia. You want to do the right thing, and you must make the decision in a memo to the chairperson of your board of directors. What will you say? What policy direction will you advocate and for what reasons? Make explicit reference to some moral theory as the basis of your decision and linking principle to action.

Macro Case 2. You are an ethicist on a panel at the National Institutes of Health that is studying guidelines for physicians nationwide concerning allowing feeding tubes to be removed from intensive care infants. These infants are in intensive care because they have some blockage that prevents them from receiving conventional nutrition. A simple operation can solve this problem, but some parents prefer to avoid the operation and to discontinue the use of the feeding tube.

The panel is currently split over several issues: (a) Should parents be allowed to make this decision, or should the state assume a paternalistic position and decide? (b) If the state should step in, then how much weight should be given to the wishes and circumstances of the parents? (c) Because the parents would normally want very aggressive treatment for their child, infants in these situations must either have a fatal disease or a serious disability. Should the state treat these instances differently? If the parents are allowed to choose, should they treat these instances differently? (d) Is there a difference in rationale for failing to save an impaired infant due to concerns over the pain it will undergo in an eventual death when it is older against the pain the parents will undergo in caring for a disabled child? (e) Do children who have a short life expectancy deserve the opportunity to live for the amount of time they have? (f) Do mentally and/or physically handicapped children deserve the opportunity to live? (g) Do parents of impaired infants have a right not to be encumbered by the extraordinary commitments (emotional, financial, etc.) such situations entail?

You are highly regarded by other members of the panel, and your opinion will carry significant weight. Write a position paper describing your views and defending them using an established ethical theory and linking principle.

Macro Case 3. You are a member of the United States Supreme Court. The Court is about to review a fast-track case concerning so-called defective infants. In this particular case, *Smith v. New York*, Ms. Jane Smith is suing to be able to remove her newborn son from a feeding tube that is keeping him alive. Ms. Smith wants the feeding tube removed because the baby has a blockage that prevents him from receiving nutrition under ordinary means. This blockage can be removed by minor surgery, but Ms. Smith does not want her son to have this operation because he is mentally retarded. She does not want a mentally retarded child. She believes that she has the right to let her child die. Why should she have to devote the rest of her life to caring for this child (either directly or by paying for his care in some type of home)?

The key question here is whether to consider this child to be defective (generally understood to be in unrelievable pain and/or with a terminal condition) and thereby subject to rules and regulations regarding defective children (who are allowed to die) or whether this child is merely handicapped, in which case federal law requires doing everything possible to save him. You want to view this question first from an ethical perspective before considering the legal aspects of the issue (not a part of this essay). Therefore, write an essay identifying the ethical issues involved and use an ethical theory to support your position.

Macro Case 4. You are the incoming administrator of the World Health Organization. The organization's policies about funding for countries that practice (a) infanticide (generally of female infants), (b) gender-based abortion, and (c) family planning–based abortion are being challenged. Some donor nations are upset because they believe the organization's standards are ambiguous. You are charged with clearing up this ambiguity. Some of your aides suggest that you opt for a political/pragmatic solution, but you believe that only an ethical solution will be accepted. Therefore, your task is to determine whether the World Health Organization should support countries that engage in any or all of these practices. What ethical issues are involved? What linking principles would you employ? Do the three different issues demand different responses? Why or why not?

Micro Case 1. Your husband is a nationally recognized journalist. He was severely injured three years ago in an automobile accident while on assignment and has been in an irreversible coma since then. As a result, he lost his reflex for swallowing and is connected to a feeding tube. Health care workers report that occasionally he sits bolt upright, utters a string of words, and then lies down again.

Your husband left no clear statement as to his wishes in such a situation. It is clear to you that he will not come out of the coma. You want to do what is right and to be able to justify your decision to your children as well as to the courts. You also want to get on with your own life. You are thirty-eight years old and have a great deal of your life ahead of you. Write an essay defending one of these positions: (a) leaving things as they are or (b) disconnecting the feeding tube.

Micro Case 2. You are a pregnant teen-aged female. You did not intend to become pregnant; obviously, you were not as careful as you should have been. Your blueprint for life includes college, graduate school, and a fulfilling job but not a child now. Having a baby will not work out with your plans.

You have missed your second period and learned at the family planning clinic that you are in the late stage of the first trimester of your pregnancy. This situation totally unnerves you. You consider suicide. Why should you bear this by yourself? Your partner, Alex, is in the state finals of the baseball championships. You have not told him; you could try to drag him into the situation, but that would not be fair to him. But is this fair to you?

Write an essay based on an ethical theory that justifies what *you* would do.

Micro Case 3. You are an eighty-two-year-old man whose wife of fifty-two years is dying of cancer. She is in great pain despite her treatments and is living in the hospice section of a nursing home. Everyone in this unit is terminal. When you visit your wife, she implores you to give her a lethal dose of her pain-killing medication. Your love her, and seeing her suffer in this way causes you considerable pain. Can killing someone be an act of love? Or is it really an act of escape so that *you* will not have to see her in this condition until the bitter end. You are perplexed. You could give in to your wife's demands, or you could leave things as they are. You could ask the physician to keep her permanently sedated, but even that could not guarantee that your wife would not endure pain and suffering.

You explore this question in your diary. Examine this question using an established ethical theory and linking principle as your guide. Make a decision as to what to do.

Micro Case 4. You are the medical representative on a mountain climbing expedition, and you have lost much of your medical gear. Your group of four has had terrible luck; it was hit by a sudden blizzard that has knocked out all communications with the base camp. Mary, one of the climbers, has been badly injured; she suffered a deep gash on her leg.

The problem is that food is running out fast. Your food supply will last little more than one day. Rescue parties could not make it in this weather, and helicopters could not land in this terrain even in perfect weather. Hope for a rescue is not realistic. You could go for help, which would probably be a three-day trip, but the food supply is a concern. Mary's leg appears to be afflicted by gangrene, and she is in great pain. You have plenty of pain killer left—more than enough for her pain. Mary knows that there is little hope for rescue and implores you to give her a lethal dose of the pain killer. You demur. She says she can inject herself if you make it available for her.

You are conflicted. Should you give Mary a lethal dose or should you make one available for her to give herself? Should you carry on and hope for a miracle? Answer this problem using a moral theory to support your argument.

Note

1   For more on macro and micro cases, see the overview on p. 58.

Genetic Enhancement

Overview: One important area of biomedical research and future treatment involves genetic engineering. Since the cloning of Dolly the sheep in 1996, the imagination and research into possible medical applications has been greatly stimulated. From diabetes to Alzheimer's disease, many biomedical researchers have sought to find treatments for diseases and chronic conditions that had previously been unavailable. However, some regard this sort of future not as promising but as menacing.

In order to sharpen your appreciation for the two essays in this section a few key terms should be elucidated. First there is the *somatic* versus *germ line* distinction. Therapy that is given to a person to cure or improve a disease or chronic condition is called somatic intervention. Somatic intervention or therapy treats the individual only. If a person has, for example, a poorly functioning pancreas, it is possible (in theory) to inject stem cells into the affected area to help the organ repair itself. This has never worked so far (in practice), but it seems possible. If it could work, it is possible that someone could be cured of diabetes. Since such an intervention fits traditional models of organ repair for health (as in heart by-pass surgery), there seems to be little controversial about somatic therapy.

Some may demur on this citing the source of the stem cells. If the stem cells come from the patient, then there is little controversy. If the stem cells come from unused fertilized eggs in an IVF clinic, some see this as an offshoot of the abortion question. These advocates view fertilized eggs in an IVF clinic as persons (even though the fertilized eggs have no developmental specialization). Neither essay in this section takes on this question. For those interested in this issue, I would suggest reading the articles on abortion.

The specialized question for this section is the issue of enhancement. Now "enhancement" is a term that is used differently by various writers. For our purposes we will adopt the definition given by Bostrom and Roache: "enhancement interventions aim to improve the state of an organism beyond its normal healthy state." This contrasts enhancement with therapy, which seeks to bring a person in a degraded state back to normal.

The argument by Bostrom and Roache is that the world would be a better place were medical research turned toward enhancement. Five key areas are highlighted: life extension, physical enhancement, mood and personality enhancement, cognitive enhancement, and selecting the best children. This sort of strategy is also called transhumanism. It seeks to improve our species so that we can control our fate and live happier, longer lives. Understandably, the authors know that there are those who disagree. Thus, much of the essay is devoted to anticipating possible objections and refuting them.

In response to some of the wide-eyed optimism of Bostrom and Roache, I provide a cautionary note. It seems to me that much of science is driven by what is called the principle of plentitude, which states "what can be known should be known," and its corollary, which is that what can be done, should be done. What is behind this imperative is a belief in unlimited scientific freedom. I argue against this position by contending that there are cases in which only unethical means can be used to pursue some scientific truths and cases in which the consequences of certain other scientific discoveries create an immoral context that harms society at large. Obviously, this cautionary note would apply to genetic enhancement. Because this would in many cases affect the germ line, a further cautionary note about unintended consequences is also in play.

Ethical Issues in Human Enhancement

Nick Bostrom and Rebecca Roache

What Is Human Enhancement?

Human enhancement has emerged in recent years as a blossoming topic in applied ethics. With continuing advances in science and technology, people are beginning to realize that some of the basic parameters of the human condition might be changed in the future. One important way in which the human condition could be changed is through the enhancement of basic human capacities. If this becomes feasible within the lifespan of many people alive today, then it is important now to consider the normative questions raised by such prospects. The answers to these questions might not only help us be better prepared when technology catches up with imagination, but they may be relevant to many decisions we make today, such as decisions about how much funding to give to various kinds of research.

Enhancement is typically contraposed to therapy. In broad terms, therapy aims to fix something that has gone wrong, by curing specific diseases or injuries, while enhancement interventions aim to improve the state of an organism beyond its normal healthy state. However, the distinction between therapy and enhancement is problematic, for several reasons.

First, we may note that the therapy-enhancement dichotomy does not map onto any corresponding dichotomy between standard-contemporary-medicine and medicine-as-it-could-be-practiced-in-the-future. Standard contemporary medicine includes many practices that do not aim to cure diseases or injuries. It includes, for example, preventive medicine, palliative care, obstetrics, sports medicine, plastic surgery, contraceptive devices, fertility treatments, cosmetic dental procedures, and much else. At the same time, many enhancement interventions occur outside of the medical framework. Office workers enhance their performance by drinking coffee. Make-up and grooming are used to enhance appearance. Exercise, meditation, fish oil, and St John's wort are used to enhance mood.

Second, it is unclear how to classify interventions that reduce the probability of disease and death. Vaccination can be seen as an immune system enhancement or, alternatively, as a preventative therapeutic intervention. Similarly, an intervention to slow the aging process could be regarded either as an enhancement of healthspan or as a preventative therapeutic intervention that reduces the risk of illness and disability.

Third, there is the question of how to define a normal healthy state. Many human attributes have a normal (bell curve) distribution. Take cognitive capacity. To define abnormality as falling (say) two standard deviations below the population average is to introduce an arbitrary point that seems to lack any fundamental medical or normative significance. One person might have a recognizable neurological disease that reduces her cognitive capacity by one standard deviation (1σ), yet she would remain above average if she started off 2σ above the average. A therapeutic intervention that cured her of her disease might cause her intelligence to soar further above the average. We might say that *for her*, a normal healthy state is 2σ above the average, while for most humans the healthy state is much lower. In contrast, for somebody whose "natural" cognitive capacity is 2σ below the average, an intervention that increased it so that she or he reached a point merely 1σ below the average would be an enhancement. As a result, an enhanced person may end up with lower capacity than even an unenhanced person with subnormal cognitive functioning; and therapeutic treatment may turn a merely gifted person into a genius. In cases like these, it is hard to see what ethical significance attaches to the classification of an intervention as therapeutic or enhancing. Moreover, in many cases it is unclear that there is a fact of the matter as to whether the complex set of factors determining a person's cognitive capacity is pathological or normal. Does having a gene present in 20% of the population that correlates negatively with intelligence constitute a pathology? Having a large number of such genes might make an individual cognitively impaired or even retarded, but not necessarily through any distinctive pathological process. The concepts of "disease" or "abnormality" may not refer to any natural kind in this context. These concepts are arguably not useful ways of characterizing a constellation of factors that are normally distributed in a population, as are many of the factors influencing cognitive capacity or other candidate targets for enhancement. A concept that defined enhancement as an improvement achieved otherwise than by curing specific disease or injury would inherit these problems of defining pathology.

Fourth, capacities vary continuously not only within a population but also within the lifespan of a single individual. When we mature, our physical and mental capacities increase; as we grow old, they decline. If an intervention enables an 80-year-old person to have the same physical stamina, visual acuity, and reaction time as he had in his twenties, does that constitute therapy or enhancement? Either alternative seems as plausible or natural as the other, suggesting again that the concept of enhancement fails to pick out, in any clear or useful way, a scientifically significant category.

Fifth, we may wonder how "internal" an intervention has to be in order to count as an enhancement (or a therapy). Lasik surgery is a therapy for poor vision. What about contact lenses? Glasses? Computer software that presents text in an enlarged font? A personal assistant who handles all the paperwork? Without some requirement that an intervention be "internal," *all* technologies and tools would constitute enhancements in that they give us capacities to achieve certain outcomes more easily or effectively than we could otherwise do. If we insist on an internality constraint, as we must if the concept of enhancement is not to collapse into the concept of technology generally, then we face the problem of how to define such a constraint. If we believe that enhancements raise any special ethical issues, we also face the challenge of showing why the particular way we have defined the internality constraint captures anything of normative significance.

Sixth, even if we could define a concept of enhancement that captured some sort of unified phenomenon in the world, there is the problem of justifying the claim that the moral status of enhancements is different from that of other kinds of interventions that modify or increase human capacities to the same effect.

Defining the therapy-enhancement distinction is a problem only for those who maintain that this distinction has practical or normative significance. Those who hold that therapy is permissible, or worthy of support, or an appropriate target for public funding, but that enhancement is not, are affected by all the difficulties mentioned above. We can call subscribers to this anti-enhancement view *bioconservatives*. *Transhumanists* (advocates of human enhancement) are unaffected by the problems associated with maintaining that there are important differences between enhancement and therapy. Transhumanists hold that we should seek to develop and make available human enhancement options in the same way and for the same reasons that we try to develop and make available options for therapeutic medical treatments: in order to protect and expand life, health, cognition, emotional well-being, and other states or attributes that individuals may desire in order to improve their lives.

In the following five sections, we briefly consider several particular areas of potential human enhancement: life extension, physical enhancement, enhancement of mood or personality, cognitive enhancement, and pre- and perinatal interventions. Our aim is not to give an exhaustive assessment of these types of enhancement; rather, by considering one or two key issues for each type, we hope to provide some insight into why they have become topics of ethical debate in recent years, and some understanding of a few key ethical concerns surrounding enhancement.

Life Extension

Human life expectancy in the Stone Age, and for present-day native "non-civilized" populations, is estimated at around 20–34 years. We might regard this as the natural life expectancy at birth for our species. Among those who survive infancy and childhood to reach the age of 15, life expectancy is about 54.[1] In recent times, Japan has consistently boasted the highest life expectancy. Those born in Japan in 2006 can expect to live 81 years (85 years for women).[2] Thus, there has been roughly a tripling of life expectancy for humans in the last few thousand years. This gain is primarily due to social and technological developments rather than any evolutionary changes in human biology: improvements in sanitation, medicine, education, and nutrition have all had a positive effect on life expectancy. This effect is significant and ongoing. Over the past 150 years, "best-practice" life expectancy (i.e., life expectancy in the country with the longest life expectancy) has increased at a remarkably steady rate of about 2.5 years per decade. If this trend were to continue, record life expectancy (for women) would reach 100 in six decades.[3]

To make further radical gains in human life expectancy, it will become necessary to slow or reverse aspects of human aging. If the processes of senescence are left unchecked, then there comes a point in each individual's life where cellular damage accumulates to such a degree that pathology and death become inevitable. Preventing and curing specific diseases can only have a limited impact on life expectancy in a population that already lives as long as people do in the industrialized world. If we cured *all* heart disease, life expectancy in the United States would increase by only about 7 years. Curing *all* cancer would result in a gain of some 3 years.[4] Curing all heart disease *and* all cancer would result in a gain less than the sum of their individual contributions (perhaps 8 or 9 years). The reason for this is that older individuals become increasingly susceptible to a wide range of sickness. If it is not heart disease today, and not cancer tomorrow, then it will be stroke the day after, or pneumonia. The aging process itself is ultimately the cause of most deaths in industrialized nations, and, increasingly, in the developing world. While the proximate cause of death may be heart failure or cancer or some other specific pathology, it is senescence that is ultimately responsible, by making us gradually more vulnerable. Were it not for aging, our risk of dying in any given year might be like that of somebody in their late teens or early twenties. Life expectancy would then be around 1000 years.

There is another reason why life extension enthusiasts particularly favor research into anti-aging and rejuvenation medicine. It is that a successful retardation of senescence would extend healthspan, not just lifespan. In other words, retarding senescence would enable us to grow older without aging. Instead of seeing our health peak within the first few decades of life before gradually declining, we could remain at our fittest and healthiest indefinitely. For many, this represents a wonderful opportunity to experience, learn, and achieve many things that are simply not possible given current human life expectancy.

Others, however, believe that dramatically increasing lifespan would deprive life of meaning and exacerbate the existing social problems associated with an aging population. These perceived drawbacks have been cited by bioconservatives like Leon Kass as reasons not to pursue life extension enhancement.[5] Let us consider whether this view is justified.

Bernard Williams, despite conceding that death is an evil and therefore an appropriate object of fear, held that an immortal life free from the prospect of death would be meaningless.[6] An immortal life, on his view, would be worse than a finite one because those projects that give one's life meaning and mark out one's life as one's own would eventually be completed or abandoned, leaving infinite years of life in which there are no remaining ambitions or desires to fulfill. Of course, one could create new projects and ambitions to replace the old; but in this case it is not clear that the pursuer of the new projects is, in the ordinary sense, the same *person* as the pursuer of the old ones: what we would end up with would not be a single, cohesive life but a series of separate but overlapping lives. Williams takes considerations like these to provide *prima facie* plausible reasons for opposing radical life extension.[7]

Transhumanists can respond to these considerations in at least two ways. First, those who oppose radical life extension on the ground that an immortal or very long-lived life is not worthwhile may advocate abandoning research into life-extension technology, and may even advocate preventing people from using it once it becomes available. However, the question of whether an extremely long-lived life would be worth living is not obviously relevant to the question of whether a life is worth saving,[8] and that there may be reasons to consider a certain type of life not worthwhile does not in itself justify preventing those who wish to live such a life from doing so. There are plenty of lifestyles led by people today that many might consider not worthwhile; for example, lifestyles entirely devoted to apparently worthless pursuits such as playing computer games or watching daytime TV, or lifestyles devoid of intellectual, social, or cultural enrichment. However, our having this belief about them is not sufficient reason for preventing those who live them from going on living them—by, for example, restricting access to life-saving medicine. Providing they are not significantly harming others, people who live in a liberal, democratic society are free to pursue whatever lifestyle they choose. That there may be reasons to believe that an extremely long-lived life would not be worthwhile, then, does not in itself justify preventing those who wish radically to extend their lifespan from doing so, if the means of doing so and the resulting extended life do not significantly harm others.

Second, whilst Williams' claim that our lives derive meaning and a sense of cohesion from the projects that we pursue during our lifetimes is plausible, his argument does not support the conclusion that no immortal or extremely long life would be worth living. In devising the sort of projects that lend meaning and a sense of cohesion to our lives, we presuppose that we will live for a certain number of years; say, until we are 80. Projects and ambitions such as mastering a musical instrument, learning a foreign language, meeting one's grandchildren, sailing around the world, and building one's own house all set challenges that can realistically be achieved within a lifetime. Projects and ambitions like mastering every musical instrument in the orchestra, writing a book in each of all the major languages, planting a new garden and seeing it mature, teaching one's great-great-grandchildren how to fish, travelling to Alpha Centauri, or just seeing history unfold over a few hundred years are not realistic: there is simply not enough time to achieve them given current life expectancy. If, like Elina Makropulos in the Karel Čapek play from whose English translation Williams' paper takes its name, one were to live for 42 years fully expecting to die in a few decades' time and then take the elixir of life and look forward to infinite existence, one could expect one's projects eventually to expire, leaving one with a choice between eternal boredom and self-reinvention. (Elina eventually chooses to stop taking the elixir, and dies.) But this is because these projects reflect a belief about when one is likely to die. If we could reasonably expect from an early age to live indefinitely, we could embark on projects designed to keep us occupied for hundreds or thousands of years. Such projects could lend to the radically extended life the sort of cohesion that more ephemeral projects lend to current lives. Indefinite life extension, far from burdening people with a choice between boredom and a disjointed existence, could represent a great opportunity for those willing to embrace this new way of thinking about their lives and what they can reasonably hope to achieve within them.

A more practical objection to radical life extension is that keeping people alive indefinitely would lead to overpopulation, and that more old people would place an unacceptable financial burden on the young.

Let us address the latter part of this objection first. One response is that, whilst the idea of extending lifespan by directly addressing the mechanism that causes us to age may be fairly novel, attempts to prolong life are all around us. Medicine, seatbelts in cars, health warnings on cigarettes, and the fluorescent jackets that roadside laborers wear are all designed to prolong the life of those who use them. If prolonging life is to be discouraged, we should not only forego enhancement, but also rethink the way we live and commit to less cautious lifestyles.

Moreover, tackling the aging mechanism may actually alleviate many of the problems that we currently associate with an aging population: many aged people alive today, being too infirm to work, are reliant on state support, and so the years that modern medicine has bought them are ones in which their economic contribution to society is negative. Life extension by delaying or reversing the aging process, in contrast, would increase healthspan, enabling old people to contribute financially and otherwise to society well beyond the 65 or so years currently expected. And, when they do finally become ill and die, there is little reason to think that the cost of their care would be any more expensive than it is today. In fact, society could benefit from being able to amortize such costs over a greater number of years.[9]

That radical life extension could lead to overpopulation has its roots in two separate worries: that overpopulation would result from existing people living longer, and that overpopulation would result from longer-lived people having more children than people today. Regarding the first worry, we can note that population growth has slowed over the past 50 years, with less developed countries accounting for 99% of current growth.[10] Researchers have found that, in general, increasing the standard of living and education of people living in poverty leads to a decrease in birth rate. Working to improve the lives of the millions living in poverty worldwide would, therefore, be a far more effective and humane means of tackling the issue of overpopulation than impeding efforts to develop life extension technology — especially when we consider that this technology is likely to be available first in developed countries, many of which are seeing their population decline.

In response to the worry that longer-lived people will have more children, increasing lifespan would not increase the number of people being born unless there is also an increase in the number of years in which people—particularly women—can reproduce. If this happened, however, it is unclear whether the net effect would be to increase the size of the population. Since 1990, the number of US women under 30 to give birth to their first child has been declining, with birth rates increasing for those over 30.[11] The average age of first-time mothers is at an all-time high. There is, therefore, a trend of postponing childbirth until later in life; a trend particularly evident among well-educated women, who choose to develop their careers before starting a family. However, since women's fertility begins to decrease after the age of 35, there is a pressure on women to have children before it is too late, and so there is a limit to how long childbirth can be postponed. Were it possible to widen the window of years in which women could conceive, this limit would be increased, and so we could expect the current trend of postponing childbirth to continue beyond the age at which fertility currently decreases for women. This might result in a reduction in the number of births per year. Along with the fact that, with enhanced people living longer, there would also be fewer deaths per year, the net effect of radical life extension on population size is far from obvious.

Whilst these considerations help to mitigate the worry that life-extension technology will inevitably lead to an overpopulated planet, it is difficult to foresee how life-extension might affect population in the long term. Even if we accept that increasing lifespan could lead to problems of overpopulation in the future, however, there are more humane ways of solving the problem than withholding life-saving medical treatments. We could, for example, consider a policy in which those who want to avail themselves of radical life-extension would have to agree to limit the rate at which they bring new people into the world.

We conclude that the arguments we have considered do not succeed in showing that radical life extension would cause any insuperable social problems, nor—as Williams believed—that it would reduce the quality of life of those who make use of it. Biogerontological research can help us prevent the diseases associated with old age, thereby increasing quality of life for everyone as our lives advance. The economist William Nordhaus has estimated that improvements in health status, and especially increased longevity, have made as large a contribution to the average standard of living in the United States in the twentieth century as all forms of consumption growth combined.[12] We may hope that research into the processes of aging will enable this trend to continue through the twenty-first century. On balance, then, we find little reason to object to enhancements that extend the healthy human lifespan, and great reason to accelerate their development.

Physical Enhancement

There are various ways in which we can currently improve what we might call bodily capacities, which include stamina, strength, dexterity, flexibility, coordination, agility, and conditioning. We can exercise, eat healthily, take dietary supplements, avoid pollution, and visit physiotherapists, massage therapists, and personal trainers.

For many, especially those who enjoy participating in sports, pursuing activities that improve bodily capacities is enjoyable, and therefore worthwhile for its own sake. For others, pursuing such activities is a time-consuming burden reluctantly undertaken as a means to achieve certain ends, such as maintaining a minimal level of health and fitness and attempting to delay the physical deterioration associated with aging. For an unfortunate few who are struggling to recover from a serious injury or illness, improving bodily capacities can be a difficult and painful feat that must be accomplished slowly and with the help and support of others. Especially for the latter two groups of people, the availability of medical interventions that could improve bodily capacities safely and conveniently would be beneficial. Increasing one's strength by taking a drug, for example, would dispense with the need to spend hours working out at the gym or exercising with a physiotherapist, freeing up time for other activities.

Those who fall into the first group mentioned, who enjoy physical activity for its own sake, could also benefit from such interventions, since improving one's bodily capacities could enhance one's enjoyment of partaking in sports. However, the issue of performance enhancement in professional sport, or "doping," is controversial. In fact, it is probably the most widely-publicized area of enhancement. In this section we shall consider some of the ethical issues raised by sports enhancement, and assess their relevance to physical enhancement generally.

The Canadian sprinter, Ben Johnson, was stripped of an Olympic gold medal following his disqualification for steroid use. Today, athletes are regularly tested for banned substances, with the chairman of the World Anti-Doping Agency (WADA) pledging to "level the playing field and protect the spirit of sport."[13]

Despite the fact that athletes found guilty of doping are condemned as cheats and punished, however, the feats that drugs enable them to achieve are sometimes impressive. The journalist David Owen wrote:

> I have a guilty secret. I think Ben Johnson's "victory" in the men's 100 m at the 1988 Seoul Olympics is just about the most exciting 10 seconds of sport I have ever witnessed. … [W]hat stood out for me mainly was the sheer bullocking power of Johnson's sprinting.[14]

Owen's comments demonstrate that—for some—physical excellence can be impressive even when achieved with the help of drugs. It is therefore not surprising that some call for performance-enhancing drugs in sport to be permitted. Doing so would remove the problem of unfairness: allowing everyone the option of enhancing would be one way of creating the level playing field sought by WADA, thereby removing one of the main concerns about illicit doping.[15] Admittedly, this is not the method of levelling that WADA has in mind, but it is arguably a more effective method than weeding out drug users.

What about the concern expressed by WADA to "protect the spirit of sport"? WADA states that "[t]he spirit of sport is the celebration of the human spirit, the body and the mind."[16] Julian Savulescu et al. observe that, in ancient times, sport was about finding "the strongest, fastest, or most skilled man"[17]: sporting contests were a test of competitors' strength, speed, and skill. Like horse and dog racing today, sport in ancient times was "a test of biological potential." If this is what the spirit of sport is about, then performance-enhancing drugs certainly go against it, since athletes can achieve things with the aid of drugs that they would be unable to achieve based on their natural potential alone. However, Savulescu et al. argue that this is not what sport today is about:

> Humans are not horses or dogs. We make choices and exercise our own judgment. We choose what kind of training to use and how to run our race. We can display courage, determination, and wisdom. We are not flogged by a jockey on our back but drive ourselves. It is this judgment that competitors exercise when they choose diet, training, and

whether to take drugs. We can choose what kind of competitor to be, not just through training, but through biological manipulation. ... Far from being against the spirit of sport, biological manipulation embodies the human spirit—the capacity to improve ourselves on the basis of reason and judgment.[18]

Since, on their view, drugs do not compromise the spirit of sport, Savulescu *et al.* argue that rather than focus on banning drugs that enhance performance, sporting authorities should focus on banning drugs that are unsafe, thus ensuring that professional sport is fair and acceptably safe for all.

Whilst human sports competitors can undoubtedly prepare for their contests using methods that are not available to horses or dogs, the biological constitution of competitors nevertheless plays a more central role in sport than Savulescu *et al.* attribute to it. Sporting contests pit competitors against others judged to be biologically similar in ways considered relevant to the nature of the competition: female adults compete in sprinting races against other female adults but not against males or children, football teams are made up of adults of the same sex and compete against similar teams, and boxers compete against those of the same sex who fall into the same weight category. Why is this?

One answer is that the impressiveness of a sporting feat is relative to the expected biological potential of the competitor. Running 200 metres in under 19 seconds is more impressive if it is accomplished by a man than by a cheetah because it is a more difficult feat for a man, given the typical biological constitution of men; and lifting 150 kilograms is more impressive if it is done by a female weightlifter than by a male weightlifter because such a feat is more difficult for a woman than for a man given their respective typical biological constitutions. In order for us effectively to compare competitors' performance in a sporting contest, then, they need to be drawn from a single biological category.[19]

Permitting the use of performance-enhancing drugs in sport would not necessarily undermine this practice of relativizing sporting achievements to biological categories. For example, permitting the use of a drug that enabled all competitors to improve their performance by 10% would not—if all competitors used such a drug—change the fact that men can generally lift heavier weights than women, or that adults can run faster than children. Nor would it by itself enable the second-best competitors to beat the best competitors. In addition, the use of such a drug would be compatible with the ancient ideal of using sport to identify "the strongest, fastest, or most skilled" competitor; it would simply be the case that the competitor in question is 10% stronger, faster, or more skilled than they would be without the use of the drug.

Whether we think that such enhancement would undermine sport depends upon exactly what role the expected biological potential of competitors plays in our evaluation of their achievements. If we are interested in testing the unenhanced biological potential of competitors, the use of drugs would indeed undermine sporting contests, though in this case we face the problem of explaining why drugs are relevantly different from other, permitted, means of improving performance, such as special training regimes and diet plans. If we are simply interested in revealing differentials—in finding the best, and in assessing competitors' performance relative to others—then a drug that gave all competitors a similar advantage would not undermine this quest. In this case, however, it is difficult to see what motivation there would be for sporting authorities to permit such enhancements, since the same differentials would exist whether or not the enhancement was used.[20] If, on the other hand, we are interested in seeing how fast, strong, or skillful we can make humans using whatever means become available, then we should actively promote performance-enhancing drugs, and expect to see competitors striving to become the first to discover the latest enhancements in order to beat their rivals.

For individual elite athletes, of course, the biggest motivation is likely none of these three; it is to win. Performance-enhancing drugs appeal to competitors for the same reason that the latest training regimes, psychological techniques, and clothing appeal to them: they hope to gain an edge over their competitors. We might say, then, that performance-enhancing drugs are attractive chiefly because they confer *positional goods*: goods whose value to those who have them depends upon others not having them. Many who oppose enhancement in sport, such as Michael Sandel, worry that permitting it would lead to an "arms race," in which competitors who refuse to enhance, or who cannot afford to do so, are left behind while those with the willingness and money to enhance strive to be the first to find new and improved drugs.[21] This would allow money, medical support staff, a physique that takes well to high doses of certain drugs, and a willingness to sacrifice long-term health to play a far more central role in professional sport than many would wish.

Whether performance-enhancing drugs should be permitted in sport ultimately depends upon what one believes to be fundamentally valuable in sport. We will not attempt to argue here for any particular conception of sport, and so we will remain agnostic about the issue of whether performance-enhancing drugs should be permitted in sport. In practice, of course, a decision to ban a particular substance in a sport would also have to take into account factors such as enforcement costs, the health effects of the drug, spectator interest, whether one might instead create two versions of the sport—one where enhancement is allowed and one where it is banned—and other complicating considerations.

It is important to note, however, that even if it turns out that physical enhancement would be a bad thing for professional sport, it may be a good thing for people in other contexts. Many tools and techniques that we find useful or indispensable in everyday life are banned from sport. Bicycles are useful even though they are banned from sprinting races. Similarly, whilst athletes are prohibited from using drugs to make them faster or stronger, improving our bodily capacities may be desirable outside the sporting arena.

The concept of positional goods can help illuminate other applications of enhancement. Generally speaking, the greater the extent to which some good is positional, the less reason there is for society to promote that good. Sports enhancements are at an extreme end where the benefits are almost purely positional. Height enhancements and cosmetic enhancements may similarly have mostly positional benefits. A taller man may gain certain social advantages from his impressive stature, but if everybody become three inches taller nobody is better off than before. Collectively, the money spent and the risks taken to effect such a change would produce no net good. This situation contrasts with some other types of enhancement. For example, health and intelligence have a positional good aspect: being healthy and smart enables a person to compete more effectively for high-status jobs and desirable mates. But health and intelligence also have important benefits aside from these competitive advantages. If we all became a little healthier or a little smarter, there would be a net benefit: we would suffer less illness and incapacity and we would be able to understand more of the world.

In practice, the benefits of many physical enhancements (except ones related to health and longevity) seem to have a very large positional component. A manual laborer might gain an important non-positional benefit from an enhancement that increases strength and stamina; but the value of such enhancement outside the sporting and cosmetic arenas is questionable. Typically, the most effective means of achieving super-human strength and stamina are through the use of "external" tools rather than physical enhancements: we increase our ability to perform hard physical jobs through the use of forklifts and jackhammers rather than anabolic steroids.

Mood and Personality Enhancement

In *Listening To Prozac*, the psychiatrist Peter Kramer describes how some of his patients who had completed a course of Prozac to relieve their depression wished to resume taking it. This was not because their depression had returned: medically speaking, they were no longer mentally ill. Rather, whilst taking Prozac, the patients had felt "better than well."[22] Prozac, as well as relieving their medical condition, had—in their view—improved various aspects of their personality which had never been classed as part of their illness: shy patients had become more outgoing and assertive, compulsive patients had become more relaxed and easy-going, and those with low self-esteem had become more confident. Is there anything wrong with prescribing a drug like Prozac for someone who is not suffering from any medically-recognized condition, but who simply wants to improve their mood or personality?

One difficulty complicating this area of enhancement is that in many cases it is not clear what would count as an improvement of mood or personality. We might think that those who are so shy that their choices in life are severely limited by the fact that they find simple social interactions highly distressing, or those who are so aggressive that they regularly come into violent conflict with others, ought to be offered personality-enhancing drugs if, on balance, these might improve their lives. However, traits like shyness and aggression are manifested in people to varying degrees, with correspondingly various effects on the way the person in question lives their life. The extent to which an intervention that, say, enabled someone who feels mild unease in unfamiliar social situations to become the life and soul of the party is an improvement or the reverse is difficult to assess, since there is no obvious sense in which a shy person is "better" than a confident one, or vice versa. This difficulty is compounded by the possibility that what the subject views—*qua* subject—as an improvement may not coincide with what those who interact with him or her judge to be an improvement: the sort of intervention described above may make the subject feel more confident and comfortable in certain situations, but others may find the resulting person less pleasant to interact with. (Alcohol can have the effect of making shy people more confident, yet most sober people interact with other sober people in preference to people in possession of Dutch courage.) Also complicating assessments about what counts as an improvement is the distinction between improvements in some particular dimension (happiness, confidence, and so on) and improvements in life generally. It is, other things equal, preferable to experience states like happiness, satisfaction, and love than states like sadness, frustration, and grief; yet experiencing undesirable states can improve our understanding of ourselves and others, and give our personalities a richness and depth that they might lack were we only ever to experience "positive" emotions.

In order to decide what changes in a person's mood or personality count as improvements, then, we must confront questions like: By what standard do we assess improvements or the reverse in cases where a person's mood or personality does not have a seriously adverse effect on their life? Is it even plausible to claim that there could be such a standard? If so, what is the best guide to what the standard is and how it applies in a particular case: the opinion of the subject, the opinions of those who interact with the subject, or something else? The importance of addressing such questions does not entail that mood and personality enhancement is impossible or inadvisable; but a certain amount of philosophical reflection and analysis is required if we are to gain genuine benefits from such technology. This need for philosophical reflection is not unique to questions relating to enhancement, but pervades everyday life. When making decisions like whether to change careers, end a long-term personal relationship, or have another cream cake, we must at least implicitly ask ourselves questions about how our decision will affect our lives, whether the benefits it brings are of the right sort given our ambitions and goals, and whether we can do without the benefits and opportunities that our decision would close off to us.

Despite these difficulties, there are many changes in mood or personality that seem, quite straightforwardly, to be improvements. Listening to a piece of inspiring music, discovering that one has an hour longer than expected in bed before the alarm sounds, and eating an excellent dinner can all lift one's spirits. An unexpected act of kindness from a stranger can lead one to resolve to be more considerate to others. Or, one may spontaneously decide to forgive an old adversary and unburden oneself of long-held anger and resentment. Most would agree that such changes are improvements: they are enjoyable to experience, they make us more pleasant for others to interact with, and they are the sort of changes that, in their small ways, make one's life go better. If we could bring about such changes using drugs, shouldn't they uncontroversially count as enhancements of mood or personality?

Even those who agree that such changes are improvements may object to the use of drugs in order to achieve them. Leon Kass expresses such a line of thought:

> In most of our ordinary efforts at self-improvement, either by practice or training or study, we sense the relation between our doings and the resulting improvement, between the means used and the end sought. There is an experiential and intelligible connection between means and ends; we can see how confronting fearful things might eventually enable us to cope with our fears. We can see how curbing our appetites produces self-command. ... In contrast, biomedical interventions act directly on the human body and bring about their effects on a subject who is not merely passive but who plays no role at all. He can at best *feel* their effects *without understanding their meaning in human terms*.[23]

By improving oneself using drugs, then, one forgoes a valuable aspect of improving oneself via more conventional means. Is this a good reason to forgo enhancement?

Well, even if we concede that certain means of achieving an improvement can add value to the end state, the end state may have value independently of the means by which it is achieved, meaning that bringing about the end state using less valuable means is better than not bringing it about at all. To use one of Kass's examples, whilst attaining an increased level of self-command may gain additional value if it is brought about by curbing one's appetites, the end state—a mastery of self-command—has value even if it is brought about using drugs. Moreover, we do not generally feel ourselves obliged always to wring as much value as possible from the process of achieving a valuable end state: we may catch a bus to get somewhere even though we recognize that there is additional value to be gained from jogging instead, or we may employ a gardener to cultivate a garden even though we recognize that there is additional value to be gained from doing it ourselves. Since, in general, we are often content to achieve a valuable end state without using the most value-adding means, additional argument is required to support the claim that the practice of improving our capacities using drugs should be subject to different standards.

One important complex of questions about the use of pharmaceutical means to influence mood and personality concerns the idea of authenticity. Kramer spent a large fraction of his book struggling with the reports of some of his patients, who claimed that Prozac had helped them to find their "true self," enabling them to be the person they really were. They identified with their on-drug persona and viewed their earlier "natural" state as a long-lasting aberration, an alien condition that they had never been able to escape. It seems possible that in some cases the use of drugs can help a person live *more* authentically. At the same time, however, we can conceive of cases in which drug-induced emotions would undermine authenticity. Sometimes it seems important that our emotions respond to life events in appropriate ways. We may want to be the kind of person who would feel deep sadness at the loss of a loved one; and if the loss should occur, we may want to experience grief. A person who used pills to disconnect her emotional life completely from what happened to her and to the people she cared about could plausibly be said to have disabled a very important part of her humanity.

Mood and personality enhancement technology, then, has the potential to make a considerable positive impact on our lives; but it is important that those who intend to make use of such technology engage with the difficult philosophical questions that surround it.

Cognitive Enhancement

There are many ways in which we try to enhance our cognitive capacities; that is, those capacities that we use for gaining, processing, storing, and retrieving information. Language, education, mastery of psychological techniques, drinking coffee or energy drinks, meditation, exercise, sleep, and taking herbal or vitamin supplements can all play a part in improving various aspects of our cognitive performance. Moreover, none of these methods of enhancement is controversial, and some—notably the acquisition of language, and education—are considered so central to living even a minimally successful life that to deny our children adequate access to them would be deemed seriously negligent.

In addition to these familiar methods, a number of novel possibilities for cognitive enhancement have emerged in recent years.[24] For example, modafinil, a drug originally used to treat narcolepsy, has memory-enhancing as well as alertness-enhancing effects.[25] Ritalin, developed to treat attention-deficit hyperactivity disorder, can improve concentration in healthy adults.[26] Transcranial magnetic stimulation (TMS) may improve some forms of motor learning.[27] Variations in some genes in humans have been shown to account for up to 5% of memory performance,[28] raising the possibility of cognition-enhancing genetic interventions in the future. Supplementation of a mother's diet during late pregnancy and three months post-partum with long-chained fatty acids has been shown to improve cognitive performance in children.[29] Given the diverse means by which we try to improve our cognitive performance for various purposes today, we can expect many to be excited by the opportunities that such novel technologies offer to improve our lives in ways previously unavailable to us. What ethical issues surround the possibility of cognitive enhancement?

Many ethical issues are familiar from our discussion of other types of enhancement. For example, enhanced intelligence, attention, and so on are – to some extent – positional goods, since they give the enhanced an advantage over others when competing for such things as places at university and certain types of job. In this respect, cognitive enhancement raises the same concerns about "arms races" as physical enhancement; and the ways of addressing these concerns are similar to those discussed earlier. However, improvements in cognitive capacities could have instrumental and intrinsic value that is far greater than that of improved physical capacities. Being able to think better would equip us to solve important political and social problems, make scientific breakthroughs, and so on; and various studies indicate that more intelligent people earn more,[30] are less likely to suffer a range of social and economic misfortunes,[31] and are healthier.[32] Moreover, being able to understand other people, appreciate great literature, make plans, be creative, and remember one's own past are non-instrumentally important for human flourishing.

Also familiar from our discussion of physical enhancement is the question of whether using such enhancement in certain contexts constitutes cheating. Just as using drugs to enhance one's strength is seen as cheating in professional sport, using drugs to improve one's memory in order to perform better in an examination could be seen as cheating. Analogous with the case of doping, whether cognitive enhancement is deemed unacceptable in the context of education depends on what we value about education, and what its "rules" are. For example, if education is primarily a competition for grades, then enhancement may be viewed as cheating if some people did not have access to it, or if its use contravened the rules. If, on the other hand, the value of education consists in equipping students with skills and knowledge that will improve their own lives and society generally, then cognitive enhancement could play an important role in education.

The medical forms of cognitive enhancement that are immediately on the horizon are likely to yield at best small to moderate improvements in memory, concentration, mental energy, and some other cognition-relevant attributes. We can speculate about radical improvements in cognitive ability that might become possible in the more distant future. Such extreme enhancements would raise some unique ethical issues that do not arise in the same way for other human enhancements. In particular, people with radically enhanced cognitive capacities might gain vast advantages in terms of income, strategic planning, and the ability to influence others; in other words, an enhanced cognitive elite may gain socially significant amounts of power.

This raises the worry, described by the geneticist Lee Silver,[33] that the enhanced, having gained cognitive abilities that far outstrip those of the unenhanced, could band together and use their superior skills to dominate and exploit the unenhanced. If the cognitive enhancements in question were brought about through germline genetic intervention, the resulting improvements could be inherited by the children of the enhanced, with successive improvements eventually resulting in the enhanced forming a new species that may prove a threat to unenhanced humans.

That enhancement might result in such a two-tier society may be rather far-fetched, however. First, biomedical cognitive enhancements tend to have the greatest benefits for those who start from a low level of cognitive functioning.[34] Intuitively this is unsurprising, since it is usually easier to correct some specific deficit that is impeding a brain's performance than to take a well-calibrated, highly-efficient neural system and boost its performance still further. As a result, far from being socially divisive, cognitive enhancement could potentially increase equality in society by enabling those with lower cognitive ability to function at a level that is closer to those with naturally high cognitive ability. Second, if people are free to pick and choose which enhancements they undergo, it is highly unlikely that society will split cleanly into two disjoint groups, the enhanced and the unenhanced. More likely, society will consist of a continuum of differently modified people, ranging from the unenhanced, through those who have undergone a small amount of enhancement, to those who have undergone major enhancement. This new spectrum of differences would be superimposed on the existing range of native capacities, educations, experiences, privileges, and unique situational advantages that already causes people to display widely varying cognitive skills. Third, we already live in a society that contains diverse groups of people who could potentially come into conflict, but often do not: short people and tall ones, males and females, healthy and sick, educated and uneducated, and so on. The existence of diverse groups in a well-functioning society does not entail that those who make up one side of the division have cause to unite and oppose everyone else. On the contrary, many believe that diversity in society can be enriching for all.[35]

Another worry is that the possibilities offered by cognitive enhancement might lead us to view those people with below-average cognitive ability as diseased, rather than as part of the normal human spectrum of abilities. In 2003, the Nobel Prize-winning biologist, James Watson, caused controversy when he suggested in a television documentary that there might come a time when we can "cure" stupidity:

> If you really are stupid, I would call that a disease. The lower ten percent who really have difficulty, even in elementary school, what's the cause of it? A lot of people would like to say, "Well, poverty, things like that." It probably isn't. So I'd like to get rid of that, to help the lower ten percent.[36]

Whilst abrasively formulated, Watson's claim raises some important issues about the treatment of people of very low intelligence. For example, whilst Watson's "lower ten percent" may have most to gain from cognitive enhancement—in that improved cognitive functioning could better equip them to participate fully in modern society—they may also be less likely than more intelligent, better informed people to pursue the possibilities that enhancement could offer them; unless, perhaps, the possibility of such enhancement is suggested to them by a doctor. This is much more likely to happen if their low intelligence is recognized as a medical disorder. In addition, included in this group of people will be those whose cognitive functioning falls so far below the average that society deems them incapable of making certain important life decisions—such as where to live and what to do with their lives—which must instead be delegated to a carer. Cognitive enhancement could enable these people to gain autonomy over their own lives; however, given their impaired cognitive abilities, it is probable that they would be deemed incapable of consenting to receive enhancing treatment. Is it right that they should be forced to forgo treatment that could give them the sort of independence that the majority of us enjoy?

That enhancing treatment should be withheld from severely cognitively-impaired people might be seen as a consequence of our current way of thinking about medicine. According to this way of thinking, it is acceptable to treat a severely cognitively-impaired person for conditions recognized as diseases or injuries, such as cancer or a broken leg, despite the fact that he or she is incapable of giving consent. Generally, we believe that such treatment is acceptable because it is in the person's best interests; whereas leaving them untreated would be contrary to their best interests. On the other hand, it is not clear that an avoidable enhancement, such as a facelift, would be in their best interests. Since very low intelligence, like having facial wrinkles, is not universally recognised as a disease state, it is questionable on the current medical model whether it serves the best interests of a cognitively-impaired person to undergo cognitive enhancement treatment.

This medical model, according to which treatment for disease is seen as necessary whereas enhancement is seen as gratuitous, is arguably outdated. To begin, we saw earlier that there are many problems associated with holding that the distinction between therapy and enhancement is practically or morally significant. In addition to this, it has been argued that decisions about what would make people's lives go best—and also, therefore, what is in their best interests—should be guided not by whether a treatment will cure a disease or heal an injury, but by whether it will increase well-being. Savulescu tells us that, "[i]t is not [disease] which is important. People often trade length of life for non-health related well-being. Non-disease [states] may prevent us from leading the best life."[37] On this view, we might conclude that, since it is acceptable to treat diseases or injuries in those who are unable to give consent, it is also acceptable to treat non-disease states in such people if the treatment would increase well-being, provided that the level of well-being we expect them to achieve is not likely to be outweighed by any stress or risks associated with the treatment. Moving away from a model that associates medical treatment with disease would enable cognitively-impaired people to receive enhancing treatment without committing ourselves to the view that such people are diseased. (It could also give these people the cognitive capacities needed to make an autonomous decision about whether they want to retain these capacities or go back to their earlier impaired state.)

Despite this argument for shifting the focus of medicine away from the treatment of disease and towards the promotion of well-being, the current system of licensing medicines exerts a pull in the opposite direction. This system was created to deal with traditional medicine, which aims to prevent, detect, cure, or mitigate diseases. In this framework, there is no room for enhancing medicine. For example, drug companies could find it difficult to get regulatory approval for a pharmaceutical whose sole use is to improve cognitive functioning in the healthy population. To date, every pharmaceutical on the market that offers some potential cognitive enhancement effect was developed to treat some specific disease condition (such as ADHD, narcolepsy, and Alzheimer's disease). The enhancing effects of these drugs in healthy subjects is a serendipitous unintended effect. As a result, pharmaceutical companies, instead of aiming directly at enhancements for healthy people, must work indirectly by demonstrating that their drugs are effective in treating some recognized disease. One perverse effect of this incentive structure is the medicalization and "pathologization" of conditions that were previously regarded as part of the normal human spectrum. If a significant fraction of the population could obtain certain benefits from drugs that improve concentration, for example, it is currently necessary to categorize this segment of people as having some disease in order for the drug to be approved and prescribed to those who could benefit from it. It is not enough that people would like to be able to concentrate better when they work; they must be stamped as suffering from attention-deficit hyperactivity disorder: a condition now estimated to affect between 3 and 5% of school-age children (a higher proportion among boys) in the US. This medicalization of arguably normal human characteristics not only stigmatizes enhancers, it also limits access to enhancing treatments: unless people are diagnosed with a condition whose treatment requires a certain enhancing drug, those who wish to use the drug for its enhancing effects are reliant on finding a sympathetic physician willing to prescribe it (or finding other means of procurement). This creates inequities in access, since those with high social capital and the relevant information are more likely to gain access to enhancement than others.

In conclusion, whilst cognitive enhancement offers real benefits, not least to those who currently lack sufficient cognitive skills to exert autonomy over their own lives, it also highlights aspects of our current medical model that need to be updated and revised. Doing so in the way that we have described would help ensure fair and equal access to enhancement, and would also help speed progress in enhancement technology by allowing pharmaceutical companies to focus on developing enhancements without also having to ensure that they can be used to treat a recognized pathogenic condition.

Selecting the Best Children

As well as helping us to improve our existing capacities, enhancement technology could also help ensure that future generations are genetically disposed to be smarter, healthier, and happier than those who have come before.

There are several ways of doing this, many of which are familiar and accepted. Most obviously, we are free to choose our sexual partners, which plays a major role in determining the genetic composition of our children. Pregnant mothers can take folic acid supplements which, whilst not affecting the genetic composition of the child, can affect the epigenetic expression of their genes. Young girls receive inoculations against rubella in order to avoid the risk of later giving birth to a child with brain damage and other problems associated with congenital rubella syndrome.

On the other hand, there are some novel and ethically controversial methods of ensuring that a child will be born with a certain genetic composition. First, there is pre-implantation genetic diagnosis (PGD). This is a technique that allows doctors to determine the sex of an embryo and its genetic disposition to diseases such as cystic fibrosis and hemophilia. Current UK legislation allows individuals with a family history of an inherited disease to select for implantation embryos found not to possess the disease gene, as part of their *in vitro* fertilization (IVF) treatment; and in Australia PGD has been used to enable couples without a history of sex-linked disorders to select the sex of their child.[38] In the future, it may become possible to use PGD to select for implantation embryos that are not only free from inherited disease, but which also contain genes likely to give rise to high intelligence, sporting prowess, musical ability, above-average height, and so on. Such selection, however, will have only weak enhancing effects, since typically there is a small number of embryos from one couple to choose from, and most desirable traits are highly polygenetic.

More effective in producing embryos with the right sort of genes would be ensuring that their biological parents have the appropriate high capacities. Human mating preferences have evolved to discriminate on the basis of traits that in our environment of evolutionary adaptation correlated with fitness. While few people are interested in overriding their natural romantic inclinations in order to achieve some conscious eugenic purpose, the issue does arise in a more plausible way for infertile couples who are reliant on donor gametes and who might have the option of selecting the source of these gametes. This opportunity has been exploited by eugenicists, without much success, as Sandel tells us:

> The Repository for Germinal Choice, one of America's first sperm banks, was…opened by Robert Graham, a philanthropist dedicated to improving the world's "germ plasm" and counteracting the rise of "retrograde humans". His plan was to collect the sperm of Nobel Prize-winning scientists and make it available to women of high intelligence, in hopes of breeding supersmart babies. But Graham had trouble persuading Nobel laureates to donate their sperm…and so settled for sperm from young scientists of high promise. His sperm bank closed in 1999.[39]

Despite these difficulties, the practice of buying gametes from donors is fairly popular, most famously in the United States, where there is no legal cap on the financial compensation that donors can receive.[40] Agencies that specialize in making donated gametes available to buyers typically target couples or single parents who wish to conceive by matching a donated gamete to one of their own, using either IVF followed by implantation of donated eggs into the female parent or a surrogate, or insemination at home or in a clinic.[41] Those wishing to buy gametes can expect to pay a premium if the donor has certain features, such as an Ivy League education.[42]

Another way of creating children of a certain genetic quality is to manipulate the genetic material of the embryo to attempt to ensure the presence or absence of certain traits in the resulting child. This sort of intervention is novel and risky, and it is currently permitted in the UK only to treat children or adults with life-threatening diseases or disorders, and by intervening only in their somatic cells (so-called "gene therapy"). In the future, it may become possible to use this technique on the germline cells of embryos, to affect a range of heritable traits not associated with disease.

Is there anything wrong with using any of these techniques to produce children with desirable qualities? Well, we might worry that some of these techniques harm the embryos. In the case of PGD, for every embryo that is selected for implantation, at least one (or, more likely, several) will be discarded, never to be allowed to develop. For those who believe that the moral status of embryos is on a par with that of fully developed humans, this amounts to murder, or at least to letting-die. The moral status of the embryo is a hotly debated topic in bioethics, and one that we do not have the space to address here. However, it is worth mentioning that, even where PGD does not take place, IVF treatment involves discarding embryos. As a result, those who do not find IVF treatment morally objectionable cannot consistently raise this objection in relation to PGD. Those who do object to IVF treatment because it involves discarding embryos should note that over half of embryos produced by sexual intercourse fail to develop; so those who object to IVF must (in the absence of an argument to show why the two cases are relevantly different) also object to unmediated procreation.

The possibility of genetic manipulation of embryos raises different issues about harm. First, there is a risk that such manipulation will have unintended effects, resulting in a child who is worse off than he or she would have been had no such intervention occurred. For this reason, it may be wise to avoid using this technology until it is advanced enough for us to be sure that the expected benefits outweigh the risks. Second, even disregarding such risks, Jürgen Habermas argues that genetic manipulation infringes the freedom of the resulting child in a way that ordinary parenting does not. Parents currently exert control over their children via the communicative, linguistic "medium of reasons," meaning that "the adolescents in principle still have the opportunity to respond to and retroactively break away from it."[43] On the other hand,

> in the case of a genetic determination carried out according to the parents' own preferences, there is no such opportunity. With genetic enhancement, there is no communicative scope for the projected child to be addressed as a second person and to be involved in a communication process. From the adolescent's perspective, an instrumental determination cannot, like a pathogenic socialisation process, be revised by "critical reappraisal." It does not permit the adolescent looking back on the prenatal intervention to engage in a revisionary learning process.

Because of this, a child whose genetic traits have been selected by his parents is denied the opportunity of being "the undivided author of his own life."[44]

Habermas's objection to prenatal interventions that do not involve the child in a communicative process, however, also applies to many practices not generally considered controversial and often considered sensible or potentially beneficial, such as taking folic acid supplements, eating healthily, and abstaining from taking drugs during pregnancy. Moreover, it is impossible completely to avoid non-communicative interventions: the environment in which very young children are raised literally shapes their nervous system in ways that they cannot later undo. Language-learning is one such process that cannot be undone; and it is, in addition, a necessary condition for entering the "medium of reasons" that surrounds what Habermas takes to be more acceptable means of controlling children.

Habermas's concern about autonomy is also misplaced. Genetic factors—along with many other influences—affect what we are able to achieve in life regardless of whether our genes have been specially selected for us. A child whose genes have been specially chosen is, therefore, no less free or autonomous than a child born with whatever genetic constitution happened to result from their conception. On the contrary, a child who, as a result of genetic manipulation, is born with improvements in capacities such as intelligence and general health is likely to enjoy more rather than less autonomy, in the sense that they will be better equipped to realize the plans and ambitions they devise for their life. As a last resort, however, we can note that a child who grows up to resent having had features like increased intelligence and better health selected for them by their parents is free to destroy their effects, for example by ingesting poisons. That it is difficult to conceive of a rational person wanting to do such a thing underlines how implausible it is to maintain that having such selected traits is unconditionally disadvantageous.

Disregarding the issue of harm to the embryo or the resulting child, some believe that there is something sinister about the very desire to create people of a certain genetic quality. Sandel, for example, believes that the desire to "remake nature, including human nature, to serve our purposes and satisfy our desires" fails to exemplify, "and may even destroy…an appreciation of the gifted character of human powers and achievements."[45] In the case of parents who wish to shape the genetic constitution of their child, Sandel believes that the desire for a child of a certain genetic quality is incompatible with the special type of love that parents have for their children. This is because "[t]o appreciate children as gifts is to accept them as they come, not as objects of our design or products of our will or instruments of our ambition."[46]

Sandel's critique of genetic engineering is not convincing, however. It is far from obvious that genetic engineering would destroy our appreciation of life or our sense of children as gifts. Sandel cites no data in support of his claim that parents would love their children less for failing to "accept them as they come"; and intuitively, as Nick Bostrom has commented, it seems plausible that "[s]ome mothers and fathers might find it easier to love a child who, thanks to enhancements, is bright, beautiful, healthy, and happy."[47] In addition, we already attempt to influence the features of our children in many ways that are universally accepted to be compatible with good, loving parenting. We attempt to improve their literacy skills by encouraging them to read. We try to develop their team spirit and social skills by encouraging them to take part in games and sport. We instil discipline and shape their behavior by using punishments and rewards. Between Sandel's extremes of accepting children as they come and viewing them as objects of our design, then, there is plenty of room for affecting the sort of people our children will become without undermining our love for them. Ensuring that children have the genes to help them do well in life, providing that we do so with their best interests at heart, plausibly falls within this acceptable middle ground.

That we need to keep the child's best interests in mind when selecting traits for him or her is an important point. On the one hand, people benefit from being more intelligent, healthier, having good social skills, and so on. It is plausible to suggest that, if we have the capability to ensure that our children are genetically disposed to have such traits, then it is desirable to make use of this capability, since doing so will benefit our children. Julian Savulescu defends a principle of "procreative beneficence," which states that IVF parents-to-be who are offered PGD to screen their multiple embryos for genetic predispositions to disease and non-disease states are morally obliged to select that child who can be expected to have the best life. For example, if they have a choice of implanting one of two embryos which are genetically identical except in that only one of them is genetically predisposed to high intelligence, the parents-to-be are morally obliged to select that embryo over the other, since a more intelligent child is likely to have a better life than a less intelligent one, other things being equal.[48]

When we use PGD to select between embryos, our choices determine which of several possible persons will come into existence. By contrast, when we genetically manipulate an embryo, we need not be determining which person will come into existence; instead our interventions affect what sort of person this embryo will develop into and what capacities she or he will have. This distinction may make an ethical difference. For example, one could hold that if an embryo with a genetic predisposition to a disability is selected for implantation, this is permissible because nobody is harmed. The embryo may grow into a person with a disability, but since this person would not otherwise have existed, they cannot be said to have been harmed by our action—at least if we assume that she or he will have a life worth living. If, however, we genetically manipulate a healthy embryo by inserting a disability-causing gene, say a gene causing blindness, then we could be accused of having harmed somebody. We have caused a particular person, who would otherwise have been able to see, to be blind. Arguably, such an act is as seriously wrong as it is to blind an infant. Even if one accepts Savulescu's principle of procreative beneficence, one might still hold (what may be termed a "person-affecting" moral principle) that the degree of moral wrongdoing is greater if we harm some person than if we merely fail to select for existence the possible child whom we expect would have the best life.

We also need to bear in mind that what may be an ethically innocuous choice for a person to make for themself—which career to pursue, whether to drink alcohol, whether to undergo a cosmetic surgery procedure—may not be ethically innocuous if a person chooses to impose it on someone else. That such choices may not be ethically innocuous has partly to do with our beliefs about personal autonomy and the having the freedom to make certain choices about one's own life; but these considerations do not apply in the case of an embryo, which does not yet have the capacity for autonomy or free choice. Instead, we can think of such choices in terms of the extent to which they are likely to improve one's life, or to be in one's best interests. A person can make a choice for themself which is likely to improve their life; but the same choice, imposed on someone else, may not improve their life, and may even have a negative effect. This is because some choices, such as the decision to pursue a career as an investment banker, are desirable for a person only in the context of their background beliefs, desires, and values, and in the context of a certain culture. Becoming an investment banker may be desirable for someone who is interested in banking; who sees a high salary as sufficient compensation for long, stressful working hours; who values the prestige associated with rising through the ranks of a successful corporation; and so on. In the absence of the appropriate context, however, such a choice is not desirable: not everyone would enjoy a career as an investment banker, and becoming one would close off certain other, more desirable choices that could have been made instead.

We should bear this in mind when selecting traits for our children. Certain traits that we would find beneficial if we had them ourselves may not be beneficial for our children. In addition, certain traits that we value today may not be valuable in the cultural context of the future. Jonathan Glover comments that "John Mackie once said to me that if human genetic engineering had been available in Victorian times, people might have designed their children to be patriotic and pious."[49] Patriotism and piety may have been valued traits in Victorian times, but they are much less valued today; at least in societies like the UK. Fluctuations in such values may be fickle, and just as we may judge it unfair of parents to push their children down a particular career path, we may also judge it unfair of them to impose their own values and preferences on their children. For this reason, when intervening in the genetic composition of a future child, the best interests of the child are more likely to be served if parents restrict themselves to shaping characteristics that are likely to benefit the child regardless of his or her eventual preferences and values, and regardless of their cultural context. Characteristics such as intelligence, happiness, and health are more likely to serve this end than characteristics like piety, competitiveness, and sporting prowess.

Another source of unease about genetic intervention are the perceived parallels between current discussions of enhancement and the coercive eugenics programs of the last century, and the idea that enhancement may foster beliefs about some people being fundamentally inferior to others (this latter concern is sometimes expressed as the concern that enhancement would undermine human dignity). Advocating enhancement, however, has no necessary link with coercive eugenics, nor with the belief that some people are fundamentally inferior to others. To address the concern about coercive eugenics first, the state-sponsored eugenics programs of the last century were objectionable because they harmed people, either by killing them or by curtailing their freedom to reproduce. Eugenics need not be coercive, exploitative, or harmful: in Cyprus, a non-coercive state-sponsored program to eliminate thalassemia has been in operation for over 20 years, and is widely supported by Cypriots. Prospective parents are tested for the disease gene, but are free to reproduce if they wish; and state-funded abortions are available if prenatal testing reveals the fetus to be predisposed to the disease.[50] The sort of genetic enhancement that we have discussed in this section would be even further removed from state intervention,[51] being available to people to make use of or not as they pleased.[52]

The concern that this sort of enhancement would undermine human dignity—by which we here mean the basis for the moral status of human beings[53]—can take more than one form. On the one hand, Fukuyama, following Silver, worries that enhancement could undermine the dignity of the unenhanced, since the enhanced could lay claim to more human rights than the unenhanced on account of their advanced capacities.[54] On the other hand, Kass worries that enhancement could rob the *enhanced* of dignity: he comments that "[t]o turn a man into a cockroach—as we don't need

Kafka to show us—would be dehumanizing. To try to turn a man into more than a man might be so as well."[55] We could respond at length to concerns that enhancement raises about the issue of human dignity (indeed, one of us already has); but in brief, it is helpful to bear in mind that, whilst having certain traits—for example, rationality and a capacity for moral action—are often judged to be constitutive of what it is to be human, our moral status is not generally held to fluctuate with our capacities in the way that seems to worry some bioconservatives. Various individuals can possess very different capacities and yet be equal in moral status. For example, whilst those who are well educated, athletic, musically gifted, or witty may have individual capacities that are superior to those who are uneducated, unfit, musically untalented, or dull, we should not infer that the moral status, or dignity, of the former group of people is thereby either superior or inferior to that of the latter. We might even say that the very idea of humans having equal dignity has its roots in a desire to prevent the stronger, more intelligent, and more powerful—that is, those with certain superior capacities—from dominating and exploiting the more vulnerable. Therefore, if we accept that all human persons who have not benefited from enhancements have the same moral status, despite their widely varying capacities, it is hard to see any justification for according a different moral status to enhanced individuals or for thinking that the existence of enhanced individuals could affect the moral status of the unenhanced.

In the light of these considerations, we conclude that there are no compelling reasons to resist the use of genetic intervention to select the best children. There are, however, important issues relating to the fact that such intervention would involve the selection of traits of a person who has no say in the matter, and for this reason it is of paramount importance to consider at all times the best interests and future welfare of the resulting children.

Notes

1   Kaplan *et al.* (2000); Godesky (2005).

2   World Factbook (2006).

3   Oeppen and Vaupel (2002).

4   Roger *et al.* (2012).

5   Kass (2003).

6   Williams (1973).

7   Williams, writing in 1973, was considering a fictional elixir rather than the sort of treatments that some scientists now see as offering real possibilities for radical life extension in the foreseeable future.

8   Or worth extending. For those who do not believe the distinction between therapy and enhancement to be morally significant, these amount to the same thing.

9   John Harris made this point in the third of his Princeton Lectures, on March 16, 2006 at the University of Oxford's James Martin World Forum 2006.

10   Population Reference Bureau (2005).

11   Martin *et al.* (2004), p. 2.

12   Nordhaus (2005).

13   http://www.wada-ama.org/en/dynamic.ch2?page Category.id=254#.

14   "Chemically Enhanced," *Financial Times*, February 10, 2006.

15   Savulescu, Foddy and Clayton make this point in Savulescu *et al.* (2004).

16   WADA Athlete Guide, third edition, p. 4.

17   Savulescu *et al.* (2004), p. 666.

18   Savulescu *et al.* (2004), pp. 666–667.

19   The way in which such categories are defined may be arbitrary to some extent. For example, Savulescu *et al.* tell us that "[b]lack Africans do better at short distance events because of biologically superior

muscle type and bone structure," yet athletes are not categorized according to their race. If we are serious about grouping competitors according to biological categories, perhaps we ought to have a separate category for black Africans. That the current way of categorizing sports competitors may not be the ideal one, however, does not undermine the general point that the expected biological potential of competitors is relevant to our evaluation of their achievements.

20 It might be deemed prudent to permit such drugs on other grounds. For example, if it would be difficult to detect whether an athlete has used a drug, it might be best to permit it so as to avoid rampant cheating.

21 Sandel (2004), p. 10.

22 Kramer (1993).

23 Kass (2003), p. 22.

24 For a more in-depth survey of cognitive enhancement and its ethical issues than is given here, see Nick Bostrom and Anders Sandberg (2009).

25 Muller *et al.* (2004).

26 Elliott *et al.* (1997).

27 Cf. for example, Pascual-Leone *et al.* (1999).

28 Quervain and Papassotiropoulos (2006).

29 Helland *et al.* (2003).

30 Salkever (1995).

31 Gottfredson (1997, 2004).

32 Whalley and Deary (2001).

33 Lee Silver (1998).

34 Cf., for example, Randall *et al.* (2005) and Muller *et al.* (2004).

35 The possibility of truly extreme forms of cognitive enhancement – such as ones involving the creation of vastly superhumanly intelligent machines – does raise special risks and ethical challenges, which we do not discuss in this chapter.

36 *DNA*, Channel 4, March 8, 2003.

37 Savulescu (2001), p. 419.

38 Savulescu (1999).

39 Sandel (2004), p. 8.

40 In the UK, donors may only claim "reasonable expenses": cf. HFEA's "FAQs for Donors" (http://www.hfea.gov.uk/cps/rde/xchg/SID-3F57D79B-0E626297/hfea/hs.xsl/1205.html).

41 Hundreds of such agencies exist. See, for example, http://www.pacrepro.com/index.htm and http://www.tinytreasuresagency.com.

42 Many US student newspapers regularly run advertisements offering thousands of dollars for donated gametes. The market for donor eggs seems to be more lucrative than that for donor sperm, perhaps because the process of extracting eggs is lengthy, laborious, and invasive whilst donor sperm can be produced quickly and painlessly.

43 Jürgen Habermas (2003), p. 62.

44 Habermas (2003), p. 63.

45 Sandel (2004), p. 5.

46 Sandel (2004), p. 6.

47 Nick Bostrom (2003), p. 498.

48 Savulescu (2001). Whilst Savulescu discusses PGD specifically, we can imagine a more general principle that applies to other means of ensuring that one's children are born with those features likely to give them the best life, such as genetic manipulation of the embryo.

49 Jonathan Glover (2006), p. 98. He made the same point in his earlier *What Sort of People Should There Be?* (Glover, 1984), in which he discussed ethical issues relating to genetic intervention before much of the technology and techniques we are familiar with today became possible.

50 Lila Guterman, (2003).

51 Save perhaps for some state-imposed restrictions to prevent parents from severely compromising the best interests of their children in choosing their traits—for example, by choosing to have a child with a disability. Such a choice was made in 2002 by lesbian couple Sharon Duchesneau and Candy McCullough, who used donated sperm from a deaf friend to have a deaf baby. Jonathan Glover discusses the ethical implications of this in chapter 1 of *Choosing Children* (Glover, 2006) as do Julian Savulescu and Guy Kahane in "The moral obligation to create children with the best chance of the best life" (Savulescu and Kahane, 2009).

52 For a defence of the right of parents to choose their children's features, see Nicholas Agar (2004). For an argument against the selection of traits, and its historical link to coercive eugenics, see Daniel J. Kevles (2001).

53 The definition of human dignity as the basis for moral status is not the only way to explicate the concept of dignity, but the only one we will consider here. For a more in-depth discussion of the concept of human dignity in relation to enhancement, see Bostrom (2005, 2007).

54 Francis Fukuyama (2002), chapter 9.

55 Kass, (2003), p. 20.

References and Further Reading

Agar, N. (2004) *Liberal Eugenics: In Defence of Human Enhancement*. London: Blackwell.

American Psychological Association (http://www.apa.org).

Bostrom, N. (2003) Human genetic enhancements: a transhumanist perspective. *Journal of Value Enquiry* 37: 493–506 (http://www.nickbostrom.com/ethics/genetic.pdf).

Bostrom, N. (2005) In defence of posthuman dignity. *Bioethics* 19: 202–14 (http://www.nickbostrom.com/ethics/dignity.pdf).

Bostrom, N. (2008) *Dignity and Enhancement*. Washington, DC: President's Council on Bioethics (available at: www.nickbostrom.com/ethics/dignity-enhancement.pdf).

Bostrom, N. and Sandberg, A. (2009) Cognitive enhancement: methods, ethics, regulatory challenges. *Science and Engineering Ethics* 15: 311–41. (http://www.nickbostrom.com/cognitive.pdf).

Elliott, R., Sahakian, B.J., Matthews, K., *et al.* (1997) Effects of methylphenidate on spatial working memory and planning in healthy young adults. *Psychopharmacology* 131: 196–206.

Fukuyama, F. (2002) *Our Posthuman Future*. New York: Farrar, Straus & Giroux.

Glover, J. (1984) *What Sort of People Should There Be?* Harmondsworth: Penguin.

Glover, J. (2006) *Choosing Children: The Ethical Dilemmas of Genetic Intervention*. Oxford: OUP.

Gottfredson, L.S. (1997) Why G matters: the complexity of everyday life. *Intelligence* 24: 79–132.

Gottfredson, L.S. (2004) Life, death, and intelligence. *Journal of Cognitive Education and Psychology* 4: 23–46.

Guterman, L. (2003) Choosing eugenics. *The Chronicle of Higher Education* (May 2).

Habermas, J. (2003) *The Future of Human Nature*. Cambridge: Polity.

Helland, I.B., Smith, L., *et al.* (2003) Maternal supplementation with very-long-chain N-3 fatty acids during pregnancy and lactation augments children's IQ at 4 years of age. *Pediatrics* 111: 39–44.

Human Fertilization and Embryology Authority (http://hfea.gov.uk).

Kaplan, H. Hill, K., Lancaster, J., and Hurtado, A.M. (2000) A theory of human life history evolution: diet, intelligence, and longevity. *Evolutionary Anthropology* 9: 156–185.

Kass, L.R. (2003) Ageless bodies, happy souls: biotechnology and the pursuit of perfection. *The New Atlantis* Spring: 9–28.

Kevles, D.J. (2001) *In the Name of Eugenics: Genetics and the Uses of Human Heredity*. Cambridge, MA: Harvard University Press.

Kramer, P. (1993) *Listening to Prozac*. New York: Penguin.

Martin, J. A. *et al.* (2004) "Births: final data for 2002." *CDC National Vital Statistics Reports*, 52/10 (2003, revised 2004).

Muller, U. Steffenhagen, N., *et al.* (2004) "Effects of modafinil on working memory processes in humans. *Psychopharmacology* 177: 161–9.

Nordhaus, W.D. (2005) "Irving Fisher and the contribution of improved longevity to living standards. *The American Journal of Economics and Sociology* 64: 367–92.

Oeppen, J. and Vaupel, J.W. (2002) Broken limits to life expectancy. *Science* 296: 1029–31.

Owen, D. (2006) Chemically enhanced. *Financial Times* (February 10).

Pascual-Leone, A., Tarazona, F., *et al.* (1999) Transcranial magnetic stimulation and neuroplasticity. *Neuropsychologica* 37: 207–17.

Population Reference Bureau (2005) 2005 World Population Data Sheet (http://www.prb.org/pdf05/05WorldDataSheet_Eng.pdf).

Quervain, D.J.F. and Papassotiropoulos, A. (2006) Identification of a genetic cluster influencing memory performance and hippocampal activity in humans. *Proceedings of the National Academy of Sciences of the United States of America* 103: 4270–4.

Randall, D.C., Shneerson, J.M., and File, S.E. (2005) Cognitive effects of modafinil in student volunteers may depend on IQ. *Pharmacology Biochemistry & Behavior* 82: 133–9.

Roger, V.L., Go, A.S., Lloyd-Jones, D.M, *et al.* (2012) Heart disease and stroke statistics—2012 update. *Circulation* 125: e2–e220.

Salkever, D.S. (1995) Updated estimates of earnings benefits from reduced exposure of children to environmental lead. *Environmental Research* 70: 1–6.

Sandel, M.J. (2004) The case against perfection. *The Atlantic Monthly* April: 1–11.

Savulescu, J. (1999) Sex selection—the case for. *Medical Journal of Australia* 171: 373–5.

Savulescu, J. (2001) Procreative beneficence: why we should select the best children. *Bioethics* 15/5/6: 413–26.

Savulescu, J., Foddy, B. and Clayton, M. (2004) Why we should allow performance enhancing drugs in sport. *British Journal of Sports Medicine* 38: 666–70.

Savulescu, J. and Kahane, G. (2009) The moral obligation to create children with the best chance of the best life. *Bioethics* 23: 274–90.

Silver, L.M. (1998) *Remaking Eden: Cloning and Beyond in a Brave New World*. New York: Avon.

WADA Athlete Guide, third edition (http://www.wada-ama.org/rtecontent/document/WADA_Athlete-Guide_ENG.pdf).

Whalley, L.J. and Deary, I.J. (2001) Longitudinal cohort study of childhood IQ and survival up to age 76. *British Medical Journal* 322: 819–22.

Williams, B. (1973) *The Makropulos Case: reflections on the tedium of immortality. In: Problems of the Self*. Cambridge: Cambridge University Press.

World Factbook (2006) (https://www.cia.gov/cia/publications/factbook/index.html).

Limitations on Scientific Research

Michael Boylan

A perennial question that arises concerning the relationship between scientific research and society is whether there should be any limitations on scientific research and if so, what are the justifications and how far do those limits extend? Over the years such prohibitions have included sanctions against dissection of cadavers, invasive surgery, and the introduction of X-rays. From a modern perspective these prohibitions seem mistaken. In the twenty-first century increasingly we are bombarded by new biomedical technologies that confront us almost on a monthly basis. Most controversial among these are: (a) scientific research trials (particularly pharmaceutical studies) that seem to offer hope for medical treatment but at the possible cost of ethically devaluing the participants, and (b) protocols that would affect the germ line of humans, animals, and plants such that we may be in the process of altering life on earth in a significant way.

We, by our actions as humans, may become one of the most significant variables in how species on our planet evolve from here on out. This is an awesome responsibility. Are we up to the task? This is the question on most people's minds as they open the morning newspaper, listen to the radio, watch television, scan the home page of their web browser, or absorb the latest tweet. How should we think about such discoveries? If we're uncomfortable, is this just a sign of intransigent, Luddite stodginess? Is our future mission on this planet one that mirrors the television show, "Star Trek:" to go forth (without restraint) and seek out new truths (civilizations) and to boldly go where no man has gone before?

In order to get a handle on how to think about this conceptual model, let us begin our interdisciplinary excursion by examining the very limits of science itself. In order to achieve a perspective on the possible ethical restraints on new science, most of this essay will cite examples in the recent history of science in order to make its point. A few contemporary examples will then be brought forward in order to match them against the derived ethical principles. The structure of our short exploration will revolve around a foundational concept called the Principle of Plenitude. This concept is fundamental to our value-directed exploration of the work of science.

The Principle of Plenitude

Many readers will be familiar with the principle of plenitude as discussed by Arthur O. Lovejoy in his classic work, *The Great Chain of Being* (Lovejoy, 1936).[1] Lovejoy intended a kind of "possibility implies normative assent" thesis. This translates to "what can be known should be known." When one applies this to the scientific realm, it rings almost like religious dogma. "Whatever can be known about the physical world should be known."

I once quizzed some scientist colleagues at the US National Institutes of Health (a national research center in biomedical research) about this principle and could not find a single objector to the proposition.

Who could argue with such a thesis? There have been some. In the seventeenth century it was an issue of contention. John Milton expresses this view in *Paradise Lost*:

> Heaven is for thee too high
> To know what passes there; be lowly wise:
> Think only what concerns thee and thy being.
> Milton, *Paradise Lost*, Bk 8, ll. 172–4

The seventeenth century was the age of scientific revolution. Entire paradigms of thinking were altering.[2] As in all changes there is an "upside" and a "downside." Some of the upside had to do with more accurate scientific theories, which had greatly expanded explanatory power. From Galileo to Newton the century was alive with discovery.

The downside had to do with the social unrest, which may have been a consequence of challenging established authority. The English Civil War and increased turbulence on the Continent are only two examples of what may be attributable to social unrest. The age of the magisterium of the Roman and English Catholic/Anglican Churches was matched by a corresponding emphasis upon the individual.[3] John Locke wrote about individual human rights that were logically prior to those that the State chose to recognize. The seeds of the American and French Revolutions were sown here.

Now many would say that such movements were very positive in the grand scope of things. They may have been. But there was much that was lost as well. Rapid change tends to reward first those opportunists who have established themselves in the vanguard. The ordinary people are often left in an onerous holding pattern (which may be worse than it was before) as things adjust.

The Limits of Science

It is characteristic of many scientists that they are consciously or unconsciously blind to the possible consequences of their actions. Since the mission ("What can be known, should be known") dangles before their eyes, they often feel that whatever it takes to get there (the means) is justified by the lofty goal (the ends). Few moral theories will say that the ends *always* justify the means. Not even utilitarianism professes this in every case (since such an action creates a precedent that, itself, can have severe negative utility).[4]

It is entirely plausible that the thesis of plenitude is not always true. There may be instances in which we should refrain from exploring certain research strategies. These include: (i) instances in which the means of obtaining the scientific ends are immoral; and (ii) instances in which the ends themselves may clearly be seen to be involved in a larger context that is itself immoral.

Let us examine these in order. First, there is the instance of *immoral scientific means*. This, in turn comes in two varieties: relative immorality and immorality per se. In relative immorality one may not have the technological means to do something humanely at the moment, but "in principle" it may be possible in the future. An example of this is the observation of human organs as they function within a living organism. In ancient times the only means available to obtain this scientific end was vivisection. Celsus reports that vivisection was performed by Erasistratus and Herophilus upon condemned prisoners.[5] The explicit purpose of vivisection (the surgical exposure of the internal organs of a live person without anesthetics of any kind) was to learn more about how the human organs functioned. This scientific end is indeed a valuable one. Under the plenitude principle what can be known should be known, ergo let's cut up another poor soul!

Of course, vivisection is cruel and inhumane—even when performed on people condemned to death. This is because inflicting severe pain upon another human at will produces (from the recipient's point of view) gratuitous suffering. Inflicting gratuitous suffering upon any human, at will, is to fail to respect their dignity. This is because tied up with dignity is a fundamental sense of rights to primary basic goods of agency (food, clothing, shelter, and freedom from dehumanizing and degrading violence; Boylan and Brown, 2012, ch. 2). All humans have a claims right to the primary basic goods of agency.[6] Thus, to fail to provide another person with the primary basic goods of agency (when it is in your power to do so) or to deny another the primary basic goods of agency, is to fail to respect their human dignity. Since all people have a moral claims right to the primary basic goods of agency, then to deny another of their primary basic goods of agency is immoral. Therefore, since performing vivisection in ancient times was an instance of denying another the primary basic goods of agency, then vivisection was an instance of failing to respect human dignity and was thus immoral.

If performing vivisection is the only means of obtaining the scientific end, then that end should be forsworn. Scientists should decide that they will *not* pursue the end (contra to the principle of plenitude) because the only way that they can do so is to employ immoral means.

However, in this instance the immoral means are relative. That is, they are relative to a particular stage of scientific development. In Galen's time up until a little more than a century ago, it would have been impossible safely and humanely to surgically examine patients in order to understand the physiology of their organs. Once the technology progressed to the point where surgery could proceed without being cruel and inhumane (and thus failing to respect the human dignity of the subjects), then surgery could become a legitimate means of pursuing the end of physiological discovery.[7]

An example of a per se immoral means would revolve around cases in which the scientific end inextricably entails pain and suffering. For example, if a scientist wished to know the stages in which a disease killed people (in a controlled setting), then the means would necessarily require taking a group of humans inflicted with a fatal disease and watch them die without providing them with any real (available) cures or significant palliative care (such as they exist at some moment in time). This is because such "intervention" might skew the pure view of the disease's progression and the effects upon humans. The researcher distances herself or himself from the project and merely observes and records people in the various agonizing stages of death.

This scenario is not too far removed from the infamous Tuskegee experiment, in which patients infected with syphilis were not properly treated so that they might be observed in their pain and suffering.[8] The scientific end of understanding the "natural" progressions of a fatal disease among a large controlled sample group is a valuable one for advancing scientific knowledge. But it can only be achieved through immoral means. Thus, the scientists should have forsworn this research plan.[9]

Similar infamous research designs were carried out in Nazi Germany, Tojo's Japan, and Stalin's Soviet Union. In each case, scientific ends that *only* could be achieved by immoral means should have been avoided. This is yet another instance in which the principle of plenitude is flawed.

Henry Beecher also brought to the fore the Jewish Chronic Disease Hospital case in which patients without known relatives or advocates were subjected to blatant deception in order to engage in research on cancer and the mechanism of transplant rejection. These patients without advocates, who did not have cancer, were injected with live human cancer cells in order to view how the human body would react. Obviously, this put these patients at risk of getting cancer. This patent disregard for research subjects is reminiscent of the Tuskegee experiment (Beecher, 1966). Ezekiel Emanuel and Christine Grady show that the most egregious violations of research ethics occur under a worldview approach of *researcher paternalism*. Under this paradigm the "what can be known, should be known" approach is unchecked. Ergo, the immoral means are allowed to go forward. The authors suggest that a check on these immoral means can occur through a mix of regulatory protectionism, participant access, and community partnership. The result is some transparent accountability (Emanuel and Grady, 2006).

A final group in this category concerns scientific discovery in realms in which double-blind testing creates an unethical context. The most common examples in this category come from the pharmaceutical industry. A key instance of this is the testing of HIV/AIDS medication in Thailand and some other Third World countries. Problems occur when trial protocols give different at-risk groups various mixtures of the AZT medication—in order to see whether lower levels of the drug might still work so that the more affluent countries of the world might save money (Stolberg, 1997). Women were given progressively lower doses in order to discover whether the standard dosage could be lowered and still work. Trials were continued even when the research subjects showed clear deleterious effects that included advancement to full-blown AIDS and death. However, proponents say that this is the only way to be sure of the exact dosage necessary. The only way to get this exact information is to fail to recognize the dignity of research subjects, which is unethical (Jacobs, 2009). In this case the means to acquiring scientific knowledge are unethical and should not be pursued in this way.

A second breach of research ethics occurred when testing HIV/AIDS vaccines. In this case a sexually active population was chosen (also in Thailand and other Third

World countries). The trials were double blind. They were continued past the point when in-progress results were not sufficiently positive to continue in the face of the demonstrable negative medical side effects to study participants (Wehrwein and Morris, 1998; Lancet, 2005; Phanuphak, 2011) as well as probable negative social side effects (Milford *et al.*, 2007).

In addition to these problems, putting research populations at risk when there is an available treatment just because they are of a lower socioeconomic class or because they reside in a Third World country and thus have no standing in compensatory law suits, is also unethical on the same grounds (Tangcharoensathien *et al.*, 2001). However, the benchmark for medical certainty (0.05 of the null set) could not be achieved except by marginalizing these women. They were treated as "means only" for the sake of a standard of medical knowledge.

It is my contention that the use of these protocols is immoral. They disregard the dignity of the human research subject. All of these aforementioned examples are centered on HIV/AIDS vaccine trials in stages I, II, and III. The information necessary to create a vaccine for a world epidemic disease seems to involve unethical research methods if full double-blind testing is used as the model. Double-blind testing is the gold standard for medical research (if one wants to achieve the most reliable results). However, early testing of AZT in the United States used a rather more informal technique of clinical trial and error. The patient population was dying of AIDS. This group of patients would search for any hope and were ready to try an experimental drug. In this case the informal trial was successful. However, in the longer term this sort of research method in this context is more expensive and less reliable—because it yields less exact scientific knowledge. However, it is this author's opinion that ethics trumps efficiency. No scientific knowledge should be obtained via unethical means (Häyry *et al.*, 2007). Less exact knowledge procured ethically is to be preferred to more exact knowledge procured unethically. This is a key limitation on scientific knowledge.

There are those who contend that some of these ethical-means problems occur because of the different roles of physician and researcher. The argument goes as follows. The physician is an advocate for the patient. However, the scientific researcher has a different imperative that is not patient centered.

It is, in fact, probably a better situation that the physician and the biomedical researcher be separate. This is because their respective missions are not identical. Physicians are concerned with the well-being of the patient and in doing no harm. Their duty is to focus upon the patient and his or her recovery. Researchers are concerned with expanding our understanding of nature and benefiting humankind. This mission may lead them in a different direction. The mission of the physician is different. When the physician and researcher are one and the same person, a conflict of mission may occur.

However, I am not advocating an absolute prohibition against the physician and researcher being one and the same person, but merely pointing out that since the missions of each are different, potential conflicts may arise. For this reason, institutional review boards (IRBs) should take this into account using the following standard: it will be assumed, prima facie, that the researcher and attending physician will not be the same individual. One would need a compelling argument to get approval otherwise.

Obviously, this sanction would not apply to medical clinical research that is observational only: a physician reporting on his or her cases under the latitude of approved patient care. Because of this latitude, some modifications of care can be published as clinical research. It is only when the course of treatment becomes experimental (beyond the standard of approved patient care) that the two roles become controversial.

Conceptually, what stands behind this limitation on scientific research is that the means to some scientific truths are unethical. If, for example, one cannot know exactly *how* one dies from syphilis without setting up a situation in which individuals are allowed to go through all the stages of the disease to death (when there are effective treatments available), or how certain sorts of cancer spread (when there are effective treatments available), or how to create an HIV/AIDS vaccine without a placebo group who will die (when there are effective treatments available), then—if this is the only way to acquire such scientific information—such knowledge should be outside our ken. It can only be acquired by unethical means. It thus stands as an exception to the principle of plentitude.

The second category of exceptions to the principle of plentitude involves instances in which the ends themselves may clearly be seen to be involved in *a larger action or context that is* very risky to the public good to such an extent that it becomes *immoral*. This second category seeks to examine the character of the proposed end of the scientific principle being explored. Fundamental to the exploration of this second category is the admission that science does not exist in a vacuum. As much as many researchers might like to think of themselves as being in a protective cocoon of pure intellectual speculation, this is really a pernicious fantasy that often blinds scientists to the actual uses of their research.

In this category I will examine two cases: (i) the proposed protocols for germ-line secondary goods enhancement, and (ii) the development of the atomic bomb.

In the first case we are involved with possible protocols for germ-line genetic secondary goods enhancement. At first blush, it might seem like genetic enhancement might be a good thing. We could create a new species, *Homo melior*. These creatures could be the best possible of all genetically engineered hominoids. So who could possibly have a problem with this? Doesn't this sound like the perfect actualization of the principle of plentitude?

Although the promise of improving humans in a number of areas sounds very fine, the devil is in the details, and the details are not as optimistic. First, one must remember that there is a difference between *somatic treatment* in which genetic engineering will seek a treatment or cure when otherwise there is no hope, and *genetic enhancement* in which the germ line is altered in such a way as to affect future generations. When the risk factor is just a single individual, the stakes are different from risking countless future offspring (potentially all of humanity over time). In genetic enhancement there is a new context that is being created. This context could be very deleterious. The reason for this is that genetics is enormously complicated. For example, what was regarded as "junk DNA sequences" just a few years ago is now seen to have some mechanical functions (though they are not very well understood). There have also been a number of unforeseen consequences in recent years during genetic therapy that have resulted in outcomes worse than those of the underlying condition or traditional treatments—including death (Englund *et al.*, 2006; Bjorklund *et al.*, 2007; Tichelli *et al.*, 2008; Amariglio *et al.*, 2009; Cyranoski, 2010; Tuffs, 2010). If somatic genetic therapy is extremely risky, think of the extended unforeseen consequences when the germ line is affected. Each mistake will be multiplied many times over.

Despite the tight controls on genetic engineering for somatic treatment, the track record has not been sterling. The principle of precautionary reason would suggest in such a situation forgoing therapy except in otherwise hopeless situations until the level of science improves—a relative prohibition (Beyleveld and Pattinson, 2001). But genetic treatment or enhancement that would affect the germ line seems to this author as having enormous risk for unintended consequences. Is this just a case of science not being up to a possible new standard where all will be possible? Or is it a case of the three-ball problem in Newtonian physics (a conundrum with per se problems due to inherent complexity that can never be solved)? No one knows for sure. Because of this uncertainty, moving forward in this arena should merit special analysis. In order to think about this let us separate two sorts of enhancements: (i) those that are concerned with "knocking out" deleterious DNA base sequences that are responsible for genetically inherited diseases, and (ii) those that seek to improve the species by adding new capacities.

In the first case, we may be in the situation of a relative prohibition (such as the prohibition of the surgical study of physiology above). The model is analogous to vaccine inoculations. Though the track record for genetic therapy has not been the best, we can imagine a future in which some skill has been acquired so that we might be able to eliminate Tay–Sachs disease, for example. This is logically possible, and it fits into the historical mission of medicine. However, because of the immense complications involved, at the very least if we are governed by the principle of precautionary reason, then we have voluntarily imposed many limitations on the principle of plenitude. This means that we must proceed at a very slow pace that follows the highest standards of research ethics. It may be the case that we will never be competent enough to pull this off. It might be that we have a case of the "three-ball problem" in Newtonian mechanics. The use of "knock-out" strategies in genetic therapy (except as an experimental last hope at this juncture in history) should be avoided. We will move forward (if at all) on the robust informed consent of those who feel they have no other options.

The second form of enhancement does not seek to protect from future harm (much on the model of vaccine inoculations), rather it seeks to improve us to *Homo melior*. The strongest case against this is that it creates a context of typology (here understood as secondary goods).[10] We seek to create preferred *types* that represent the "perfect" person. This drive toward homogeneity is radically against the acceptance of diversity among peoples and against the viability of those who have various forms of disabilities (now defined as against the perfect phenotype). Will everyone have a certain facial construction, skin color, sexual orientation, and brain configuration (including values and tastes)? Such a social context would be radically against diversity (considered by biologists to be essential to evolution and by some ethicists to be a key element in social justice; Boylan, 2004, ch. 5). Therefore, genetic enhancement for the sake of improving the capabilities of the species (as opposed to knocking out deleterious genetic diseases) is a valid instance of a per se limitation on scientific knowledge.

The second case of a per se resultant immoral context concerns the research into weapons of mass destruction. In the United States, the former Soviet Union, and many smaller countries around the world there has been research into chemical and biological warfare (Cirincione et al., 2005; Spiers, 2010). Sometimes the country says to its scientists that they are investigating ways of deploying nerve gas or anthrax as a defense against such weapons that might be used against them. This is the ploy of many leaders: We only want to create an effective *defense*. No one wants to admit that they are engaged in anything that might be construed as *offensive*. When Nazi Germany invaded Poland it was on the pretext that they were responding to earlier injustices. Later conquests were likewise linked to past grievances that needed to be settled. Likewise, with so many other countries, the US invasion of Iraq, various conflicts in the Middle East, wars in south central Africa, unrest between Pakistan and India, among other—all of these were sold to their peoples as being somehow defensive.

Which leader, after all, is going to approach their people and say, "Today we are about to engage in a grand offensive land/property heist because I, as your leader, think it my manifest destiny to garner as much money and power as possible because that is my personal mission in life?"

A classic case that covers the essential elements in the weapons of mass destruction scientific paradigm is that of the Manhattan Project. If you were a scientist asked to head the atomic bomb project in the early 1940s, what *would* you say, and what *should* you say?

On the one hand, you might think that here is a chance to be funded to perform basic research that will alter how particle physicists understand the nature of matter. What a grand opportunity! We now have a chance to demonstrate that the very word "atom" (meaning in ancient Greek "uncuttable") is wrong. The atom can be split, and you are on a research team that will do it. This is a chance to extend the boundaries of science: to know whatever can be known (the principle of plenitude).

On the other hand, you might realize that this research is for the purpose of creating a bomb that can have no other purpose but to kill civilian non-combatants—in unthinkable numbers.[11] This bomb is so devastating that it could never be used in accordance with the recognized "rules of war" that assert that armies only attack armies. Non-combatants and civilians are not fair game in the rules of war. But since the atomic bomb's effects were so pervasive, it would not be possible to deploy it without violating these rules of war. Whenever it was used, it would be a weapon of mass destruction. As such, it would be a vehicle of killing that would redefine warfare. The way warfare would be redefined is through the inclusion of mass killing of civilians on a scale that the world has never known before. What this means is this:

1. Warfare is morally justified only on the principle of generalized self-defense— Assertion.
2. Self-defense is defined as committing minimal effective force against an aggressor to protect oneself—Fact.
3. In the case of war, the aggressor consists of the attacking army and/or those civilians actively engaged in fabricating armaments—Assertion.
4. Warfare only morally justifies the killing of combatant soldiers in the army and/ or those civilians actively engaged in fabricating armaments—1–3.
5. Civilians living in the countries engaged in war are (except for armament workers) materially separated from the act of aggression—Assertion.

6. Anyone materially separated from an act of generalized aggression is to be considered innocent—Fact.
7. Civilians living in the countries engaged in war are (except for armament workers) morally innocent—5,6.
8. *Murder is defined as the killing of an innocent without just cause—Fact.*
9. The killing of soldiers or civilians engaged in armament fabrication can be morally justified in a defensive war, but the killing of other civilians is murder—4,7,8.[12]

The practical end of the Manhattan Project was to create a weapon of mass destruction. A weapon of mass destruction will necessitate the deaths of thousands of innocent civilians. This entails that the practical end of the Manhattan Project was murder (according to the argument set out above). Is being a part of the Manhattan Project as a contributing physicist something that *you*, as a scientist, should accept? You may pretend that you do not see the real end, but it is there nonetheless. One possible reason a scientist might blind himself or herself to this intersubstitution of ends in the causal chain is because the scientist may view the proposition as opaque. However, this does not wash because we are not talking about mere substitution of terms, but of logical relationships that exist when anyone enters a causal process.[13] This point can be illustrated by the following example. If Mary is an accountant for a pharmaceutical company (that is adulterating its products with impotent fillers in order to make more money), and if Mary knows this (or could have reasonably figured it out), then she cannot throw up her hands and claim innocence when someone dies from taking the medication. She cannot say that all she was doing was keeping the books according to the highest standards of accounting practice and that one cannot connect her to the ultimate end because the context is opaque. No; Mary is responsible for understanding that she acts in a context and bears some responsibility for the reasonably foreseeable outcomes of that context. If the end leads to a foreseeable immoral outcome, then scientists should not join. On this line of analysis (instances in which the ends themselves may clearly be seen to be involved in a larger action that is, itself, immoral), no scientist should have signed on to the Manhattan Project (or other like projects that had immoral ultimate ends). Following this line of argument, the second limit of science is not to participate in research projects that will or probably will create an immoral context in their implementation.

There are, however, two rejoinders to my argument:

A. What if the immoral ends are less immoral than some other end?
B. What if an individual joined the project that had an immoral end with the purpose of sabotaging it?

Both of these suggestions are challenging. Let us address each in order. The first suggestion is that there are gradations of unethical conduct. If one were to do x (where x is an unethical action), then x might be *less* unethical than some other consequence, y. In this situation, one might be confronted with a dilemma situation (meaning that without any prior wrongdoing on the agent's part he or she might be put in the situation in which they must perform an unethical action). If one holds that dilemma situations can occur, then performing the lesser of two evils may be the most moral alternative. In order to enter this style of reasoning we have to consider all lives as equally at risk: combatants and non-combatants. Under standard accounts of just war theory combatants in war are fair game while non-combatants are not. But under this rejoinder, that sort of reasoning is rejected.

Returning to our example, if creating an atomic bomb that will kill more than 300 000 people,[14] is compared to a land invasion that will mean the aggregate deaths of two million people, then (if human life is additive) it would be better to drop the atomic bomb than to attempt a land invasion.

This style of analysis is highly dependent upon a consequentialist calculation that ignores the distinction between combatants and non-combatants. It assumes that the rightness or wrongness of any given human action depends upon the net result of utility consequences as seen over a reasonable time period (Boylan, 2009, ch. 12). Some would see this as an instance of the Trolley Problem. In the Trolley Problem one is asked whether it is more ethical to kill a fewer number of people than a greater number of people.[15] This speaks to the question of whether human life is additive or whether it is not. If human life is additive (and if the additive assumptions are correct, viz., that non-combatants and combatants are to be viewed as equally viable military targets), then clearly dropping the atomic bomb is morally justified. But if human life is not additive (meaning that it is just as horrific to kill one immorally as to kill ten immorally) or if there is a hard and fast distinction between combatants and non-combatants, then there are no moral criteria to justify dropping the atomic bomb.

One might effectively ask whether any scientist recruited at the beginning of the Manhattan Project would have the sort of information that President Franklin Roosevelt cum President Harry Truman did when Truman made the executive order to drop the bombs. For all these scientists might have known, the death toll could have been in the tens of millions. All they knew was that they were engaged in the creation of weapon of mass destruction. How many people might be murdered or killed in violation of the rules of war was entirely unclear. Also, it is unclear how many soldiers would have been killed if the United States had adopted another strategy. In 2001 during a faculty ethics seminar I co-ran, one participant was a former general in the Air Force who said that she had studied a US military-generated account of an alternate strategy of setting an extended siege and conventional bombing campaign against military targets in natural-resource-poor Japan before setting forth on a land invasion. The number of American soldiers to be killed under this strategy was less than 100 000—far fewer (even under the aggregative strategy) than with dropping the two atomic bombs.[16]

Thus, if even the best argument for the development and deployment of the atomic bomb is suspect, the scientists must have seen what they were doing as either an instrument of very shocking evil or else as part of a marginal call (at best). Be this as it may, the first rebuttal against the sanction of scientists on the Manhattan Project would be one of consequential comparative advantage.

The second rebuttal centers around a person who joined the project with the purpose of sabotaging it (at least from the most evil excesses). This sort of "fifth column" approach works like this. Mr X is invited to be a part of the Manhattan Project. He knows that though the proximate guise of the project is to extend basic research in physics, the ultimate goal is the creation of a weapon of mass destruction.

Mr X believes that the creation of a weapon of mass destruction is an immoral ultimate goal. But he also realizes that if he checks out of the project, there will be many others who are anxious for admittance. These others may be morally blind to what they are doing. They may be so wrapped up in the proximate ends of advancing fundamental knowledge in physics (the principle of plenitude) that they do not contemplate the implications of what they are ultimately doing (viz., creating a weapon of mass destruction). Because of this moral blindness, such scientists may allow the worst possible scenarios to occur. If the team contains at least a few people of good faith (i.e., ethical scientists who are sensitive to how their research is being put to use), then it is possible that—even if bad politicians try to misuse the atomic bomb—the scientists of good faith (members of the fifth column) might be there to sabotage the process.

The fifth column approach has been occasionally used in the political sphere. In one prominent case, Dietrich Bonhoeffer (a Protestant Christian theologian) pretended to be a Nazi in order to join a plot to kill Adolf Hitler. Unfortunately for Bonhoeffer, the plot failed and Bonhoeffer was executed (Bonhoeffer, 1997; Bethge and Barnett, 2000).

The problem with the fifth column approach is that (at least in the short run) a person participates in and supports a system that has an immoral end. Because of this the saboteur is in the position of having to defend that which is really evil. He or she works and helps bring about evil. And if they, like Bonhoeffer, are unsuccessful in their act of sabotage, then the net effect of their action is actually to have promoted evil.

This can be particularly troubling in cases in which there is a significant resistance movement that has taken it as their mission to work *outside* the system in order to bring about its demise. If the resistance movements are almost effective, but need just a few more committed individuals, then the fifth column advocates deny the resistance fighters their point of critical mass In the Manhattan Project, J. Robert Oppenheimer might be called a fence-sitting fifth column advocate. Oppenheimer forever felt some conflict about his role as scientist and as a man of conscience who might engage in a fifth column effort to abort the project (Oppenheimer, 1989).

This author would say that there may be situations in which the strategy of the fifth column may seem to be the only way to overturn the immoral system (or research program). But it is a highly risky tactic that has many inherent drawbacks.

In the contemporary context, some of these principles can be readily applied. For example, instances of relative immoral ends might include the cloning of whole humans. Because the present (2013) state of cloning of whole organisms is so crude, it would be immoral to saddle an infant with the probability of a quick and painful death simply to satisfy the principle of plentitude. It is possible that some time in the future this approach will be perfected on other animals such that the application to humans no longer poses such risks. In this event, cloning may simply be another (albeit very costly) option for infertile couples or single women. This is a case of "relatively" immoral ends that are relative when measured against our current state of knowledge.

When one envisions the cloning of another person (generally a twin of a sibling needing a vital organ) merely as a means of saving a brother or sister when that sacrifice entails the cloned donor's own death, then we are engaged in a per se immoral end. If we all agree to the principle that all people count equally, then to bring a new person into the world solely to harvest his or her organs for the sake of a sibling is to fail to respect the donor's basic rights. Just as in the Tuskegee case, the end is absolutely immoral and therefore should not be pursued. Protocols that seek to explore this sort of organ transplant strategy ought not be pursued.

In conclusion, though the principle of plenitude is very alluring because it appeals to the mind's eternal quest for knowledge, it is not conclusive. There are moral constraints upon the quest for scientific knowledge. These include (i) instances in which the means of obtaining the scientific ends are immoral; and (ii) instances in which the ends themselves may clearly be seen to be involved in a larger context that is, itself, immoral. Both of these situations dictate that scientists should take the advice of Odysseus, who ordered his men to stop their ears with beeswax and bind him to the mast of the ship as they passed the region of the Sirens. Odysseus knew that knowledge had its limits and though he was compelled to listen to the melody, he took precautions against his ability to act.[17] Odysseus knew that there are limits to the principle of plenitude. Modern scientists must also learn this lesson.

Notes

1 My exposition of the principle of plenitude is not meant to be a faithful representation of Lovejoy's intent in his expression of the principle. Rather, I am taking his principle and applying it to the issue of how scientists view their mission in their activity in the context of Lovejoy's principle.

2 There has been much written about scientific revolutions. One starting point is with Thomas Kuhn (1962). Two prominent critiques of Kuhn's notions are by Imre Lakatos and Alan Musgrave (1970) and Karl Popper (1965, pp. 232 ff).

3 The rise of individualism and its corresponding corollaries (such as the depiction of private property) has been documented by Matthew H. Kramer (1997).

4 Unless one is an extreme act utilitarian.

5 "Herophilus and Erasistratus acted in by far the best way: they cut open living men—those who were condemned criminals released by the king for such purposes. These prisoners were observed while they still breathed: their body parts previously hidden were now exposed…to cut open a living man is cruel and unnecessary, but to cut open the dead is essential for medical students" (Celsus, 1915, *Prooemium* 23, 74 [my trans.]).

6 The word "primary" here denotes one subclass of the basic goods of agency. The primary goods of agency are universal and can be defined scientifically according to the parameters of human necessity. For example, humans generally die when their core temperature drops below a certain temperature for a given interval. Humans also, for the most part, die when they do not receive x calories per kilogram of bodyweight. Likewise, humans generally lose their ability to maintain mental health when they are subject to y amount of gratuitous violence and fear. All of these can (within certain ranges) be defined for all humanity. A second level of basic goods is relative to each society. These are the goods necessary to be an effective agent within that society. For example, in the United States today it is hard to be an effective agent without a certain level of education and the protection of basic human rights (including the right not to be used as a means only). For more discussion on this see Boylan (2004) and Boylan (2011).

7 Of course, as further advances in technology have occurred, investigators have been able to use even less invasive techniques so that patient risk has dropped substantially. This is always important, since risk to patient health is a relative snapshot of the state-of-the-art that researchers should always strive to improve.

8 Two contemporary discussions of the Tuskegee experiment that fill out the horrific details are those of James Howard Jones (1993) and Susan Reverby and James H. Jones (2000).

9　There are, unfortunately, many such examples. The United States asked military personnel to act as guinea pigs during atomic bomb testing in order to determine the effect of radiation upon unprotected human subjects. This was an inhumane and immoral action comparable to the vivisection cases discussed earlier. Similar atrocities have been committed against citizens of many different countries who have tested biological and chemical warfare agents upon their own citizens.

10　Secondary goods are those goods that are less necessary for basic human action than are other sorts of goods. For a discussion of this see Boylan (2004) and Boylan (2011).

11　This is because the atomic bomb is not a *target bomb*. It cannot be used surgically against a particular target, but instead is broad in its effects, killing and destroying everything within a given radius.

12　This argument depends upon an understanding of traditional just war theory. For a survey of some important issues at stake see Walzer (1977), Miller (1991), Coates (1997), Kamm (2004), McMahan (2004), Rodin (2004), Coady (2004), and Miller (2009).

13　Most philosophers consider the work of Willard Van Orman Quine to be pioneering with respect to opaque contexts. Basically, an opaque context is created when a construction resists the substitutivity of identity. Quine uses the example: (1) "'Tully was a Roman' is trochaic." (1) is a true proposition. Now Tully is identical to Cicero, so it would seem as if

you could create the proposition (2) "'Cicero was a Roman' is trochaic." But (2) is false since "Cicero" is a dactyl. For a more complete discussion see Willard Quine (1960, pp. 141 ff).

14　According to the *Encyclopedia Americana* (1995) the number of people killed at Hiroshima was 271 000 and at Nagasaki 71 000. For further background on this devastation see Hershey (1989), Lifton and Mitchell (1996), and Selden and Selden (1997).

15　The situation of the Trolley Problem is this: you are the engineer of a trolley and the trolley has gotten almost out of control. You cannot stop your trolley. You are approaching Lincoln Junction. On the right track is a school bus filled with children. On the left track is a homeless person whose poorly fitting shoes have caught in the track. As the engineer, you have the choice of moving your lethal train from the right track to the left. This is your only choice. What do you do? Is there an ethical justification for your choice?

16　The numbers of civilian Japanese casualties would have been miniscule. Even including the deaths of Japanese combatants, this strategy would have killed the fewest number of people. Yet, few know about this option.

17　Of course there are some who believe that the sin of Odysseus was thirst for knowledge. Alfred Lord Tennyson frames his poem "Ulysses" upon the thesis that the lack of self-control toward the acquisition of new knowledge was the cause of Ulysses' long journey home.

References

Amariglio, N., Hirshberg, A., Scheithauer, B.W., *et al.* (2009) Donor-derived brain tumor following neural stem cell transplantation in an ataxia telangiectasia patient. *PLoS Medicine* 6(2): 1000029.

Beecher, H. (1966) Ethics and clinical research. *New England Journal of Medicine* 274: 1354–60.

Bethge, E. and Barnett, V.J. (eds) (2000) *Dietrich Bonhoeffer: A Biography*. Philadelphia: Fortress Press.

Beyleveld, D. and Pattinson, S. (2001) Precautionary reason as a link to moral action. In: M. Boylan (ed.), *Medical Ethics*. Upper Saddle River, NJ: Prentice Hall; pp. 39–52.

Bjorklund, A., Aschan, J., Labopin, M., *et al.* (2007) Risk factors for fatal infectious complications developing late after allogeneic stem cell transplantation. *Bone Marrow Transplantation* 40(11): 1055–62.

Bonhoeffer, D. (1997) *Letters and Papers from Prison* (ed. E. Bethge). New York: Macmillan.

Boylan, M. (2004) *A Just Society*. Lanham, MD, and Oxford: Rowman & Littlefield.

Boylan, M. (2009) *Basic Ethics*, 2nd edn. Upper Saddle River, NJ: Prentice Hall.

Boylan, M. (2011) *Morality and Global Justice*. Boulder, CO: Westview.

Boylan, M. and Brown, K.E. (2012) *Genetic Engineering: Science and Ethics on the New Frontier*, 2nd edn. Oxford: Wiley-Blackwell.

Celsus (1915) *Prooemium*. In *De Medicina* (ed. F. Marx). Leipzig: Teubner.

Cirincione, J., Wolfisthel, J.B., and Raikuman, M. (2005) *Deadly Arsenals: Nuclear, Biological, and Chemical Threats* (revised edn). Washington, DC: The Carnegie Endowment for Peace.

Coady, C.A.J. (2004) Terrorism, morality, and supreme emergency. *Ethics* 114(4): 772–89.

Coates, A.J. (1997) *The Ethics of War*. Manchester, UK: University of Manchester Press.

Cyranoski, D. (2010) Strange lesions after stem-cell therapy. *Nature* 465: 997.

Emanuel, E.J. and Grady, C. (2006) Four paradigms of clinical research oversight. *Cambridge Quarterly of Healthcare Ethics* 16: 82–96.

Encyclopedia Americana (1995) Danbury, CT: Grolier.

Englund, J.A., Boeckh, M., Kuypers, J., *et al.* (2006) Brief communication: fatal human metapneumovirus infection in stem-cell transplant recipients. *Annals of Internal Medicine* 144: 344–9.

Häyry, H., Takala, T., and Herissone-Kelly, P. (2007) *Ethics in Biomedical Medical Research: International Perspectives*. Amsterdam: Rodopi; pp. 1–6.

Hershey, J. (1989) *Hiroshima*. New York: Vintage.

Jacobs, A.J. (2009) *The Guinea Pig Diaries*. New York: Simon and Schuster.

Jones, J.H. (1993) *Bad Blood, The Tuskegee Syphilis Experiment*. New York: Free Press.

Kamm, F.M. (2004) Failures of just war theory. *Ethics* 114: 650–92.

Kramer, M.H. (1997) *John Locke and the Origins of Private Property: Philosophical Explorations of Individualism, Community and Equality*, Cambridge: Cambridge University Press.

Kuhn, T. (1962) *The Structure of Scientific Revolutions*. Chicago: University of Chicago Press.

Lakatos, I. and Musgrave, A. (eds) (1970) *Criticism and the Growth of Knowledge*. Cambridge: Cambridge University Press.

Lancet (2005) The trials of tenofovir trials. *Lancet* 365: 1111.

Lifton, R.J. and Mitchell, G. (1996) *Hiroshima in America: A Half Century of Denial*. New York: Avon.

Lovejoy, A.O. (1936) *The Great Chain of Being*. Cambridge, MA: Harvard University Press.

McMahan, J. (2004) The ethics of killing in war. *Ethics* 114: 693–733.

Milford, C., Barsdorf, N., and Kafaar, Z. (2007) What should South African HIV vaccine trials do about social harms? *AIDS Care* 19: 1110–17.

Miller, R.B. (1991) *Interpretations of Conflict: Ethics, Pacifism, and the Just War Tradition*. Chicago: University of Chicago Press.

Miller, S. (2009) *Terrorism and Counterterrorism*. Malden, MA, and Oxford: Blackwell.

Oppenheimer, J.R. (1989) *Atom and Void: Essays on Science and Community*. Princeton, NJ: Princeton University Press.

Phanuphak, P. (2011) Ethical issues in studies in Thailand of the vertical transmission of HIV. *New England Journal of Medicine* 338: 834–5.

Popper, K. (1965) *Conjectures and Refutations: The Growth of Scientific Knowledge*. New York: Harper & Row.

Quine, W.v.O. (1960) *Word and Object*. Cambridge, MA: MIT Press.

Reverby, S. and Jones, J.H. (eds) (2000) *Tuskegee's Truths: Rethinking the Tuskegee Syphilis Study*. Chapel Hill, NC: University of North Carolina Press.

Rodin, D. (2004) Terrorism without intention. *Ethics* 114: 752–71.

Selden, K. and Selden, M. (eds) (1997) *The Atomic Bomb: Voices from Hiroshima*. Armonk, NY: M.E. Sharpe.

Spiers, E.M. (2010) *A History of Chemical and Biological Weapons*. London: Reaktion.

Stolberg, S.G. (1997) U.S. AIDS research abroad sets off outcry over ethics. *New York Times* (Sept. 18), A 32–3.

Tangcharoensathien, V., Phoolcharoen, W., Pitayarangsarit, S., *et al.* (2001) The potential demand for an AIDS vaccine in Thailand. *Health Policy* 57: 111–39.

Tichelli, A., Bhatia, S., and Socié, G. (2008) Cardiac and cardiovascular consequences after haematopoietic stem cell transplantation. *British Journal of Haematology* 142: 11–26.

Tuffs, A. (2010) Stem cell treatment in Germany is under scrutiny after death of 18 month old child. *British Medical Journal* 341: 960.

Walzer, M. (1977) *Just and Unjust Wars*. New York: Basic Books.

Wehrwein, P. and Morris, K. (1998) HIV-1-vaccine-trial go-ahead reawakens ethics debate. *Lancet* 351: 1789.

Evaluating a Case Study
Applying Ethical Issues

You are finally at the last stage of the process of evaluating case studies. By this point, you have (a) chosen a practical ethical viewpoint (including the choice of an ethical theory and practical linking principles, whose point of view you will adopt), (b) listed professional and ethical issues, and (c) annotated the issues lists by examining how imbedded each issue is to the essential nature of the case at hand. What remains is the ability to come to an action decision once these three steps have been completed. The final step is to discuss your conclusions.

To do this, you must enter an argumentative phase. In this phase, I suggest that you create brainstorming sheets headed by the possible courses of action open to you. Prepare an argument on each sheet to support that particular course of action utilizing the annotated charts you have already prepared. Then compare what you believe to be the pivotal issues that drive each argument. Use your chosen ethical theory to decide which issue is most compelling. Be prepared to defend your outcomes/action recommendation.

Let us return to the case of contraception in the less-developed countries. As you may recall, the case was as follows.[1] You are a regional director at the World Health Organization. One of your duties is to supervise the distribution of birth control devices to less-developed countries. The product of choice has been the intrauterine device (IUD), which has proved to be effective and inexpensive.

The problem is that in the United States, several hundred users of the IUD have contracted pelvic inflammatory infections that have been linked to use of the IUD.

As regional director, you must decide whether to continue to supply IUDs to women in less-developed countries.

Remember that in this case, the professional practice and the ethical issues were both deeply imbedded, which creates an intractable conflict; there is no simple way to justify one instead of the other.

What you must do is (a) consult your worldview and see what it dictates that you do, and (b) consult the ethical theory of your deepest convictions and see what it would dictate that you do. Is there a synonymy between these? If not, then engage in a dialogue between your worldview and the professional practice. Let each inform on the other. In the end, you should be able to come to some resolution.

One step in this direction is to examine the arguments that support each. What are the critical premises in these arguments?[2] In any argument, there is a conclusion. If you want to contrast two arguments, you must begin by contrasting two conclusions. Conclusions are supported by premises that (logically) cause the acceptance of the conclusion. Therefore, what you must do is to create at least two arguments that entail different conclusions. To do this, create brainstorming lists on the *key issue(s)* involved in the argument. The key issue is that concept that makes the difference. This case has a number of key issues. Let us try to construct arguments that are both for and against the position.

Sample "Pro" Brainstorming Sheet for the Position

Position to be supported. Continue to sell IUDs in less-developed countries.

Key Thoughts on the Subject

1. As a public health professional, you are enjoined to benefit the greatest number of people possible in your health policy.
2. It is a fact that in less-developed countries, millions die of starvation each year. The simple cause of starvation is too many people for the available food. When you decrease the number of people (given a level food source), more people can eat.
3. There are "blips" to any project. In this case, it is a few hundred or so cases of pelvic inflammatory infection. These casualties pale when compared to the number who will benefit from continuing to provide IUDs.
4. Utilitarian ethical theory dictates that the general good supersedes any individual's good.
5. In less-developed countries, the general good is advanced by continuing to distribute IUDs since more people (by far) benefit than are hurt.

Argument

1. In countries that have a limited amount of food that would feed only a certain population (n), increases in population ($n + x$), will result in x not having enough food to live—fact.
2. Many less-developed countries experience the condition mentioned in premise 1—assertion.
3. In many less-developed countries, x increase in population will result in x number of people starving to death—1,2.
4. Many children who are born are not planned—assertion.
5. If one subtracts the number of unplanned births from the total birth rate, the number of births decreases significantly—assertion.
6. If all children were planned, the number (more than x) of births would decrease significantly—assertion.
7. If all children were planned, less-developed countries would not experience starvation (given constant crop production)—3–6.
8. The IUD is the most effective birth control device in the less-developed countries—assertion.
9. The imperative of professional conduct in public health is to help as many people as possible—fact.
10. Public health professional standards dictate that the IUD should be provided to women in less-developed countries—7, 8.

11. The IUD poses potential health risks to some women (less than 5 percent)—fact.
12. The ethical imperative of Utilitarianism dictates that the right ethical decision is to advance the cause of the common good—fact.
13. Distributing IUDs helps more people in less-developed countries than it hurts—fact.
14. Utilitarianism dictates that the IUD should be provided to women in less-developed countries—11–13.
15. The regional director must continue the distribution of IUDs to less-developed countries—10, 14.

Sample "Con" Brainstorming Sheet Against the Position

Position to be supported. Stop selling IUDs in less-developed countries.

Key Thoughts on the Subject

1. As a public health professional, you are enjoined to benefit the greatest number of people possible in your health policy.
2. It is a fact that in less-developed countries, millions die of starvation each year. The simple cause of starvation is too many people for the available food. When you decrease the number of people (given a level food source), more people can eat.
3. There are "blips" to any project. In this case, it is a few hundred or so cases of pelvic inflammatory infection. These casualties pale when compared to the number who will benefit from continuing to provide IUDs.
4. Human life is precious. No amount of practical gain that can weigh against one human life.
5. Ends do not justify the means. One may have a very good end in mind, but unless the means to that end are just, the end cannot be willed.

Argument

1. In countries that have a limited amount of food that would feed only a certain population (n), increases in population ($n + x$) will result in x not having enough food to live—fact.
2. Many less-developed countries describe the conditions mentioned in premise 1—assertion.
3. In many less-developed countries, x increase in population will result in x number of people starving to death—1, 2.
4. Many children who are born are not planned—assertion.
5. If one subtracts the number of unplanned births from the total birth rate, the number of births decreases significantly—assertion.
6. If all children were planned, the number (more than x) of births would decrease significantly—assertion.
7. If all children were planned, less-developed countries would not experience starvation (given constant crop production)—3–6.

8. The IUD is the most effective birth control device in less-developed countries—assertion.
9. The imperative of professional conduct in public health is to help as many people as possible—fact.
10. Public health professional standards dictate that the IUD should be provided to women in less-developed countries—7,8.
11. The IUD poses potential health risks to some women (less than 5 percent)—fact.
12. The ethical imperative of Deontology dictates that knowingly jeopardizing the essential health of any person is absolutely impermissible no matter what the practical advantage—assertion.
13. It is absolutely ethically impermissible to provide IUDs to women in less-developed countries when the devices have been shown to be deleterious to the health of Americans—10, 11.
14. In cases of conflict, an absolute ethical imperative trumps an absolute professional standards imperative—assertion.
15. The director must halt the distribution of IUDs to less-developed countries—10, 13, 14.

Obviously, the crucial difference in these two arguments is the choice of an ethical theory and the way each is interpreted. Thus, whether a person takes a pro or con position is a function of the underlying value system that person holds. The way a person chooses a value system and the broader practical viewpoint is through the person's worldview and its accompanying baggage.

You must determine how to apply your practical ethical viewpoint. This requires careful attention to the theory and the linking principles you have chosen and the way they affect your evaluation of actual cases. To be an authentic seeker of truth, you must engage in this dialectical process. To do less is to diminish yourself as a person.

You are now ready to evaluate a case study.

Macro and Micro Cases[3]

Macro Case 1. You are the head of a major state university's genetic research facility. A large multinational company, Perfecta, Inc., has contacted you about a grant related to developing a germ-line therapy to promote growth. Simply put, this therapy would turn families with genes for short adults into families with genes for tall adults. "Think of the market," the president of Perfecta said. "We'll make billions! We also have plans for gene therapy to correct 'imperfect noses' and other undesirable features. The sky is the limit on this one," the president added.

The facts are these. Your laboratory could do the work that Perfecta wants, and a segment of the public will buy genetic enhancement for their future children. You will not be breaking any laws (at least in the way Perfecta has the research setup). Research monies are difficult to obtain, and you are responsible for obtaining grant funding. If you turn down the grant for any reason, other laboratories will do the work and take the money that is now offered to you.

You must respond to Perfecta in three days in the form of a report that will be copied to the president of the university and the chairperson of the board of trustees. What will you say? How will you defend your position?

Macro Case 2. You hold an endowed professorship at an important school of agriculture and are the head of the school's planning committee that is reviewing the school's strategic direction for the future. To be an outstanding research and graduate program, the school must be at the cutting edge of developments. An issue facing the school is cloning, not of sheep but of cattle. People in the United States have been turning away from beef as a staple food over the last decade because of concerns about fat and cholesterol. Now there is the opportunity to create a new breed of cattle that will be more healthy to eat and be more disease free (no more "mad cow disease!").

Such a project would entail a partnership between the school of agriculture and the university's biological research facilities. You have talked with the head of the genetic program, and she made several observations. If you are successful and the industry link (one of the largest in the world) is able to sell the new technique, the school will have made a significant impact on the cattle industry in the United States and around the world. Such success will bring the university (especially the biological research program and the school of agriculture) tremendous amounts of money, which can allow them to extend their mission and their programs. It is also possible, she notes, that moving ahead on this project before more preliminary tests have been conducted to determine the consequences to future filial generations could create a number of negative outcomes, such as a decrease in the genetic diversity in the cattle population that could render them less fit for environmental changes. Also, they might become susceptible to new disorders and/or diseases that had been held in check by mechanisms that this project would change. Other possible threats to the equilibrium of the cattle population could, in time, threaten their very existence (because all mechanisms of genetics and how they operate are not fully understood).

These comments are important to you because you want to help lead your school in the right direction for the future. No one wants to be accused of rushing and thereby causing great harm to cattle and humans alike. Likewise, no one wants to be too timid to boldly move forward when an opportunity exists. One of your teachers once said to you, "What can be known, should be known." This is very suggestive to you—yet you are also bothered by some of the things your colleague shared with you. However, you know that agriculture schools have worked on selective breeding for years in an effort to produce the perfect cow. How is this proposal any different?

The time to make your recommendation to the planning committee is at hand. As head of the committee, you are a *very* influential member. Should you recommend accepting or rejecting the project? Write a report stating your decision and presenting your reasons for it.

Micro Case 1. You are a single woman with no intention of ever marrying. However, you like children and have often thought about either adopting a child or conceiving a child through artificial insemination. The problem for you with both of these alternatives is that you never know about the genetic material of the parents (in the case of adoption) or of the father (in the case of artificial insemination). This lack of control on such a crucial point has always bothered you to the point of preventing you from moving forward.

Now you have been contacted by a friend of a friend who knows your dilemma. Your contact is about to work on cloning humans on an island laboratory in the Caribbean. He wants to use a technique to activate one of your eggs and then to implant that egg into your uterus so that you will go through a normal pregnancy and bear your own child who will be genetically identical to you.

This satisfies a number of worries that you have had about "undesirable" genes from other people. Now you can be in total control. Your baby will be genetically identical to yourself. You are inclined to go ahead with the project but want to seek some advice before proceeding.

Write a dialogue between yourself and another person. In this dialogue, explore issues in favor of and opposed to proceeding. Conclude by making a choice and presenting your reasons for it.

Micro Case 2. You are a physician meeting with a couple expressing concerns about starting a family. First, both the man and the woman come from families of short people. Being short has always been a problem for them; they feel that society discriminates against them because of their size. They would like something better for their children. They have heard that a new company, Perfecta, Inc., now offers a procedure that promotes height. They know that the procedure is still experimental and may have some unforeseen effects.

Basically, what this couple wants is advice. The man and woman want to have children, and they want their children to have every opportunity to succeed in this world (and it is their opinion that being tall could help).

Your task as a physician is to advise them about the benefits and risks of such a procedure. What should you tell them and why? What responsibilities do you have toward these people in your professional capacity? What are your ethical duties?

Notes

1 I have heard that many of the structural problems with the IUD that caused pelvic inflammatory infection have not been rectified. I am not competent to comment on this; nevertheless, for this case, let us assume that these problems still obtain.

2 See my book, *Critical Inquiry* (Boulder, CO: Westview, 2010; part 3), on the details of this process.

3 For more on macro and micro cases, see the overview on p. 58.

6
Healthcare Policy

Most of the essays in this book have focused upon clinical ethics. Clinical ethics is the domain of patient and healthcare provider. The setting is private and the discussion is personalized to that individual. Though most instances of healthcare interaction do occur in this setting, it is not by any means the exclusive domain. The second domain, of healthcare is the public domain which refers to public health policy and implementation. Some people mistakenly think that public health is only about prevention and response to infectious disease in the general population. While it is true that public health *is* interested in prevention and response to infectious disease in the general population, it is not true that that's the entire extent of its purview. As we saw in the three essays in Chapter 2, health can be construed very broadly. This allows public health a wide berth as well.

If we return to examples mentioned in Chapter 2, such as smoking and obesity, we can see how clinical versus. public health concerns can contrast. Cigarette smoking and obesity are proven to be unhealthy to the point of moving individuals to terminal diseases (such as lung cancer and uncontrollable diabetes). For years since the 1964 US Surgeon General's report on the dire health effects of smoking, a clinical approach to cure people of their cigarette smoking habit proved generally unsuccessful. The total numbers of people smoking declined only slightly. Then there was a public policy shift. The focus of attention became a public health approach. This included advertising in schools and in the media on smoking, using all the persuasive techniques that good ad-makers know how to employ. It was the public health campaign that proved to be successful. We are in a similar situation in the United States on obesity. Clinical approaches have failed, so a public health campaign is even now (at the writing of this overview) being set in place.

Three public health policy issues concern: the right to healthcare, the sort of allocation formula used to distribute scarce organs for life-saving transplantation, and issues in global public health.

Medical Ethics, Second Edition. Edited by Michael Boylan.
© 2014 John Wiley & Sons, Inc. Published 2014 by John Wiley & Sons, Inc.

A. The Right to Healthcare

This section begins with the late John David Lewis's (1955–2012) argument against the universal right to healthcare. Lewis begins by exploring what rights are. Citing Jefferson, Lewis believes these fundamentally are the right to *pursue* life, liberty, and happiness. This pursuit is to be free from coercion. This position is generally termed libertarianism. The libertarian believes that the only rights are so-called negative rights. These consist in not being interfered with unless one is unduly interfering with someone else. When this occurs or when person A harms person B, then A owes compensation to B proportional to the harm.

The three Jeffersonian rights can be combined into the right to liberty and the right to pursue happiness. The focus on the procurement of these rights is the individual her or himself. No one else has a duty to provide for others what they cannot provide for themselves (unless one wishes voluntarily to be charitable). Thus, the fact that there are people who are in need of welfare goods does not, in itself, create a rights claim. These so-called positive rights have no proper grounding. Most proponents of positive rights, Lewis claims, have altruism deeply embedded into their system. This is the real source of positive rights. But altruism has never been proven to be more descriptive of the human condition than egoism. Thus, positive rights stand on shaky ground. If we assume the more intuitively plausible egoistic position, then the assertion that there is a positive right to healthcare is tantamount to pitting person X's need for healthcare (that he cannot provide by himself) against person Y's liberty to pursue happiness as she sees fit (which probably won't include paying for X's healthcare). To make Y pay for X is to pit two equal claims for the pursuit of liberty and happiness against each other. There is no moral way to decide between two equal claims, thus there is no entitlement for healthcare against the state and its citizens.

Lewis provides a powerful argument from a consistent philosophical position. However, in my essay I disagree with Lewis on the nature of rights and this leads to a different conclusion about whether or not there is a moral right to healthcare. Unlike Lewis, I hold that there are both positive and negative rights. How do I get there? The key argument for my position is "The Argument for the Moral Status of Basic Goods." This argument sets out a conjecture that human nature is about wanting purposively to act in order to fulfill our vision of what is good. If we examine the implications of this, we find that on a species level everyone has the same needs and wants to fulfill all the preconditions for action. Among these are basic healthcare (seen as being connected to the right to protection from unwarranted bodily harm—level-one Basic Good in the Table of Embeddedness). If an individual were to claim that only they should get the goods necessary to fulfill their human nature—the ability to commit purposive action in order to do what they see as good, then that individual would be asserting idiosyncratic preference. Because all people are morally equal, claims for idiosyncratic preference are illogical (and therefore wrong). Readers assessing these two different positions should think carefully about the starting point and whether there are both positive and negative rights or merely negative rights.

The rest of my essay looks at the right to healthcare in light of the 2010 bill passed by the US Congress.

B. The Organ Allocation Problem

It is a fact that there are more people who want vital organs (lungs, livers, kidneys, etc.) than there are available organs for transplant. This creates a distributive justice problem: how do we decide who gets the heart or liver necessary to maintain life? Before 1984 when regulations were established governing the allocation of human organs for transplantation, organs were given to surgeons who could pass them on to their patients who needed them. To create a more equitable system, the US Congress passed the National Organ Transplant act of 1984 that created the United Network for Organ Sharing (UNOS). Since 1986, UNOS and its 66 regional organ procurement organizations have carried out the intentions of the 1984 act.

The list of organs that can be transplanted is always increasing, but transplanted kidneys head the list followed by hearts, pancreases, livers, hearts-lungs, lungs, and intestines. Not every regional transplant center transplants every organ; most handle kidneys but limit other organs to their specialty. Obviously, the scarcity of donor organs along with their perishable life means that the life-and-death decisions concerning their allocation must be well-conceived.

Various people have suggested different standards to apply. The two essays in this section refer to most of these approaches. Rosamond Rhodes' article presents the standard position of seeing organ allocation as an instance of distributive justice. The principle of allocation is based on the greatest need for the longest time. Rhodes also discusses whether free riders (those who have not elected to be organ donors themselves) are entitled to a transplant. She also discusses the "right" to new organs.

Brian Smart takes a different approach. He suggests that a principle of rectificatory justice be adopted. Under this system, a person who has not taken care of her or his body would be penalized in placement on the waiting list. In this case, Smart takes pains to argue that his system is not against people who have mistreated their bodies, but is for those who have led healthy lifestyles.

The section closes with a short story by Felicia Nimue Ackerman concerning a person who wants a transplant to live, but needs to satisfy a requirement of having a family (a utilitarian criterion to insure that the general happiness is increased by the allocation of said organ). But this family connection is a problem for the protagonist, Yvonne Sibley. She has no living parents and her sister disowns her. So she needs a fiancée. There is one person she has in mind, Nick, but this leads to a tricky ethical conundrum of its own. The problem develops as the possible phoney fiancée has to decide whether he will go along or not.

The use of fiction in teaching applied ethics is very powerful and most students enjoy it.[1] I would heartily recommend that classes use this story as sort of a capstone for this section.

C. International Public Health Policy and Ethics

The last part of this section addresses traditional public health problems of controlling disease. The twist is that in two of the essays there is a distinctly international emphasis (while the other is relevant to both the national and international perspective). Certainly, these are crucial issues for our time. As more bacteria become resistant to antibiotics, former diseases that we thought were tamed or extinct, have resurfaced in mutated forms that threaten the health of the world's population. These are problems that won't go away. We can either prepare for them and create a plan or wait for pandemic death.

The essay has Margaret P. Battin, Charles B. Smith, Leslie P. Francis, and Jay A. Jacobson's article explores the notion of "a comprehensive global effort for the eradication, elimination or control of infectious disease," with particular attention to the ethical issues that arise. This is to "think big" about disease control efforts that are now often done in piecemeal ways. This essay identifies five tracks along which such efforts need to be pursued: (1) national and international organizations and the development of a collective will; (2) epidemiological and healthcare infrastructure; (3) scientific development; (4) religious, social, and cultural considerations; (5) legal and social protections for individuals and groups. Each of these poses significant ethical issues which, the authors argue, should be viewed in a comprehensive way, to ensure that practice, research, and policy in each of these areas understands the person with communicable infectious disease as both a victim and (potential) vector.

Rosemarie Tong explores the territory of an influenza pandemic. She describes the process of shaping ethical guidelines for an influenza pandemic in this century, comparing efforts of the past to today. As Tong sets out the ways in which influenza would be spread, be treated, and hopefully contained, she also sets out the ways in which one becomes ethically prepared for an influenza pandemic (including the challenges to incorporating ethical guidelines in preparations). Tong also addresses the role of a duty/obligation/responsibility to work by healthcare personnel, the role of volunteers, and when healthcare personnel may refuse to treat someone. Also taken into consideration are such issues as the distribution of food and vaccines, quarantines, work stoppage, both physical and social infrastructure, the role of military and police forces, and the effect of a pandemic, isolation, and quarantine on various industries. Tong shows the complicated nature of working on a task force and the complexity of incorporating ethics into logistical planning.

In the last essay Michael J. Selgelid, Paul M. Kelly, and Adrian Sleigh discuss the new strains of tuberculosis that are drug resistant and the effect upon global health. The essay first establishes the importance of focusing international public health policy on containing this new strain of tuberculosis and its ethical impact. Second, the essay documents the current neglect in medical ethics of discussing tuberculosis and its possible effects. Third, the essay maps the terrain of ethical issues involved with tuberculosis, and finally the authors advocate a moderate pluralistic approach to the ethical issues associated with tuberculosis.

Note

1   See my co-authored empirical study on this: Michael Boylan, Felicia Nimue Ackerman, Gabriel Palmer-Fernandez, Sybol Cook Anderson, and Edward Spence, (2011) "Using Fictive Narrative to teach Ethics/Philosophy" *Teaching Ethics* 12: 61–94.

A. The Right to Healthcare

There Is No "Right" to Healthcare

JOHN DAVID LEWIS

The greatest motivation behind calls for government control of medicine today may be found in the idea that medical care is an individual right, to be provided by the state. Such a claim is powerful precisely because it is moral in nature; it demands that doctors, other medical professionals, and taxpayers accept the moral duty to provide medical care to others because they need it. As Speaker of the House of Representatives Nancy Pelosi put it, on the night that the vote was taken to pass the Patient Protection and Affordable Care Act, so-called "Obamacare":

> Today we have the opportunity to complete the great unfinished business of our society and pass health insurance reform for all Americans that is a right and not a privilege.[1]

If medical care is a right, then every member of the medical profession is bound—and may be required by law—to provide such care, at terms set by the government, whether they agree or not. Further, every citizen of means will be bound to finance such care for others, through taxation. But is this moral claim correct? Those who oppose such government interventions generally see medical care not as a right, but as a personal responsibility for each individual, to be purchased voluntarily from willing producers. If so, then no one may properly demand medical services as a right—or be coerced into providing such services.

These two positions are in deep conflict in America today. This essay will expand upon each, and show how they are founded upon diametrically opposed views of individual rights, which are at moral and conceptual odds with each other. A conclusion follows: claims to medical care as a right are historically recent, are not consistent with the rights set forth either in the Declaration of Independence or the US Constitution, and are logically contradictory. Acceptance of these claims, however, has greatly empowered the growth of the welfare state, and has hastened the decline in freedom for everyone all the while dramatically increasing medical costs.

Rights as Freedom of Individual Action

What is a "right?"[2] If there is any consensus about the many differing conceptions of rights, "it is that the concept of a right is essentially distributive, that is, rights are ascribed to and possessed by each individual or entity in a group separately rather than collectively."[3] I start with a particular claim about the concept of rights: a right is a *moral principle* that identifies and prescribes the freedom of the individual in a society under law. A right defines the scope of individual freedom against which others may not infringe. The grounding of rights is found in the nature and identity of the individual, not in wishes or needs belonging to a group.

The *Oxford English Dictionary* presents, as its first meaning of rights, the right to act: "The standard of permitted and forbidden action within a certain sphere; law; a rule or canon." As clarified by John Locke in 1690, reason teaches "that being all equal and independent, no one ought to harm another in his life, health, liberty, or possessions." No one, Locke continues, may "take away, or impair the life, or what tends to the preservation of the life, the liberty, health, limb, or goods of another."[4] Historically, rights began with the right to maintain one's own life, free of coercion by others. Each person is properly free and autonomous; their only obligation is to refrain from harming others. There is no right to forcibly redistribute the labor or property of one person on behalf of another—even if that other person desperately needs it.

The American Founders enshrined these fundamental rights in the Declaration of Independence. "All men," the Declaration asserts, are "endowed" with "certain unalienable rights," and "among these" are the "right to life, liberty, and the pursuit of happiness." The right to "pursue" one's happiness is precisely that: the right to act as one deems necessary to achieve one's own happiness. There is no guarantee that one will actually attain happiness; a proper government does not try to guarantee a good outcome, it rather establishes the conditions whereby each person may pursue personal happiness free of coercion by others. The rights of doctors, and of all medical professionals, are anchored in their capacity to think and to act freely, in pursuit of their own values.

This view is deeply Aristotelian in nature. It was Aristotle who identified the goal of life as "successful living" or "flourishing" (*eudaimonia*), often translated as "happiness."[5] The processes of life—the actions that constitute being alive—are the essence of life itself. Life *is* action, and to say that a person may act (in thought and in deed) is to say that a person may live. One may test this hypothesis by considering how a doctor knows that someone is dead. The key indicator is the absence of action: no muscle movement, no response to stimulus, no metabolic activity, no heartbeat, no brainwave activity. The flatline of inactivity indicates death. Life is action, and individual rights allow one to live a fully human life in the company of others.[6]

The right to liberty is the ability to act free from the coercive restraints of others. Suppose one lived on an island that was deserted of other human beings. One would need many things, but would have no "right" to receive a hot meal, a new home, or the alleviation of an ailment. The universe would not be beholden to fulfill such needs—rather, a need would be a motivation for the individual to think and to act. The same goes for life in a free society—each person is at liberty to pursue the values that make life possible, but no one has the "right" to demand that others satisfy them. No doctor, who has spent years learning his or her craft, has a duty to fulfill the needs of others because they wish it—for this would infringe upon the doctor's liberty to pursue his or her own values and happiness, and would undercut their own efforts to excel as a doctor.

These two rights—the rights to liberty and the pursuit of happiness—shed light on the meaning of the "right to life." Each person has the right to live life as he or she sees fit, constrained only by the fact that others have rights as well. The vital core of this conception of rights is that every individual is a rational being, who must be left free to think and act in pursuit of the good life. The essential purpose of rights is to define the proper scope of freedom when living with others. In a fuller definition, "a 'right' is a moral principle defining and sanctioning a man's freedom of action in a social context."[7] To "define" the scope of proper action is to identify it conceptually; to "sanction" it is to defend each individual's right to act within that defined scope.

Examples of the requirement for freedom of thought and action abound: readers could not understand this essay if they were told in advance that they must agree with the author. Students could not learn if they were told that they must think what their teacher thinks. A wage earner whose money is expropriated and redistributed is to that extent not free. And a doctor, told what form their career must take, what patients they must see and under what terms, and what treatments are approved, is not free to act on their own judgment (nor is their patient).

The purpose of government, it follows in the Declaration, is "to secure these rights." The American Constitution put forth a plan of government limited to this purpose. The freedoms in the Bill of Rights—to speak, to practice one's religion (or none), to assemble, and to bear arms—all uphold the liberty to act. Other amendments set limits to the actions of government officials, such as prohibitions against unreasonable search and seizure and the quartering of soldiers, in order to preserve the freedom of each individual from coercion. One searches the Constitution in vain for institutions, akin to the modern departments of Health and Human Services, Agriculture, Commerce, Labor, or Energy, that are empowered to provide largesse forcibly collected by the government.

There is no right to medical care, because there is no right to coerce medical professionals to provide it.[8]

Rights as Entitlements to Goods and Services

There is a different view of rights accepted today: that rights are entitlements to things and services that other people have a duty to provide. Returning to the *Oxford English Dictionary* entry, the second meaning attached to a right is: "that which is proper for or incumbent on one to do; one's duty."[9] President Franklin Roosevelt codified this understanding of rights with his statement of the Four Freedoms, which invoked new claims to rights not formerly recognized as such.[10] For instance, "freedom from want" means that certain goods are due to every person. On an international scale, it was the United Nations that put forth a "Universal Declaration of Human Rights" in 1948.[11] Article 22, for instance, establishes new "rights" to which every person is "entitled":

> Everyone, as a member of society, has the right to social security and is entitled to realization, through national effort and international co-operation and in accordance with the organization and resources of each State, of the economic, social and cultural rights indispensable for his dignity and the free development of his personality.

The grounding for such claims can be found in human needs, which, proponents claim, impose duties on those who can satisfy them. Each of us certainly has many needs, beginning with food, clothing, and shelter, and without the satisfaction of these essential needs, life would be impossible, or at best dreary (and short). Would we want to live in a society in which people are left starving in the streets? Perhaps the government should ensure that such people get care, at no cost to them if they are poor.

But such needs—which exist in some form for all living beings, rational or not—do not describe what in our nature allows us to satisfy them. Back on a desert island, the fact that we need food will not bring it to us—only our capacity to think and to act can do that. In the company of other people, even a rich playboy relies on someone in the past who took the responsibility to create and manage the wealth he inherited. A claim that a need constitutes a right means that those who are able to satisfy that need must accept, as a moral requirement, the duty to subordinate their lives, liberty, and pursuit of happiness to others. In the end, every individual will have a claim on the life of every other individual, because each of us has needs that others can satisfy.

Each individual is due these benefits, advocates claim, so there must be some guarantee that they will be available. Rejecting voluntary charity as the last source of such goods—which would allow people to request aid, but not to demand it as a right –the government becomes the guarantor of such largesse, given its power to coerce through taxation. Those who uphold this conception of rights often see the US Constitution as an evolving document by which rights are created by legislative and popular fiat. The Constitution's "general welfare" clause, for instance—"to … promote the general welfare"—becomes a wide-open invitation for any powerful official to do anything he or she thinks is required for the general welfare. The so-called "living constitution" is thus in constant flux, serving not to limit the power of government but rather to empower officials to address any need through laws and regulations.

The modern welfare state is greatly energized by the moral nature of such claims, which motivate people to do what they think is the right thing by increasing the reach of government programs. At every step these programs have grown in response to claims of need, as have the duties imposed upon those people able to finance them. Given that the federal budget is now nearly 4000 billion dollars annually and the national debt over three times that amount, history suggests that, once morally asserted and institutionalized, there is little possibility of enacting effective limits to the expansion of entitlement programs. The moral claims trump political and economic realities. Doctors, caught in the middle, find themselves saddled with increasingly complex reams of regulations, threats of lawsuits, and economic controls.

The Moral Foundations of Rights: Egoism Versus Altruism

The two versions of rights embody two very different ethical conceptions, egoism and altruism. They differ fundamentally, especially with respect to the proper beneficiary of a moral action.[12]

"Egoism," according to the *Internet Encyclopedia of Philosophy* (IEP), "is the theory that one's self is, or should be, the motivation and the goal of one's own action."[13] The first conception of rights outlined above was egoistic: every individual has the right to act for their own sake, exercising their own liberty and pursuing their own happiness as he or she judges best. A young doctor builds a career based on her or his own abilities, values, and choices, and offers their services to others in a non-sacrificial way. The doctor does not presume to force others to satisfy her or his own needs—to do so would imply that others may in turn force the doctor to act against her or his own judgment. The doctor is free to donate time and money to charities, for instance, but no one can force her or him to do so.

Egoism would not allow a person to prey on others by force or fraud, for this would deny that others have their own lives to live, and would leave one open to their predations in turn. Such an idea is not a valid social principle. Hedonism fails as well, the idea that one should go by feelings to gain pleasures for the moment. Egoism rather means pursuing one's own happiness and exercising one's own liberty in order to live one's own life in a rational way, meaning, without violating the rights of others.

In contrast, the conception of rights as the satisfaction of needs or wishes is based on altruism, the idea that each individual should act primarily for the sake of others, placing others above self. As the IEP states, "An ultimate motivation of assisting another regardless of one's direct or indirect self-benefit is necessary for it to be altruistic in the ordinary sense— for what we might call *moral altruism*."[14] In these terms a moral action would mean something like "providing the goods needed by others." Implemented politically, such a program has motivated citizens and officials alike to strive for moral goodness by empowering ever-growing political institutions to redistribute the goods of a nation's citizens.

Moral deontologists, consequentialists (usually utilitarians), and virtue ethicists base their systems largely on an altruist conception of ethics. Deontologists, such as Immanuel Kant, start from duties. "Duties" are first and foremost those actions that are "due" to others categorically, as an unalterable rule. They are to be done solely because they are duties, regardless of outcomes. If an action results in death or destruction, a deontologist may claim, the action is still moral, if done from duty alone. No hint of self-interest should taint the performance of such a duty, and no benefit should accrue to the actor for it. Thus a deontologist may claim that doctors—or prosperous citizens—have categorical duties to others, which must be performed for the sake of the duty alone, regardless of rights, even if the plan fails.

Utilitarians—often deriving their systems from Jeremy Bentham or John Stewart Mill—focus on the consequences of moral action rather than duties.[15] "The greatest good for the greatest number" is the principle behind such a system. Bentham understood that utilitarianism was not compatible with rights, which he called "nonsense on stilts."[16] Once again, the moral foundation here is altruistic, in that the "greatest good for the greatest number" demands that those who can provide the goods subordinate their interests to the greater number of others. Healthcare policy-makers may calculate that more people will benefit by the creation of a national healthcare system than will be harmed by it, and may proceed accordingly.

So-called virtue ethicists focus on virtues (and their opposites, vices) as observed in the human character. Classical Greeks such as Aristotle claimed to find the good by observing good men doing good things. This of course begs the question as to how he knew those men were good, or that the things they were doing were good things. Aristotle's answer was that human beings should pursue "flourishing" (*eudaimonia*), and that those character traits that allowed people to flourish were proper because they allowed people to live well. Virtues are those habituated actions that in fact foster successful living.

An altruistic interpretation of such positions dominates moral discourse today. Each position may base its moral claims—and its understanding of rights—upon the premise that people with needed skills must provide them to others, either from duty, for the good of the greatest number, or because it is virtuous to do so. Given human needs, the rights of individuals must either be subordinated to duties owed to others, or denied outright as "nonsense on stilts." Under such an impetus, doctors may find themselves increasingly divorced from control of their own values and career goals, precisely because they are able to satisfy the needs of others for medical care.

The Failure of Entitlement "Rights"

A critical argument can be raised against an egoistic conception of rights given that real needs—at times, desperate needs—can cause immense suffering. Shouldn't those who have personal wealth or skills assume the responsibility of caring for others? In a free society a person may of course choose to do so, by exercising the right to give to charity or to offer free services. But should this be made an inescapable duty? Should the government forcibly collect and redistribute the wealth of some citizens in order to alleviate the needs of others?

Those who answer "no" to these questions may point out that such a plan institutionalizes what economist Frederic Bastiat called "legalized plunder."[17] This is the forcible taking of wealth (primarily through taxation) for redistribution to others. Not only does this violate the maxim against taking property, it also violates the maxim that no group of individuals may delegate to the government any power that an individual alone does not have the right to. Such a policy has led to an endless creation of duties, and to ever-increasing government control over the lives of citizens, precisely because there is no end to the needs that one person may demand that others satisfy.

To claim a right to medical care is to claim nothing less than a right to run the lives of those who must provide the care. The "duties" invoked may be in direct opposition to the goals of doctors and other medical professionals, each of whom made a commitment to pursue medicine as a career across decades. It is *because* they made this commitment that they are now to be placed under state control. This highlights the deep opposition between the egoistic conception of rights as freedom from coercion, and the altruistic conception of rights as imposing duties on others. The significant reduction in liberties that follows is demanded by the morality of duty that lies at the heart of the altruistic conception of rights.

From a logical perspective, to hold that the right to life justifies the right to demand that others provide the needs of life introduces a contradiction in the very concept of rights. It pits one person's right to life against the liberty of another, thus fostering conflict. To the extent that a person acts egoistically—by pursuing their own interests—he or she fails to follow the altruistic command to place others first, and may be considered immoral. To the extent that they truly place others first—above their own interests—they fail to pursue their own happiness. Given this conceptual conflict, it is easy to forget that doctors' self-interest lies in the successful performance of their craft, which aligns with the self-interest of their patients who want to regain their health.

An egoistic conception of rights would not allow doctors to become the political means to maintain the lives of others, but rather the providers of a valuable service whose rights are respected. For patients, access to medical care could be greatly improved by eliminating government barriers to purchasing medical care and insurance, especially state laws that restrict the carryover of insurance across state lines. Those who are genuinely unable to satisfy their own needs could appeal to others for help based on choice rather than coercion. Those others, freed from onerous taxation and bureaucratic rules, would have more money than they do today to contribute to such charities or to do pro bono work—but they would not be forced to do so.

Most of all, no person would have the right to demand that others provide such services under threat of political coercion. There is no "right" to medical care, because there is no "right" to violate the rights of others.

Healthcare Policy and Ethics

In the United States today, government policy is most consistent with altruistic moral systems, which provide the moral foundations and the motivations for redistribution programs. For nearly three generations now American lawmakers, with the support of many constituents, have added entitlements at every identification of a need, and have accepted that redistribution from the prosperous to the needy is a proper function of government. At every step, under Democratic and Republican administrations, the federal government has expanded its scope in response to moral claims that those who are affluent have a duty to provide for those who are not.

But those concerned with ethics as a prescriptive field need not agree that such a claim is correct. One should ask whether one person's flourishing demands the violation of liberty for others, whether one person's pursuit of happiness requires others to forego their own pursuits, or whether the right to life means that some people must be coerced into maintaining the lives of others. One should also think carefully about the social and political implications of such a system, as enforced by the power of the state over a nation of millions.

Those interested in the practical application of ethics should also ask whether the growth of this system has had good economic effects. The US government today has an annual budget nearly one-third the size of the gross domestic product. Entitlement spending is the single largest item in this budget, and projections of such programs show future shortfalls in the tens of trillions of dollars. The growth of healthcare costs correlates directly with the increased government spending that followed the Great Society programs of the 1960s. The federal government today controls about half of all healthcare expenditures in the United States—and the costs continue to skyrocket. The result has been unsustainable federal programs, thousands of pages of dense regulations, massive debt, and a federal budget lurching towards bankruptcy.

Absent the economically distorting effects of multi-hundred-billion-dollar government programs, it is arguable that we would no more see outrageously increasing prices in medical services than we do in other industries. People would not want to see others bleeding in the street, so they would establish insurance companies and charities to pay for the remission of such tragedies—as they have done today. The insurance companies, however, would not be required to spend millions of dollars in order to meet thousands of pages of often contradictory government regulations on state and federal levels.

But the foundation of the entitlement state is not economic—it rests on moral foundations. The altruist morality provides a powerful impetus to redistribute wealth from the prosperous to the needy. The contradiction this introduces into rights—between a person's own (egoistic) right to their own life, liberty, and pursuit of happiness, versus (altruistic) duties imposed on them by coercion—is embodied in a contradiction in American politics, between the self-interested pursuit of profit and the altruistic demands to expropriate and redistribute that profit. The moral duties imposed upon each one of us take the economic form of spiraling costs. From this perspective, one may claim that there is a right to medical care, but the fact remains that this is a claim on the time, efforts, and lives of those forced to provide the services that constitute this care.

Notes

1 PR Newswire: http://www.prnewswire.com/news-releases/pelosi-today-we-have-the-opportunity-to-complete-the-great-unfinished-business-of-our-society-and-pass-health-insurance-reform-for-all-americans-88793287.html [accessed February 26, 2013].

2 Works consulted here: A. Brett, *Liberty, Right, and Nature*, Cambridge: Cambridge University Press, 1997. T. Campbell, *Rights: A Critical IntroductionI*, London: Routledge, 2006. W. Edmundson, *An Introduction to Rights*, Cambridge: Cambridge University Press, 2004. W. Hohfeld, *Fundamental Legal Conceptions*, W. Cook (ed.), New Haven: Yale University Press, 1919. D. Ivison, *Rights*, Montreal: McGill-Queen's University Press, 2007. J. Narveson, *The Libertarian Idea*, Peterborough, Ontario: Broadview, 2001. R. Nozick, *Anarchy, State and Utopia*, New York: Basic Books, 1974. G. Rainbolt, *The Concept of Rights*, Dordrecht: Springer, 2006. H. Steiner, *An Essay on Rights*, Oxford, Blackwell, 1994. L. Sumner, *The Moral Foundations of Rights*, Oxford: Oxford University Press, 1987. B. Tierney, *The Idea of Natural Rights*, Atlanta: Scholars Press, 1997. J. Waldron (ed.), *Theories of Rights*, Oxford: Oxford University Press, 1984.

3 C. Wellman, "Rights: systematic analysis," in Reich (1995), vol. 4, p. 2306.

4 *The Oxford English Dictionary*, 2nd edn. Oxford: Clarendon Press, 1991; p. 922. Found in Bede's *Ecclesiastical History*, circa AD 900. John Locke (1980), sect. II.6.

5 Aristotle, *Nicomachean Ethics*, I.6, in Aristotle (1984), p. 1730.

6 "Life is a process of self-sustaining and self-generated action; the right to life means the right to engage in self-sustaining and self-generated action" (Rand, 1967, pp. 321–2).

7 Rand (1967), pp. 320–8.

8 As used by rights theorists, such rights are often called "negative rights." "A positive right is one that implies a positive duty to some second party, a duty to do some sort of action; a negative right imposes a negative duty, a duty not to act in some specific manner." C. Wellman, "Rights: systematic analysis," in Reich (1995), vol. 4, p. 2308. Wesley Hohfeld called these "liberty-rights," which imply no duties by others. See Jones (1994), pp. 12–25.

9 Found in Alfred's *Gregory's Pastoral Care* (circa AD 897).

10 Franklin D. Roosevelt Presidential Library, "FDR and the Four Freedoms speech," available at: http://www.fdrlibrary.marist.edu/fourfreedoms [accessed February 26, 2013].

11 United Nations, "The Universal Declaration of Human Rights," available at: http://www.un.org/en/documents/udhr/index.shtml [accessed February 26, 2013].

12 On egoism, altruism and rights, see Smith (1995), ch. 3.

13 Internet Encyclopedia of Philosophy, "Egoism," available at: http://www.iep.utm.edu/egoism/ [accessed February 26, 2013].

14 Internet Encyclopedia of Philosophy, "Altruism and group selection," available at: http://www.iep.utm.edu/altr-grp/ [accessed February 26, 2013].

15 There are different forms of utilitarianism. "Act" utilitarianism is based on the performance of actions with little regard for principles or rules that connect a series of actions. "Rule" utilitarianism is concerned primarily with certain rules by which one can determine the best action.

16 J. Bentham (1987), pp. 46–76.

17 F. Bastiat (1990), pp. 20–3.

References

Aristotle (1984) Nicomachean ethics (trans. W.D. Ross, rev. J. Urmson). In: J. Barnes (ed.), *The Complete Works of Aristotle: The Revised Oxford Translation*. Princeton: Princeton University Press.

Bastiat, F. (1990) *The Law* (trans. D. Russell). New York: Foundation for Economic Education.

Bentham, J. (1987) Anarchical fallacies. In: J. Waldron (ed.), *Nonsense upon Stilts: Bentham, Burke, and Marx on the Rights of Man*. London: Methuen.

Jones, P. (1994) *Rights*. New York: St Martin's Press.

Locke, J. (1980) *Second Treatise of Government* (C.B. Macpherson, ed.). Indianapolis: Hackett.

Rand, A. (1967) Man's rights. In: *Capitalism: The Unknown Ideal*. New York: Signet.

Reich, W.T. (ed. in chief) (1995) *Encyclopedia of Bioethics, Revised Edition*. New York: Simon & Schuster and Prentice Hall International.

Smith, T. (1995) *Moral Rights and Political Freedom*. Lanham, MD: Rowman & Littlefield.

Waldron, J. (ed.) (1984) *Theories of Rights*. Oxford: Oxford University Press.

The Moral Right to Healthcare: Part Two[1]

Michael Boylan

All of us sometime will need healthcare due to illness or accident. In one sense the availability of healthcare is an "invisible" commodity because it is not really apparent to us until we need it. Advances in medical science in the last 75 years mean there is ever more that can be done for us by modern medicine. All of this has a price tag. And the price tag is staggering. But not all Americans have actual access to healthcare. ("Actual access" means the ability to utilize appropriate healthcare providers for the remedy of health conditions.[2]) This lack of actual access is generally due to lack of insurance, and health insurance is not cheap. Therein lies the genesis of the problem. If healthcare is a right, then it is not presently actually accessible to all, and the reason is tied to costs that we are willing to bear. The Patient Protection and Healthcare Affordability Act of 2010 (hereafter referred to as the Healthcare Affordability Act) is one approach to this problem in the United States. Other countries have instituted solutions of their own.[3] But because among the wealthiest nations in the world the right to healthcare is a controversial issue only in the United States, this essay will therefore confine itself to discussing the problem from that perspective.

Because the healthcare industry is over 15% of the United States' economy (thus constituting a large market segment) and because virtually every business is confronted with the health insurance problem, some careful thinking on these issues is very important. The purpose of this essay is:

1. To outline the strengths and weaknesses of the current healthcare system and the system as potentially modified by the Healthcare Affordability Act.
2. To sketch the ethical arguments on human rights and healthcare.
3. To argue that everyone has a right to healthcare consistent with the "ought implies can" doctrine.
4. To admit that the entitlement of health insurance may bring about conditions requiring rationing and to suggest a meta-principle of justice to guide such rationing.

Strengths and Weaknesses of the Present System within the United States

When my grandfather was in medical school, around the turn of the twentieth century, there were still classes that used Galen as their basis. I am a great admirer of Galen, but the medical world that Galen knew depicted the physician as one who set broken bones, helped deliver babies, prescribed diet/exercise, and suggested herbs to balance the four humors of the body.

With the advent of the twentieth century, Galenic medicine became a thing of the past. Medicine advanced rapidly on two fronts: (i) pharmacology, and (ii) surgery. The former was stirred by advances in specialized medical research and the latter by advances in technique (including ways to keep the patient alive both during and after an operation) and biomedical technology (including diagnostic tests, prosthetics, and improved surgical equipment and monitoring apparatus). The "new medicine" enabled miracles to be performed that were thought to be impossible in my grandfather's medical school days.

With the new medicine came a greater price tag. Most of this price tag was associated with hospitalization. To enable people to be able to afford expensive hospitalization, medical insurance was promoted. Originally health insurance was designed for catastrophes. (Insurance often works best when it protects its policyholders against an unlikely catastrophe—as in homeowners' insurance.)

In the post-World War II period American companies began buying health insurance policies (hospitalization and/or major medical) for their employees as a *fringe benefit*. Other countries in the post-World War II period began various other strategies, ranging from national health services, to single payer health plans, to subsidized national health insurance as a public-private endeavor. These other countries began with the community worldview conviction that the sort of good that healthcare represented was very dear, indeed. However, in the United States, since the delivery system was an employer-purchased *fringe benefit*, the community worldview of health insurance was of a luxury item—kind of a *bonus* for work done. As a bonus, it was rather an optional commodity. Those without health insurance could pay what they could to their family physician, and the physician would personally make up the difference (generally not a lot of money). Those who couldn't even do this were set to meet their maker sooner rather than later. This community worldview has stuck in the United States and is the origin of our intuitive attitudes on just what health insurance and healthcare are.

From its bare beginnings in hospitalization policies and major medical supplements, health insurance gradually began adding other features to its coverage: pregnancy and childbirth, office visits, and prescription drugs. At the same time medical advances were increasing rapidly. Hospitals bought new and expensive machines that had to be paid for by each and every patient who entered the door—whether he or she needed those services or not. Medical accountability also rose as the litigious climate heated up. Each and every time that things "went badly," it had to be "somebody's fault" (meaning a malpractice suit). This created a climate in which both physicians and hospitals had to establish careful guidelines about what the "prudent practitioner" would do in such and such situation (i.e., standards of professional practice). If anyone varied from this, then they were liable for malpractice. This led to defensive medicine in which expensive tests were ordered that were not medically necessary to the patient at hand, but whose absence might be a part of a malpractice lawsuit. Hospitals had to add layers of administrative staff to comply with the demands of high accountability. This meant an increasingly larger price tag.

Insurance companies, which had routinely paid every bill presented to them in the 1950s and 60s, were now auditing bills more carefully for mistakes and fraud. This also increased the costs.

The good news is that healthcare in the United States has enabled many people to live longer lives.[4] The bad news is that this aging population has greatly increased healthcare needs. Medicare was established to help meet these needs, but Medicare pays far less for procedures than what physicians generally get on the open market from insurance companies.[5] This means that younger patients (and their insurance companies) are forced to subsidize the difference. It is an invisible tax. The same holds true for Medicaid, which provides some coverage for critical care among those living around the poverty line (young and old)[6]

The late 1980s saw an explosion of health insurance costs that was caused by a similar rise in healthcare costs. More people were getting knee and back operations instead of hobbling around as their parents had. The survival rate for heart by-pass surgery moved past 50%. Americans were using their health insurance as they never had before because it really improved the quality of their lives.

By the 1990s health insurance was too expensive for many Americans. Most companies no longer paid the full cost of coverage. Most employees paid a portion of the single rate leaving the costs for dependants to be met by the employee. Family coverage was often as costly as the rent or mortgage. The *fringe benefit* luxury item became for many a luxury they could not afford. For many there was no choice. They could not afford the high premiums and went without coverage. This gamble works so long as you don't need to go to the hospital. But if you do, then you can find yourself forced to go to public hospitals that are overcrowded and often without the latest medical equipment.[7]

The systems of allocation of healthcare in the United States revolve around two principles: (i) equal care for those who are in need and (ii) unequal care depending upon one's ability to pay. The first is an offshoot of an egalitarian system of distribution while the second treats healthcare in the neo-Lockean capitalist mode of one's private property being completely at one's disposal to garner whatever is available to it (more on this in "Rationing Scenarios" below).

The Healthcare Affordability Act attempts to remedy this situation. The law requires everyone to have health insurance or pay a fine. Thus, in the abstract, there should be universal coverage. The primary venue for health insurance will still be through employers (though since it is mandated it will no longer conceptually be a fringe benefit but a *quasi-entitlement*). Small employers who cannot afford to offer health insurance to employees are eligible for bridging grants. Thus for most Americans the dollars and cents of health insurance will not change. What will change is: (i) insurance companies will no longer be able to decline coverage or claims because of *pre-existent conditions*; (ii) insurance companies will no longer be able to create annual or lifetime limits for coverage; (iii) there is some definition as to what will constitute a basic medical insurance plan (particularly for the individual market, aka state/federal insurance exchanges); (iv) a requirement that insurance companies cover a wide array of preventative medical tests; (v) a requirement that 80% of monies received go to patient care (and not overhead expenses); and (vi) students can stay on their parents' plan until their 26th birthday (adding 1.8 million previously uninsured individuals). There are other cost containment features particularly regarding Medicare and managed care.

For those individuals who are self-employed or whose companies are too small to offer coverage, there is the mandate that states create insurance exchanges that will replace the current individual insurance marketplace (or else give way to a federal exchange marketplace). This provision will be enacted state by state. For those who do not qualify for Medicaid, sliding subsidies will be made available to purchase health insurance up to as much as three times the poverty level.

This is a market-based solution to providing healthcare. It fits into the model of private/public partnership (which is one of the international models found in France, Germany, and Japan). This approach is meant to fit into the market-oriented American community worldview. It was first proposed by Republicans as an alternative to President Clinton's healthcare proposal for a more government slanted system (which did not pass). A version of this approach was later adopted in Massachusetts as proposed by Republican governor Mitt Romney.

Though it is difficult to assess the success of the Healthcare Affordability Act, since many provisions of the law do not begin until 2014 (and it is not fully implemented until 2018), it is estimated that the 49 million uninsured Americans will be trimmed to 17 million.[8] This is not universal health insurance, but if it works as advertised, it will bring health insurance coverage to 95% of all Americans. At time of writing, there are 14 states that have lawsuits against implementation of this bill. This reveals deep division among a portion of the American populace on this policy strategy to lessen the number of uninsured from 16% to 5%. The source of this disagreement comes because objectors do not view the good of basic healthcare as a human right but rather as an optional commodity that people may purchase if they have the money—along the lines of an automobile. As I've argued, I believe that this classification comes about because of the way the community worldview in the United States viewed healthcare just after World War II (as a fringe benefit—a sort of bonus for good work).

Ethical Arguments on Human Rights and Healthcare

Obviously one important part of the healthcare debate is whether or not a citizen or resident of a country has a right to healthcare.[9] If he or she does, then it is the government's correlative duty to provide this good to the individual.[10] Thus, if all citizens have a right to basic healthcare, then the government has the correlative duty to provide it (either directly or via a public/private partnership).

Therefore, it is an important question whether or not individuals have a right to basic healthcare.[11] This brief exposition does not attempt to fully explore this issue, but merely raises some important issues and points to the way that the question might be answered. This essay will address the question from the point of view of a rights-based deontological theory. It will be my contention that a strong argument can be made to support a moral right to basic healthcare for people (subject to the "ought implies can" caveat).

There are a number of versions of deontological rights-based theories. Some follow from a natural rights tradition.[12] What concerns us here is a form of the theory that states that there is some characteristic that all people possess that justifies their claim to that good as a right. This good is thus claimed solely on the basis of the claimant's status as a human being (or in some cases an "adult" human being).

There are several persuasive writers in the natural rights tradition that, at least, began with John Locke (if not earlier). The principal problem with this tradition is being able to ground a theory of rights upon some intersubjective principles. I have made this general argument:[13]

The Argument for the Moral Status of Basic Goods

1. All people, by nature, desire to be good—Fundamental Assumption
2. In order to become good, one must be able to act—Fact.
3. All people, by nature, desire to act—1,2.
4. Whatever all people desire before anything else is natural to that species—Fact.
5. Desiring to act is natural to *Homo sapiens*—3,4.
6. People value what is natural to them—Assertion.
7. What people value they wish to protect—Assertion.
8. All people wish to protect their ability to act beyond all else—5–7.
9. The strongest interpersonal "oughts" are expressed via our highest value systems: religion, morality, and aesthetics—Assertion.
10. All people must agree, upon pain of logical contradiction, that what is natural and desirable to them individually is natural and desirable to everyone collectively and individually—Assertion.
11. Everyone must seek personal protection for their own ability to act via religion, morality, and/or aesthetics—5,8–10.

12. Everyone upon pain of logical contradiction must admit that all other humans will seek personal protection of their ability to act via religion, morality, and/or aesthetics—10,11.

13. All people must agree, upon pain of logical contradiction, that since the attribution of the Basic Goods of Agency are predicated generally, it is inconsistent to assert idiosyncratic preferences—Fact.

14. Goods that are claimed through generic predication apply equally to each agent and everyone has a stake in their protection—12,13.

15. Rights and duties are correlative—Assertion.

---

16. Everyone has at least a moral right to the Basic Goods of Agency and others in the society have a duty to provide those goods to all—14,15.

From the moral status of Basic Goods a more robust picture of human rights can be constructed—all based upon their proximity to the foundations of human action. My depiction of these relations is shown in Table 6.1.

What is the justification for this classification? Let us start at the beginning. I have parsed the Basic Goods into two levels. The first level is the most deeply embedded. On this level there is an appeal to the *biological* conditions of agency. What does every human need in order to act from a biological point of view? Every person needs so many calories (based on a number of different variables such as body mass and metabolic rate, etc.) on a regular basis.[14] Without this requisite number of calories the individual will not be able to act, but instead will become sick and eventually die. Clean water and sanitation are equally important.[15] The same is true with the second two categories of clothing and shelter. These are for the sake of maintaining a core body temperature and protecting the individual from the ravages of nature. In more temperate climates, there is less of a need for clothing, but generally some need, nonetheless, for shelter (to protect the individual from storms and high winds). Finally is the related item of protection from unwarranted bodily harm. If a person lived in the forest without any shelter, there are many predators (large and small) that may attack him or her. This causes post-traumatic stress disorder. It biologically inhibits action. One cannot live this way for long (much less commit purposive action). When we sleep we are vulnerable to attacks of all sorts. If we are totally unprotected, it is probable we will suffer. Finally, accident, injury, and sickness also constitute a sort of unwarranted bodily harm (in most cases). Thus basic healthcare would fall here as well—due to its primacy to committing human action.

The other goods are presented according to their order of embeddedness to the conditions of human action. According to the earlier argument our claims for the goods of agency are stronger as they involve more deeply embedded goods and weaker for less embedded goods.[16]

Clearly, when our bodies are assailed by microbes (disease) or by accident, we have been subject to unwarranted bodily harm. Since the protection from such is a Basic Good of Agency, there is a strong rights claim for the same against all members of the society to provide basic healthcare (subject to the "ought implies can" caveat).

Now some might object on the grounds that certain types of lifestyles might make "unwarranted" bodily harm actually "warranted" bodily harm. This is a controversial

Table 6.1 Moral goods and their accompanying levels of embeddedness

Category	Level of embeddedness	Examples
Basic goods	Level One: Most deeply embedded* (that which is absolutely necessary for human action)	• Food • Clean water/sanitation • Clothing • Shelter • Protection from unwarranted bodily harm (including basic healthcare)
	Level Two: Deeply embedded (that which is necessary for effective basic action within any given society)	• Literacy in the language of the country • Basic mathematical skills • Other fundamental skills necessary to be an effective agent in that country (e.g., in the United States some computer literacy is necessary) • Some familiarity with the culture and history of the country in which one lives • The assurance that those you interact with are not lying to promote their own interests • The assurance that those you interact with will recognize your human dignity (as per above) and not exploit you as a means only • Basic human rights such as those listed in the US Bill of Rights and the United Nations Universal Declaration of Human Rights[†]
Secondary goods	Life-enhancing: Medium to high-medium embeddedness	• Basic societal respect • Equal opportunity to compete for the prudential goods of society • Ability to pursue a life plan according to the personal worldview imperative • Ability to participate equally as an agent in the shared community worldview imperative
	Useful: Medium to low-medium embeddedness	• Ability to utilize one's real and portable property in the manner one chooses • Ability to gain from and exploit the consequences of one's labor regardless of starting point • Ability to pursue goods that are generally owned by most citizens, e.g., in the United States today a telephone, television, and automobile would fit into this class
	Luxurious: Low embeddedness	• Ability to pursue goods that are pleasant even though they are far removed from action and from the expectations of most citizens within a given country, e.g., in the United States today a European vacation would fit into this class • Ability to exert one's will so that one might extract a disproportionate share of society's resources for one's own use

*"Embedded" in this context means the relative fundamental nature of the good for action. A more deeply embedded good is one that is more primary to action.

[†]It should be noted here that this hierarchy has been questioned by some at this point. Marcus Düvel has suggested that basic liberty should be a level-one basic good and criticizes my categorization. See his claim and my response in Gordon (2009).

argument that some pose.[17] There is one sense that it is correct. If x does P and P happens to be detrimental to x, then x is responsible for her or his ailment. In this case, it would seem as if "unwarranted" should be revised to "warranted" (and thus outside the sphere of moral obligation).

However, for the most part, I would demur. Generally, behavioral lifestyles are either entered into consciously or via an opaque context. In the case of conscious choices, it would be my contention that most who choose a deleterious behavior do so out of ignorance. For example, many in the United States engage in exercise. It is presented as a healthy lifestyle. But this author is a living example of how exercise (long-distance running) can lead to multiple knee and back operations. A friend of mine who heads one of the largest orthopedic surgery practices in the Washington DC area told me that sports and exercise have combined to substantially increase his practice over the years. Most of these patients thought they were engaging in something healthy, but it turned out to be otherwise. By intention these individuals believed that they were engaging in healthy behavior. There was good scientific evidence to support this belief. However, in fact, they were planting the seeds of their own injury. They were ignorant of the actual state of affairs. This is a classic case of ignorance mitigating culpability.[18]

The second category concerns opaque contexts.[19] In this case, the agent does not understand that what they are doing is actually hurting them (another form of ignorance). This is because she or he does not properly make intersubstitutable connections. For example if Jane drinks whiskey, she knows (a) that whiskey gives her pleasure and (b) that whiskey will damage her liver. However, when Jane considers drinking she does not say to herself, "I will now drink whiskey in order to damage my liver." This is because the context is opaque. Jane does not make the requisite substitution, and thus only sees the proposition, "I will now drink whiskey in order to receive pleasure." Since an opaque context is another instance of ignorance, it is my contention that it, also, is not fully culpable. Because of this, medical personnel should feel secure in fulfilling their professional obligation of beneficence without regard to the behavior of their patient.[20]

Thus, from the point of view of the above deontological theory, all people have a claims right to level-one Basic Goods of Agency. This is not an endorsement of universal access to medical procedures that concern Secondary Goods (such as cosmetic surgery). It merely says that for sickness and injury involving well-being that is situated as a level-one Basic Good, all people may properly claim this as a human right and (on the basis of the correlative nature of rights and duties) all other people in the society have a duty to provide them this good.[21] (The nature of international claims is beyond the scope of this essay.[22])

Many would disagree about there being a right to healthcare because it seems tantamount to writing a blank check to the healthcare industry. This would require a considerable increase in taxation to pay the bill. However, if the taxation were on a progressive principle (aka graduated on the ability to pay), then we have a clear case of wealthy individuals complaining about their loss of level-three luxury goods against poorer people's claim to level-one Basic Goods. As I have argued there is an important sense in which the general good should be accommodated even when it is individually inconvenient.[23]

However, it is still possible that accommodating all the claims for level-one Basic Goods (even in a wealthy country such as the United States) might prompt pharmaceutical and medical technology companies to open the throttle on research and development with the result that sooner or later the bill will be too much to pay—for everyone. In this scenario it seems that rationing of some sort will be necessary.

Rationing leads us to the Kantian doctrine that "ought implies can."[24] Under this doctrine no one can be said to have a binding moral duty to perform something that it is practically impossible for him or her to do. This maxim is important to Kant for without it, his theory is doomed to inconsistency.[25]

But what lies behind this "can"? Does the can mean (i) "logically possible," or (ii) "practically possible," or (iii) "comfortable to implement," or (iv) "may be implemented without raising taxes or cutting other programs," or (v) "politically easy to bring about"? Obviously the answers to these interpretations of "can" are different. Therein lies a large part of the practical implementation of any healthcare reform.

Assessing the "Ought implied Can" Restriction on Universal Health Coverage

If you ought to do something it implies that you can.

The Healthcare Affordability Act has been attacked as being a huge expense that the United States cannot afford. It was very difficult to pass. It is not difficult to sketch some of the reasons for this. First, there are the vested interests that will be disturbed. These include: (i) hospitals, (ii) doctors, (iii) pharmaceutical companies, (iv) insurance companies, (v) the myriad of medical support facilities, and most importantly (vi) the opposition political party (the Republicans). President Obama did what he could early on to get groups i–v on his side so that there might be a different dynamic than when President Clinton's plan was defeated. But there was nothing President Obama could do about factor 6. Even though this plan originated at a Republican think tank (as an alternative to Clinton's plan) and was enacted first in Massachusetts by Mitt Romney, a Republican governor, the perceived *ownership* of the bill became the President's such that the popular name for it was "Obamacare." It is a political fact that entrenched interests are difficult to overcome in a democracy. This is one aspect of the "can" described in the last section.

A second element of the "can" equates to "economically afford." This, in turn, requires a specification of "afford." Clearly this word implies a value system that ranks alternatives. Most Americans live paycheck-to-paycheck. Few really believe that comprehensive coverage can be obtained without raising taxes significantly. And healthcare is an odd sort of commodity because it is invisible until you need it. When pressed with buying groceries, filling up the automobile with gasoline, and buying junior some new shoes, most families are always looking for ways to cut costs. Abstract concepts like insurance seem to many like low-hanging fruit. There are many self-employed Americans (especially younger Americans) who are willing to gamble that they won't need health insurance so they are against the mandate to buy it. But this ignores that already more than 15% of all monies spent in the United States are on healthcare. The Healthcare Affordability Act will actually drive down long-term costs because of cost containment measures—particularly in Medicare. But for most people it is difficult to think in the long term. John Maynard Keynes is reputed to have said, "In the long term we are all dead." It is quixotic justification for most people. This is because it requires one to move away from the personal present into a future that might not benefit the self but instead might benefit others. The individualist anti-community perspective shudders at the thought of public policy that might only help others. This is at the heart of this affordability version of "ought implies can."

The third sense of "can" involves what sort of healthcare we want. Do we desire everyone to have access to the "best available care" or will we settle for a rationing formula? If so, then what sort of formula? If the rationing formula is too restrictive, then it may not be an improvement over what we presently have (more on this later).

Again, the "can" is involved in people making a conscious decision about whether they believe "best available care" is an integral part of their well-being (or at least a more integral part of their well-being than a second car, boat, or summer home).

The last sense of "can" involves *who* will pay for it. At time of writing this essay, the most popular candidate in the United States is still business. When healthcare was inexpensive, it became a standard fringe benefit of most employers. As health insurance became more and more costly, employees have taken on an increasingly greater share of the premium payments.

There is often a false sense among individuals that if payment for some good does not come directly out of their pockets, then they are not paying for it. Thus, government and big business are thought to be able to provide fringe benefits "free of cost" to the average person. This, of course, is untrue. The government depends upon taxes for its revenue, and business passes on its expenses to consumers. We all pay. Again, recognition of this echoes back to how we understand our sense of community. Those who want to pretend that they are individuals doing everything in life by themselves without any community help are leery of cooperative social public policy.

Whether healthcare is provided through a private enterprise system, a modified private system, a single payer system, or a government-run system is, in one sense, beside the point. It has been argued above that there are many false guises for the "ought implies can" caveat in fulfilling moral duties. Only real cases of practical impossibility should count. In the current US economy, the argument presented above supports universal coverage for all in the country (by whatever policy model can best deliver it). At our present moment in history there is no "can" so powerful that it can overcome the moral ought. Those who seek to repeal the Healthcare Affordability Act are wrong. *Almost* universal health coverage ought to be allowed to roll out over eight years as intended to become an actualized reality in the United States. However, this is not the end of the story.

Rationing Scenarios

The last section argued for a universal right for all to healthcare subject to the "ought implies can" restriction. Several senses of "can" were examined and rejected for the United States (even in a recession) as merely being alibis for those unwilling to sacrifice their less embedded goods of agency to help others obtain their more deeply embedded goods.

If the Healthcare Affordability Act continues until its full implementation in 2018, it is my conjecture that there will come a time when healthcare rationing will become necessary. This is because when we declare to the healthcare industry that the nation is behind in providing the "best available care" to all, the pharmaceutical companies and the biomedical technology companies will take this as an opportunity to pour millions into research and development because the promise of return will seem so certain (i.e., backed by a guarantee of the United States of America, the richest nation on earth). Very soon "best available care" will become too expensive for us to afford—even if we put it on a par with national defense. In this case, rationing will become a necessity for those covered under the basic insurance plan (when money is the issue). Rich people will still be able to buy more expensive plans or pay out-of-pocket for overly expensive treatments. However, when the issue is not money—such as human organs—then money should not be the issue. All people—those on the basic plan or those on the gold-plated plan—should be treated equally regarding organ transplants. Rationing will thus become a reality for all people though American culture is loath to admit it.[26]

But what should be our principle of medical rationing? If one were a utilitarian, the answer would be to create a rationing system based on aggregate utility. But would that mean instrumental utility to the nation (thus favoring the gifted and the young) or treating all people as one? This is not clear. The argument could go either way. Some have suggested criteria that look like favoring the young over the old and the productive over the non-productive.[27]

Since I am not a utilitarian, this option is not open to me. The dynamics of this case seem similar to the Trolley Dilemma in which (according to one version) the driver of an out-of-control trolley has the choice of killing one man on the siding or a school bus full of children. In the Trolley Dilemma, I believe that from a deontological rights-based system there are no moral criteria to choose between killing the few or the many.[28] This does not mean that there are no criteria at all, but merely no moral criteria for the case at hand. In some particular case the individual seeking an answer to his or her quandary should turn to other values in their worldview, among which are aesthetic and religious norms.

However, this is not the end of the story. Cases of public health require considerations of justice.[29] Social policy depends upon principles of justice for its proper genesis and implementation. In the case of rationing, the principle of justice I would bring forward is egalitarianism. Egalitarianism is a normative rule of distributive justice. Thus, in the case of healthcare rationing, it seems to me that since we are choosing among a large number of equally strong rights claims we should base policy criteria upon egalitarian standards according to the level of one's distress. The reason for treating all with equal regard is that each person has the same strength of claim for best available healthcare. This means that among rationing criteria, certain candidates that do not exhibit egalitarian characteristics based upon one's level of distress would be discarded. Equal regard would require some sort of oversight.[30]

From the perspective of level-one Basic Goods all people are identical.[31] It is at this level that our human similarity is most evident. Thus, it is entirely appropriate that on this level all people on the basic plan are treated equally. Since I'm not a utilitarian, this would mean some sort of lottery. When we only have enough money for x number of procedures and we have $x+n$ number of claimants, then the only fair decision procedure is chance. Given that we have created a decent minimum plan that covers basic medical care (normal sickness/accident physician visits, prenatal care, most categories of chronic care—such as diabetes, extraordinary care, home healthcare, etc.),[32] expensive operations, transplants, and expensive experimental care will have to be rationed. A lottery under a rights-based deontological system is the only fair way to do this (when there are limited resources).

When considering the one versus the many, it is a little more complicated. If we must ration between a single person needing expensive treatment and a thousand poor mothers needing important prenatal care, then if they all deserve equal consideration, and if equal consideration means dividing up the dollar equally for each, then it is probable that though (deontologically) all have an equal claim, the procedure in an ought-implies-can scarcity will be for the many to be given treatment. This is not because of some aggregation calculation but because equal consideration divides the available money equally, with the probable result that the pregnant women get their care and the patient needing extraordinary, expensive treatment is left in the lurch.[33] Creating a basic set of medical procedures that all can expect must be the cornerstone of any designed national healthcare policy.

All people's level-one Basic Goods are on a par, but given a situation of rationing based upon the "ought implies can" caveat, a policy based upon a meta-principle of justice that is supported by the Table of Embeddedness (Table 6.1) (such as egalitarianism) is the only fair way to distribute critically scarce resources.

Conclusion

It is my opinion that one may create an argument for the universal moral right to healthcare based upon the rights-based system sketched in this essay. This right incurs an immediate correlative duty upon us (and all societies) to provide it subject to the ought-implies-can caveat. But though this caveat can be misinterpreted, marketplace realities being what they are will necessitate the creation of a split entitlement: basic care for all and a rationed care for very expensive life-saving procedures. Those who can afford gold-plated plans will get whatever their money can pay for (short of human organs for transplants). The rest of society will have to make do with a lottery for these more expensive life-saving procedures. This is a hard reality. The explosion of options in the healthcare industry has dramatically raised the ceiling of what is possible and the price tag is astounding![34] Given this quandary, a social allocation system that is based upon egalitarianism and degree of need is the best principle of justice to guide our society through the difficult choices ahead.

Notes

1   This essay is called "Part Two" because it expands upon my previous essay in the first edition. I have also lectured on this topic. This is my latest take on this issue.

2   In this context, "Actual access" means access to healthcare that involves the Basic Goods of Agency (as set out later in this essay). There is no argument for access to health services that were designed to enhance Secondary Goods. I have made this argument more completely in Boylan and Brown (2002, part 3).

3   For a general survey of these see Cummiskey (2008).

4   This good news is not distributed evenly. Those who have been discriminated against, for example, African-Americans, have a statistically significantly greater mortality rate than European-descent Americans; see Grant and Boylan in Chapter 3, this volume, and Boylan and Grant (2007).

5   This is evidenced by the recent wave of insurance companies that have left the Medicare Health Maintenance Organization (HMO) marketplace. Companies cannot make money on Medicare

patients unless they engage in the practice of "skimming" (meaning that they take only the healthiest patients) or they have a very large client base that includes enough healthy patients to compensate for those who need care the most. It has been said that in the last months of life a typical patient may require a cost outlay equal to his or her entire life combined. Thus it is that private insurance companies shy away from Medicare unless forced to do so by legislation.

6   At the time of writing the US Supreme Court upheld the Affordable Healthcare Act except the section that permitted the federal government to punish states that did not extend Medicaid to 133% of the poverty line. Instead, a rather perverse result may occur if a state refuses to define Medicaid eligibility in this way. For example if state A says they will set eligibility at 50% of the poverty level—as some do now—then there will be a gap in coverage from 50% of poverty to 133% of poverty—at which point the federal government will subsidize individual plans. This could sabotage the intent of almost universal coverage in those states that act this way. This will be a contentious issue in the years ahead.

7   Some county hospitals that are accustomed to provide healthcare to all needy individuals are in desperate shape. One prominent example is D.C. General Hospital in Washington, DC, which has recently been closed as a full service hospital. Many other such hospitals are in deep financial trouble since the public has little inclination at present to support costly hospitals that serve the disenfranchised of society.

8   Center for American Progress, April, 2010.

9   Because of the special context of this essay around the United States of America, I have focused my attention there. But I have argued in Boylan (2011, ch. 8) that this is a basic human right to be viewed from a cosmopolitan perspective against all the nations of the world.

10 This idea of correlative rights is derived from Wesley N. Hohfeld (1919). In that work Hohfeld describes a "claims right." A claim is a right with a specific correlative duty of the form "x has a right to y against z in virtue of p." In this case x and z are individuals. Z has a duty to give x some good, y, because of p (some institution that validates the transaction). Thus, if x lends $10 to z, then because of the institution of paying debts, x has a right to that $10

at some specified time from z. In this way, rights and duties are correlative. A right of one agent is identified as the duty of some other agent. A right is a duty seen from another standpoint.

11 Of course this is not the only concern. Brock (2000) has argued that concentration upon the *right* to healthcare obscures the inevitability of rationing and also makes opaque the plight of the poor. I agree with this to the extent that any argument about the right to healthcare should include these discussions, as well.

12 Some timeless discussion on this controversy includes: Boylan (1979, 2004a, 2011), Hart (1955), Buckland (1912, 1925, 1963), Villey (1957, chapters 11 and 14); Benn and Peters (1959), Melden (1977), Maritain (1942), Pound (1959), and Singer (1999); see also J. Reiman's commentary on Singer's article (Reiman, 1999).

13 I make this argument in Boylan (2004a, 2011). For a discussion of my argument see Seumas Miller (2009) and Dale Jacquette (2009).

14 The United Nations has set three levels: (a) survival needs—500 calories a day; (b) minimum effectiveness—1000 calories a day; and (c) basic effectiveness—2000 calories a day (Boylan, 2011, ch. 7).

15 Boylan (2008a).

16 Tong in Gordon (2009) asserts a place for feminist ethics (see pp. 29–38).

17 For a discussion of some of these issues see Rhodes (1994) and Smart (1994).

18 Ignorance is generally held to be a mitigating factor in calculations of culpability. For a discussion of the philosophical foundations of this position see "Introduction" in Boylan (2000).

19 Most philosophers consider the work of W.V.O. Quine (1960) to be pioneering with respect to opaque contexts. Basically, an opaque context is created when a construction resists the substitutivity of identity. Quine uses the example: (1) "'Tully was a Roman' is trochaic." (1) is a true proposition. Now Tully is identical to Cicero, so it would seem as if you could create the proposition (2) "'Cicero was a Roman' is trochaic." But (2) is false since "Cicero" is a dactyl. For a more complete discussion see Quine (1960), pp. 141 ff.

20 The foundation of medicine is compassion for those in need. The Hippocratic duty to do no harm and to act for the well-being of the sick should thus be an act, *simpliciter*, without regard for blame, which (at the very least) is a tortured judgment.

21 I should note that not everyone who views the problem in terms of rights agrees with my conclusion that there is a firm right to healthcare. For example, Beauchamp and Faden (1979) conclude that "the major issues about right to health and healthcare turn on the justifiability of social expenditures rather than on some notion of natural, inalienable, or preexisting rights." Others such as Charles Dougherty (1984), Rashi Fein (1990), L.O. Gostin (2001), and J.C. D'Oronzio (2001) argue for interpretations that are consistent with the one I am advocating. Recently, the debate on the right to healthcare has taken a particular turn toward child-based rights. For a flavor of this discussion see Callahan (2001), Brock (2001), Kopelman and Mouradian (2001), and Kopelman (2001).

22 I argue that the right is the same for all people around the world—a cosmopolitan obligation (Boylan, 2011, ch. 8).

23 Boylan (2004a, 2011).

24 This doctrine has its own controversies. For a discussion of these see Christine Korsgaard's fine treatment (Korsgaard, 1985).

25 The inconsistency is this: on the one hand one may have a duty to do x, yet on the other hand it is impossible to do x. Thus the individual is put in the position of a moral dilemma. No matter what one does, one is immoral. If one tries to do one's duty and fails (which must happen if doing one's duty is impossible), then one is immoral. If one ignores one's duty, then one is immoral. For a discussion of the consequences of moral inconsistency for Kant (or similar systems) see Donagan (1977, ch. 5).

26 Mongan et al. (2008).

27 Lawrence J. Schneiderman has an argument that looks a lot like this (though he denies it) (Schneiderman and Jecker, 2011).

28 Boylan (2000), pp. 85–6.

29 Boylan (2004b).

30 Arrow et al. (2009).

31 In this respect, our attention should be directed toward the disenfranchised in society. As part of the rationing formula, we must recognize that at the perspective of level-one Basic Goods, all are identical. This means that the poor cannot be shuttled away from the public vision. No one's claims to level-one goods should become invisible.

32 Emmanuel (2002).

33 For example, if there were 10 000 women needing care that cost 1500 a piece ($15 000 000) and 10 people needing a heart transplant costing $75 000 ($750 000), and if the total available were $14 000 000, then if the pot were divided equally among all 10 010 it would amount to $1398 apiece. This would almost provide the women with what they need, but would not allow enough money for the heart transplant recipients.

34 See Boylan (2008b).

References

Arrow, W., Auerbach, A., Bertko, J., et al. (2009) Toward a 21st century health care system: recommendations for health care reform. *Annals of Internal Medicine* 150: 493–5.

Beauchamp, T.L. and Faden, R. (1979) The right to health and the right to healthcare. *Journal of Medicine and Philosophy* 4: 118–31.

Benn, S.I. and Peters, R.S. (1959) *Social Principles and the Democratic State*. London: George Allen & Unwin.

Boylan, M. (1979) Seneca and moral rights. *The New Scholasticism* 53: 362–74.

Boylan, M. (2000, 2008) *Basic Ethics*. Upper Saddle River, NJ: Prentice Hall.

Boylan, M. (2001) Justice, community, and the limits of autonomy. In: J.P. Sterba (ed.), *Social and Political Philosophy: Contemporary Perspectives*. London and New York: Routledge; pp. 187–202.

Boylan, M. (2004a) *A Just Society*. Lanham, MD, and Oxford: Rowman & Littlefield.

Boylan, M. (2004b) The moral imperative to maintain public health. In: M. Boylan (ed.), *Public Health Policy and Ethics*. Dordrecht: Kluwer/Springer; pp. xvii–xxxiv.

Boylan, M. (2008a) Clean water. In: M. Boylan (ed.), *International Public Health Policy and Ethics*. Dordrecht: Springer; pp. 273–88.

Boylan, M. (2008b) Medical pharmaceuticals and distributive justice. *Cambridge Quarterly of Healthcare Ethics* 17 (Winter): 32–46.

Boylan, M. (2011) *Morality and Global Justice: Justifications and Applications*. Boulder, CO: Westview.

Boylan, M. and Brown, K. (2002) *Genetic Engineering: Science and Ethics on the New Frontier*. Upper Saddle River, NJ: Prentice Hall.

Boylan, M. and Donahue, J.A. (2002) *Ethics Across the Curriculum*. New York and Lanham, MD: Lexington Books.

Boylan, M. and Grant, R.E. (2007) Distributive justice in hospital healthcare. In: D. Micah Hester (ed.), *Ethics by Committee: A Textbook on Consultation, Organization, and Education for Hospital Ethics Committees*. Lanham, MD, and Oxford: Rowman & Littlefield; pp. 231–48.

Brock, D.W. (2000) Broadening the bioethics agenda. *Kennedy Institute of Ethics Journal* 10: 21–38.

Brock, D.W. (2001) Children's right to health care. *Journal of Medicine and Philosophy* 26: 163–77.

Buckland, W.W. (1912) *Elementary Principles of the Roman Private Law*. Cambridge: Cambridge University Press.

Buckland, W.W. (1925) *A Manual of Roman Private Law*. Cambridge: Cambridge University Press.

Buckland, W.W. (1963) *A Text-Book of Roman Law from Augustus to Justinian* (reprint). Cambridge: Cambridge University Press.

Callahan, D. (2001) Health care for children: a community perspective. *Journal of Medicine and Philosophy* 26: 137–46.

Cummiskey, D. (2008) Health care justice: the social insurance approach. In: M. Boylan (ed.), *International Public Health Policy and Ethics*. Dordrecht: Springer; pp. 157–74.

Donagan, A. (1977) *The Theory of Morality*. Chicago: University of Chicago Press.

D'Oronzio, J.C. (2001) A human right to healthcare access: returning to the origins of the patients' rights movement. *Cambridge Quarterly of Healthcare Ethics* 10(3): 285–98.

Dougherty, C. (1984) The right to healthcare: first aid in the emergency room. *Public Law Forum* 4: 101–28.

Emmanuel, E. (2002) Preface. In: M. Danis, C. Clancy, and L.R. Churchill (eds), *Dimensions of Health Policy*. Oxford: Oxford University Press; p. viii.

Fein, R. (1990) Entitlement to health services reappraised. *Bulletin of the New York Academy of Medicine* 66: 319–28.

Gewirth, A. (1978) *Reason and Morality*. Chicago: University of Chicago Press.

Gordon, J.-S. (2009) *Morality and Justice: Reading Boylan's A Just Society*. Lanham, MD, and Oxford: Roman & Littlefield/Lexington.

Gostin, L.O. (2001) Beyond moral claims: a human rights approach in mental health. *Cambridge Quarterly of Healthcare Ethics* 10(3): 264–74.

Hart, H.L.A. (1955) Are there any natural rights? *Philosophical Review* 64: 176–7.

Hohfeld, W. (1919) *Fundamentals of Legal Conceptions*. New Haven, CT: Yale University Press.

Jacquette, D. (2009) Justification in ethics. In: J-S. Gordon (ed.), *Morality and Ethics: Reading Boylan's A Just Society*. Lanham, MD, and Oxford: Lexington/Rowman & Littlefield; pp. 55–70.

Kant, I. (1948) *Groundwork of the Metaphysics of Morals* (trans. H.J. Paton). London: Hutchinson.

Kopelman, L.M. and Mouradian, W.E. (2001a) Do children get their fair share of dental care? *Journal of Medicine and Philosophy* 26: 127–36.

Kopelman, L.M. and Mouradian, W.E. (2001b) On duties to provide basic health and dental care to children. *Journal of Medicine and Philosophy* 26: 193–209.

Korsgaard, C. (1985) Kant's formula of the Universal Law. *Pacific Philosophical Quarterly* 66: 24–47.

Maritain, J. (1942) *Les droits de l'homme et la loi naturelle* (reprint). New York: Editions de la Maison Français.

Melden, A.I. (1977) *Rights and Persons*. Berkeley, CA: University of California Press.

Miller, S. (2009) Justification in ethics: desiring to be good and ethical communication. In: J-S. Gordon (ed.), *Morality and Justice: Reading Boylan's A Just Society*. Lanham, MD, and Oxford: Lexington/Rowman & Littlefield; pp. 39–54.

Mongan, J.J., Ferris, T.G., and Lee, T.H. (2008) Options for slowing the growth of healthcare costs. *New England Journal of Medicine* 358: 1509–14.

Pound, R. (1959) *Jurisprudence*. St Paul, MN: West Publishing Co.

Quine, W. (1960) *Word and Object*. Cambridge, MA: MIT Press.

Reiman, J. (1999) Commentary on Beth Singer. In: M. Boylan (ed.), *Critical Essays on Action, Rationality, and Community*. New York: Rowman & Littlefield.

Rhodes, R. (1994) A review of ethical issues in transplanting. *Mount Sinai Journal of Medicine* 61: 77–82.

Schneiderman, L.J. (2011) Rationing just medical care. *American Journal of Bioethics* 11: 7–14.

Schneiderman, L.J. and Jecker, N.S. (2011) *Wrong Medicine: Doctors, Patients, and Futile Treatment*, 2nd edn. Baltimore, MD: Johns Hopkins University Press.

Singer, B. (1999) Community, mutuality, and rights. In: M. Boylan (ed.), *Gewirth: Critical Essays on Action, Rationality, and Community*. New York: Rowman & Littlefield.

Smart, B. (1994) Fault and the allocation of spare organs. *Journal of Medical Ethics* 20: 26–31.

Villey, M. (1957) *Leçons d'histoire de la philosophie du droit*. Paris: Vrin.

B. The Organ Allocation Problem

A Review of Ethical Issues in Transplantation

ROSAMOND RHODES

Traditional medical practice cleaves to the principles of doing no harm, acting for the good of patients, and caring for all who come in need. The ethical practice of organ transplantation sometimes requires the thoughtful surgeon to violate each of these central moral tenets. From this alone it is clear that the moral conflicts raised by organ transplantation are complex, compelling, and deserving of especially careful consideration. Unavoidable characteristics of the transplant surgeon's practice require difficult moral judgments which are peculiar to this field. The two major areas of moral quandary are organ procurement and organ allocation. This paper outlines the key ethical issues in transplantation and draws attention to some of the recent literature that argues these issues in greater detail [1–5].

Organ Procurement

Obviously, an organ for transplantation must be harvested from either a recently dead cadaver or a living donor. Taking organs from a cadaver violates certain traditional religious and social attitudes which require us to show respect for the dead by not mutilating the corpse. Taking an organ from a living donor violates the medical dictum "do no harm." Removing a vital organ from a healthy person puts the donor at risk of serious harm from anesthesia, intraoperative complications, and postsurgical complications. The procedure itself is also certain to harm the donor with disfigurement.

The preservation or the significant enhancement of life can justify overriding the moral imperatives that would otherwise prohibit dismembering corpses and harming healthy individuals. However, even though we may decide that organ transplantation can be a morally acceptable practice, we still have to answer many weighty ethical questions about organ harvesting. How should death be defined? What other criteria must be met before organs can be taken from a corpse? Must the consent of families be obtained? Can cadaver organs be purchased from the family of the deceased like other inherited property? Should we allow people to sell their own duplicate organs? When can a living donation be accepted? Can we use organs from the nearly dead or the hardly human?

"A Review of Ethical Issues in Transplantation," by Rosamond Rhodes, was originally published in the *Mount Sinai Journal of Medicine* 1994; 61(1): 77–82. Reprinted with permission of the publisher.

Brain death and cortical death

There has been a religious and historical tradition of identifying death with a permanent cessation of heart beat and the absence of respiration. But now there are artificial means for keeping hearts beating and lungs working. The technology that makes it possible to keep alive those who would otherwise be dead leaves us with uncertainty about when someone can be called dead. This becomes a crucial issue in transplantation because transplant organs must be kept viable until harvested by keeping the donor body on life support until the organs are removed. Yet it is immoral to kill someone in order to transplant his or her organs. So, if discontinuing life support is killing, then the organs cannot be harvested from those who are on life support.

Brain death has been used as a new medical standard for defining death. According to the new criteria, when brain function has terminated, death is declared, and organs may be taken even though heartbeat and respiration continue. Does this new criterion reflect what is in fact ethically permissible? Brain death has not been accepted as the standard in Japan, so no cadaveric transplants can be performed there. Is brain death too broad a standard, or is it actually too narrow? Perhaps confirmation of the death of the cerebral cortex is a sufficient moral standard for declaring that artificial life support could be discontinued and that organs could be taken for transplantation. Only if cortical death were the accepted standard could the organs of anencephalic new borns and also of those in persistent vegetative states be used [6–10].

Arguments about the acceptability of the brain-death standard reflect broader moral positions on personhood and life. Someone who holds life itself to be sacred is inclined to resist any laxity in the death standard. Those who associate personhood or autonomy with the demand for respectful treatment readily accept the new standard because, once the brain is dead, the individual can no longer make choices or act with deliberation or from principles as an autonomous person could. According to those with a commitment to autonomy, we do not have obligations to the brain dead that we do have to those who can still think and autonomously make choices for themselves [11, 12].

Required request, presumed consent, and required donation

Regardless of whether brain death or cortical death is the accepted standard, decisions will have to be made about whether other criteria have to be met before usable organs can be removed from the deceased for transplantation. Currently in the United States *1.* we follow the "required request" policy. The next of kin must be asked to donate the organs of the deceased, and their consent must be given before organs can be removed. Some other countries function under a "presumed consent" rule. On this model it is *2.* assumed that viable organs will be used for transplantation, although families are given the right to refuse. A third approach (employed for example in Austria) treats the *3.* corpse as property of the state and takes all viable organs for transplantation.

Because of the serious shortage of transplant organs, many in the United States have argued for moving from "required request" to "presumed consent" or even to required donation. Although the latter two policies are expected to make more organs available for transplantation, defenders of the "required request" status quo argue that the other policies conflict with our historical commitments to individual liberty and religious freedom and cannot be accepted in our society because the population does not sufficiently trust the medical establishment. Following our present policy leaves about two thirds of those who need transplants without organs and so increases the impetus for accepting organs from living donors [13–17].

Using living organ donors

Physicians consider that they should act for the good of, and should avoid harm to, their patients. If they also consider the psychological benefit to a donor from saving a loved one, or significantly improving a beloved's quality of life, or avoiding the guilt of not trying to help, it will be apparent that donating an organ could be good for the donor. From this perspective, even though subjecting someone to the risks of surgical complications and the certainty of mutilation can never be good, in the context of the totality of what is being achieved, accepting an organ from a living donor could be better than the alternative.

In accepting someone as an organ donor, the most crucial considerations are the seriousness of the recipient's need, the likelihood of avoiding serious complications for the donor, and the quality of the donor's consent. The more pressing the need of the recipient, the greater the reason to do some harm to another. The slimmer the chance of serious harm to the donor and the more autonomous the donor's choice, the greater the acceptability of the donation.

Autonomous donor consent is a basic consideration in taking an organ from a donor because it would be an assault to take an organ from someone without her or his consent. Furthermore, in light of the clear harms that will be done, unless the person declares that the donation would be an overall good, there is no reason to presume that it will be. However, since respect for autonomy is one of the most crucial moral imperatives, cooperating with someone's autonomous choice to give provides a prima facie reason for accepting her or him as an organ donor [18].

Unfortunately, the one who can donate an organ for transplantation—who has an organ that suits the recipient's needs—may not be autonomous. Small children, the demented, and the insane cannot make such decisions for themselves. The autonomy of other prospective donors (including adolescents and those who are being pressed to donate by family members) may be questionable. When you are acutely aware of the moral dimension of taking an organ from a living donor, the ethical acceptability of each prospective donor must be carefully assessed. Furthermore, because the ethical acceptability of living donation relates directly to the likelihood of taking the organ without causing serious harm, the minimum requirement is that each prospective donor must have her or his own medical advocate who is committed to considering the donation only from the perspective of the good of the donor [19–22].

Organ sales

If organs for transplantation can be taken from dead and also from living donors, can organs be sold? The marketplace serves as an incentive. Since we need more transplant organs to save and improve lives, is it permissible to allow the market to operate and thus increase the available pool?

One argument against organ sales has been that it would result in unjust distribution of organs—the rich would be able to buy what they needed and the poor would be left without. However, a system could easily be devised to avoid this problem. The United Network for Organ Sharing (UNOS), the national organ distribution network, could be the only buyer and could continue allocation of what would be a more adequate supply, following principles that would not discriminate against the poor. If the distribution of purchased organs were just, would organ sales be acceptable? Those still opposed argue that body parts are the kinds of things that should be given and not sold, that using money as the incentive would deprive people of the opportunity to be generous, and that offering money for organs would offend more people than it would inspire. Furthermore, they point out that offering a financial incentive would be unjust to the poor because it would be more likely to coerce them than to affect the decisions of the well-heeled.

Those in favor of allowing organ sales to increase the supply of transplantable organs claim that taking organs from the deceased without financial reimbursement is unfair to the family that might be happy to receive some compensation (for instance, burial costs) for their property. It is also argued that refusing to allow the living to sell their own duplicate organs fails to respect their autonomy by refusing to allow people to act on the choices they think are best for them. Those who argue against a prohibition on organ sales point to the inconsistencies in our attitudes. We do allow people to take much greater risks for financial compensation (boxing, playing football), and we do allow and even praise people who donate without compensation for taking the same risk [23–33].

Organ Allocation

Once transplant organs are obtained, careful consideration must be given to how they should be allocated. Meeting the needs of all patients is impossible because there are not enough organs for everyone who needs one. And whenever someone is chosen to receive an organ, those who are passed over and have to wait longer are being harmed as they get sicker and in some cases die. Justice and fairness must be considered in the distribution of the limited supply, but the allocation that would be just and fair is not obvious. Complex issues are subtly interrelated, making theoretical answers hard to reach and harder still to spell out in the individual cases that must be addressed [34].

Distributive justice

Should everyone who needs a vital organ to live or to live a significantly better life be treated the same way, or are there some considerations that need to be given special weight in distribution? Should social grounds be taken into account, or only medical factors? Which factors should be counted, and how much? Should people be given no more than one organ? Two? Three?

In organ allocation, UNOS—the national distribution system—now gives priority to urgency of need and then to length of time on the list. However, if urgency is always and without qualification the primary consideration, people with the least likelihood of surviving, including some in serious danger of losing a transplanted organ, are the most likely to receive a transplant. But because fewer patients would survive transplantation if such a policy were adopted, some alternative scheme would better maximize the effective use of organs.

In listing potential recipients, transplant centers typically pay most attention to the medical features of gravity and the likelihood of long-term success. Including benefit in their focus improves the overall utility of the distribution system. However, we can still ask whether it is just to overlook considerations like the patient's previous contribution to society or the patient's future prospects of depleting or contributing to the stock of social resources. If the supply of transplant organs does not increase, and if the demand for organs continues to increase, we will be pressed to justify not paying more attention to such social considerations in organ distribution [35–38].

Free riders

Beyond these most obvious considerations about the characteristics of individual organ recipients, a host of questions arise about whether certain categories of individuals should be excluded from the pool of possible organ recipients. Should free riders— those who are not eligible to donate and those who would not be willing to donate—be denied access to the limited supply of transplant organs? Or should free riders be allowed to benefit from the kindness of strangers without being willing or able to give anything in return? For example, should foreign nationals or those with religious convictions that would rule out donations be eligible to receive organs through UNOS [39]?

Duties and debts

The discussion of justice in organ allocation can be understood as an attempt to understand who has a right to transplantation. However, rights are often associated with duties. If some people have the right to a transplant, what does "the system" owe them? In other words, when a society declares its commitment to providing transplantation as one form of medical therapy, what are patients entitled to expect? What are the duties of the system to the recipient?

By creating, regulating, and funding UNOS, and by funding the research that has made organ transplantation into a viable therapy for organ failure, our government has implicitly proclaimed its acceptance of an obligation to provide this therapy. Since government's support is drawn from the common pool of social resources, and since the cadaveric organs are donated through a national distribution network, all (citizens, taxpayers, residents) should have equal access to the beneficial therapy. According to this argument, those without the financial wherewithal to pay for transplantation nevertheless have the right to equal access because they are part of the society that has supported its development. Furthermore, because organ harvesters would not refuse cadaveric organ donations from those without health insurance and financial means, monetary considerations should also be irrelevant in organ distribution. So far our society has not acknowledged its obligation to provide for equal access to transplantation; some people cannot get organs because they cannot pay. Unless there is an argument to show why it is just for the poor, who can give organs and who may vote their support of transplantation research, to be ethically denied the opportunity to get organs, we must respect everyone's right to equal access.

Besides the government, individual health care facilities also have duties to their transplant patients.

Certainly the institution is obligated to have facilities and staff adequate for performing the surgery and managing the postsurgical care. They should also have the ability to provide pretransplant and posttransplant education and necessary psychological and social support. A transplant program is also obliged to treat patients with respect by providing sufficient information about the institution's policies, the usual experience of living with a transplanted organ, and about the particular complications of their individual case, so as to allow patients to make autonomous choices about their own lives.

As in other areas of doctor-patient communication, the extent of "informing" that counts as satisfying the obligation to inform is imprecise. Before transplantation, must a patient be informed about the policies of the institution, particulars of the donor's age, life, and death, the cold ischemia time, the condition of the organs, the sources of blood for transfusion, the surgical experience of members of the transplant team, and other details? What must patients be told about their own case shortly after the surgery and then throughout the complications that ensue? The rule of respect for autonomy requires patients to be given all of the information which would be relevant to their immediate and future decisions. Thoughtful and imaginative assessment must go into determining the parameters of that requirement [40, 41].

Since special rights usually come with special duties, do those who get the right to an organ transplant also get special obligations? In other words, once people are accepted as organ recipients, do they then owe anything to "the system"? To get an organ, must you also be willing to donate your transplantable organs if you should die? Must you be willing to commit yourself to acting as an advocate for others to donate organs? Must you be willing to authorize an autopsy if your transplant should fail, so that something might be learned to help others who come later? Although no center demands that patients fulfill these duties, potential recipients should be made aware of them and encouraged to pay their moral debts.

Research

Research raises other questions about organ allocation. Should the goals of improving transplantation success in the current patient population or extending the treatment to patients who are currently considered untreatable be a consideration in organ allocation? If likelihood of success is an important consideration in distribution, is there a place for trying new or modified therapies on patients for whom success is now not likely? Given the generally accepted duty of medicine to pursue new therapies, research that could produce new medical knowledge would justify some overriding of considerations of utility, benefit, and need. The competing concerns of maximizing effective organ use and advancing transplantation must be prudently balanced in allocating transplant organs. An increasing degree of scarcity may impose increasingly strict limitations on those research projects designed to extend the treatment to a greater pool of patients and, at the same time, relax the restrictions on research that would hold a promise of somehow augmenting the organ supply, including split liver transplantation [42], xenografts [43], procuring organs from non-heart-beating donors [44].

Summary and Conclusions

Organ transplantation can save and improve lives. So physicians who are obliged to try to save lives and to act for the good of their patients are morally committed to offering this valuable treatment option to those who can benefit from it. Unfortunately, the serious shortage of organs for transplant leaves our society and the medical community to map out and navigate the obscure moral terrain of ethically procuring and allocating organs. The task in this time of organ scarcity is to draw the moral lines with creative and thoughtful consideration of all those who need transplantation, so that those who must decide can courageously go to the edge in trying to do the right thing. And because of the ethical complexity of the situation, those who must act in this uncomfortable moral position must often remember to ask themselves, "Did we do the right things?"

References

1. Childress JF. Ethical criteria for procuring and distributing organs for transplantation. *J Health Politics Policy Law* 1989; 14(1):87–113.

2. Diethelm AG. Ethical decisions in the history of organ transplantation. Ann Surg 1990; May:505–520.

3. Singer PA. A review of public policies to procure and distribute kidneys for transplantation. *Arch Int Med* 1990; 150:523–527.

4. Annas GJ. The transplant odyssey. *Second Opinion* 1989; 12:33–39.

5. Thomasma DC. Ethical issues and transplantation technology. *Cambr Q Healthcare Ethics* 1992; 1(4): 333–344.

6. Rothenberg LS. The anencephalic neonate and brain death: an international review of medical, ethical, and legal issues. *Transplantation Proc* 1990; 22(3):1037–1039.

7. Churchill LR, Pinkus RLB. The use of anencephalic organs: historical and ethical dimensions. *Milbank Q* 1990; 68(2):147–169.

8. Berger DH. The infant with anencephaly: moral and legal dilemmas. *Issues Law Med* 1989; 5(1):67–85.

9. Davis A. The status of anencephalic babies: should their bodies be used as donor banks? *J Med Ethics* 1988; 14:150–153.

10. Cutter MAG. Moral pluralism and the use of anencephalic tissue and organs. *J Med Philosophy* 1989; 14:89–95.

11. Veatch RM. The impending collapse of the whole-brain definition of death. *Hastings Center Rep* 1993; 23(4):18–24.

12. Olick RS. Brain death, religious freedom, and public policy: New Jersey's landmark legislative initiative. *Kennedy Institute of Ethics J* 1991; 1(4):275–292.

13. Prottas JM. The organization of organ procurement. *J Health Politics Policy Law* 1989; 14(1):41–55.

14. Spital A. Sounding Board—The shortage of organs for transplantation: where do we go from here? *N Engl J Med* 1991; 325(17):1243–1246.

15. Veatch RM. Sounding Board—Routine inquiry about organ donation—an alternative to presumed consent. *N Engl J Med* 1991; 325(17):1246–1249.

16. Caplan AL, Virnig B. Is altruism enough? Required request and the donation of cadaver organs and tissues in the United States. *Crit Care Clin* 1990; 6(4):1007–1018.

17. Ross SE, Nathan H, O'Malley KF. Impact of required request law on vital organ procurement. *J Trauma* 1990; 30(7):820–824.

18. Kluge EHW. Designated organ donation: private choice in social context. *Hastings Center Rep* 1989; 19(5):10–15.

19. The Partnership for Organ Donation. The American public's attitudes toward organ donation and transplantation. Princeton, NJ: The Gallup Organization, 1993.

20. Tomlinson T. Infants and others who cannot consent to donation. *Mt Sinai J Med* 1993; 60(1):41–44.

21. Rhodes R. Debatable donors: when can we count their consent? *Mt Sinai J Med* 1993; 60(1):45–50.

22. Hunter J. Consent for the legally incompetent organ donor: application of a best-interest standard. *J Legal Med* 1991; 12:535–557.

23. Rhodes R, Burrows L, Reisman L. The adolescent living related donor. *Healthcare Ethics Committee Forum* 1992; 4(5):314–323.

24. Essig B. Legal aspects of the sale of organs. *Mt Sinai J Med* 1993; 60(1):59–64.

25. Dworkin G. Markets and morals: the case for organ sales. *Mt Sinai J Med* 1993; 60(1):66–69.

26. Altshuler JS. Financial incentives for organ donation: the perspectives of health care professionals. *JAMA* 1992; 267(15):2037–2038.

27. Peters TG. Life or death: the issue of payment in cadaveric organ donation. *JAMA* 1991; 265(10):1302–1305.

28. Pellegrino ED. Families' self-interest and the cadaver's organs: what price consent? *JAMA* 1991; 265(10):1305–1306.

29. Harvey J. Paying organ donors. *J Med Ethics* 1990; 16:117–119.

30. Dickens BM. Human rights and commerce in health care. *Transplantation Proc* 1990; 22(3):904–905.

31. Brecher B. The kidney trade: or, the customer is always wrong. *J Med Ethics* 1990; 16:120–123.

32. Brecher B. Buying human kidneys: autonomy, commodity and power. *J Med Ethics* 1991; 17:99.

33. Sloan FA. Organ procurement: expenditures and financial incentives. *JAMA* 1993; 269(24):3155–3156.

34. American Medical Association Council on Ethical and Judicial Affairs. Report 49: Ethical considerations in the allocation of organs and other scarce medical resources among patients. *Code of Med Ethics Reports* 1993; 4(2):140–173.

35. Rhodes R, Miller C, Schwartz M. *Transplant recipient selection: peacetime vs. wartime triage.* Cambridge Q Healthcare Ethics 1992; 1(4):327–332.

36. Veatch RM. Allocating organs by utilitarianism is seen as favoring whites over blacks. *Kennedy Institute of Ethics Newsletter* 1989; 3(3):1–3.

37. Cohen C, Benjamin M. Alcoholics and liver transplantation. *JAMA* 1991; 265(10):1299–1301.

38. Moss AH, Siegler M. Should alcoholics compete equally for liver transplantation? *JAMA* 1991; 265(10):1295–1298.

39. Davis DS. Those who don't give. *Mt Sinai J Med* 1993; 60(1):59–64.

40. Schanzer H. Child-donor kidneys. *Mt Sinai J Med* 1993; 60(1):52.

41. Moros D. Cases and doubts: panel discussion. *Mt Sinai J Med* 1993; 60(1):55–58.

42. Serge M, et al. Partial liver transplantation from living donors. *Cambridge Q Healthcare Ethics* 1992; 1(4):305–326.

43. Nelson JL. Transplantation through a glass darkly. *Hastings Center Report* 1992; 22(5):6–8.

44. Younger SJ, Arnold RM. Ethical, psychosocial and public policy implications of procuring organs from non-heartbeating cadaver donors. *JAMA* 1993; 269(21):2769–2774.

Fault and the Allocation of Spare Organs

Brian Smart

There has been much useful discussion over the allocation of spare resources between patients who are not at fault for the scarcity of healthy organs. The debate here has been over the criteria for the fair distribution of such resources. Should the choice

"Fault and the Allocation of Spare Organs," by Brian Smart, was originally published in the *Journal of Medical Ethics* 1994; 20: 26–30. Reprinted with permission of the BMJ Publishing Group.

between those who are to receive spare organs and those who are not to receive them be made by lot, by social usefulness, by quality adjusted life years (QALYS) or by appeal to the 'good innings' criterion [1]? For our present purposes I shall assume that we have an answer in the 'distributive justice criterion' (DJC). The DJC gives us an order of priority between innocent parties. The question is: should the DJC be restricted to allocations involving innocent parties or should it apply to those responsible for the scarcity too? Should the allocation of spare organs ignore all questions of fault, or should considerations of rectificatory justice enter when at least one of the patients in need is responsible for the scarcity? Rectificatory justice covers both punishment and reparation for wrongs, and in law is to be found both in the criminal and civil law, for example in torts and contract [2].

Historical Fault

There are those who hold that the DJC should command all allocation simply on the ground that the question of responsibility never arises. Michael Lockwood, for example, expresses scepticism about free will: '... we are all of us victims of our genetic inheritance, upbringing and so forth, and ... it is not true that people who bring certain kinds of health care needs on themselves—for example by driving dangerously, overeating, smoking or abusing drugs or alcohol—really *could*, in the final analysis, have acted any differently' [3]. This is not the place to discuss the issue of free will and responsibility. But, whether we believe in free will or not, we need to discuss its *implications*, and Lockwood has not addressed these. Our everyday practice of morality and law certainly does distinguish between people who are at fault and those who are not. The cloth out of which that everyday practice weaves culpability is made up of intention and foresight, knowledge of right and wrong, rationality, control over one's actions and emotions, beliefs about the circumstances of the action and a capacity to exercise reasonable care about others. For those who wish to reserve judgement on free will our question still stands: *if* a person is responsible for a shortage of healthy organs, should their access be determined wholly by distributive criteria or should rectificatory justice (punishment or reparation) be involved?

In a recent article proposing a complete criterion of allocation, Michael J Langford distinguishes between past fault, which his proposed criterion excludes as ground for allocation, and a present or future condition, for example alcoholism, which could ground allocation 'if it rendered the medical prognosis poor' [4]. However, he does not provide any reason why past fault should be excluded. Now for our purposes it may just be the case that Langford has successfully delineated *the* DJC. Indeed, exclusion of historical fault would be definitionally required, for it would exclude questions of rectificatory justice. But it would plainly beg the question arbitrarily to exclude rectificatory criteria from a complete criterion of allocation: that requires argument.

It is, however, possible to reconstruct a line of reasoning that may have influenced Langford. He believes that a principle of equality should govern his criterion, and, he claims 'that certainly looks like a deontological principle' [4], by which he means 'one that relates to rights and duties that are alleged to apply regardless of the consequences' [5]. However, it emerged that he is not defending a deontological principle since he is elaborating a principle to which deontologists, utilitarians (who are interested in only the consequences) and those uncommitted to an ethical theory may subscribe [4]. But there is no such neutral principle. It is only utilitarianism which, at base, wholly rejects the moral significance of the past. It is only utilitarianism which would find no possible role for historical fault in a complete principle of allocation: deontology and ordinary morality commonly base judgements of desert, entitlement and liability on past fault of one of the parties involved.

It might also be the case that Langford believes that including rectificatory criteria turns scarce resource allocation into punishment. To that argument I now turn.

A Non-Punitive Principle of Restitution

The idea that historical fault should play a key role in the allocation of health care is vigorously rejected by John Harris. He writes:

> 'We all, of course, have a duty to encourage and promote morality, but to do so by choos-
> ing between candidates for treatment on moral grounds is to arrogate to ourselves not
> simply the promotion of morality but the punishment of immorality. And to choose to
> let one person rather than another die on the grounds of some moral defect in their
> behaviour or character is to take upon ourselves the right not simply to punish, but cap-
> itally to punish, offenders against morality' [6].

We need to distinguish here between at least two different ways of choosing between people for treatment on moral grounds. The first way is where we give preference to one on grounds of her superior moral character or behaviour, but where neither party is in any way responsible for the scarcity of resources. To decide in this way is to include morality in the DJC: it is not addressed to rectifying any wrong, for the problem of scarcity is neither party's fault. Harris may be right not to include morality in the DJC, but that is another matter. The second way of choosing between people for treatment on moral grounds is where the need to choose is the fault of one of the parties in need of treatment. However, the most obvious cases of such choices are not cases of punishment at all, but cases of self-defence and other-defence.

Consider a case of other-defence in which an unprovoked attack has been launched on Kurt by Charles. Kurt cannot retreat or restrain Charles but you have the power, at no risk to yourself, of intervening by killing Charles. Suppose you do this on the ground that Charles is at fault for causing the dilemma. There is a scarcity of resources, since you do not have the power to save *both* Kurt *and* Charles, only the power to save *either* Kurt *or* Charles. A just case of other-defence would be one in which you choose between these two on moral grounds, not on grounds of general character blemishes but on the ground that Charles is at fault for causing the scarcity of resources and so should bear the cost. This ground needs elaboration. Kurt is not at fault, and so not only should he not have to bear the cost, but Charles *should be forced to make restitution* to Kurt: in other words, Charles should be forced to restore Kurt to the position he rightfully enjoyed before Charles's attack endangered his life [7].

Here we have all the ingredients of a preferential choice between lives on moral grounds. But does it constitute the punishment of immorality, or, in this case, capital punishment? I suggest not. First of all, there is no account of punishment which licenses the treatment justified by self-defence. If Charles is killed for launching an unsuccessful attempt on Kurt's life, that is not because it is a suitable punishment but because it is the minimal reasonable force to defend Kurt: as punishment it would exceed even the harsh limits imposed by the *lex talionis* (an eye for an eye …). If all that was needed to defend Kurt was for you to give Charles a slap on the cheek or a harsh frown then that would hardly be a punishment to fit the crime of attempted murder, but it would be all that would be licensed by other-defence. In cases of self-defence and other-defence where the aggressor survives, we can distinguish more clearly between the treatment licensed by defence and the treatment licensed by punishment: the question of punishment obviously does arise in cases of unsuccessful murder even when the aggressor has received the harm that was minimally necessary for a successful defence of the victim.

Self-Inflicted Harm Is Not a Crime

A second reason for rejecting preferential treatment as punishment lies in the fact that self-inflicted harm is not a crime. Damaging one's own heart or lungs by smoking is not forbidden by law: it would be legal paternalism if it were. So the justification, if there is one, for discriminating against a smoker when only one healthy spare set of heart and lungs is available must be non-punitive. And that justification lies in restitution. For suppose that what the smoker who is at fault must do is to restore to others what was rightfully theirs before the commission of the fault. True, the smoker has inflicted harm on only himself. But this ceases to be true if he does not forfeit equality of entitlement to a spare set of heart and lungs. For example, if there is no forfeiture of equality then, the one non-smoker in need of a transplant has a $1/2$ chance of acquiring the spare set rather than a $1/1$ chance. Without differential treatment according to fault the nonsmoker would be denied his rightful opportunity. By forfeiting his own right to equality the smoker restores the nonsmoker to her rightful *status quo*.

Interestingly, much of this argument applies to someone who damages another's healthy heart or who vandalises one of the two healthy spare sets of organs available [8]. The obvious difference is that a crime has now been committed—harm to the person or damage to property: punishment is a matter for the criminal courts. But, in addition to the crime, we have the same kind of situation that arose with self-inflicted harm: there is a scarcity of resources. By harming another's heart, or by vandalising a spare set of organs on their way to the theatre, the person at fault has forfeited his right to equal priority with the innocent patient. The innocent patient is owed restitution of his $1/1$ chance of access to healthy organs that he possessed before the fault occurred. Restitution and reparation is a matter either for the civil courts or may be settled out of court.

It might be thought that self- and other-defence are sufficiently unlike choice between lives caused by a shortage of resources to provide a useful insight into the nature of that choice. After all, self- and other-defence involve an aggressor who is a current threat to the victim. For this reason, Langford's distinction between historical fault and current condition might explain why he could justify self- and other-defence. And it might also explain why Harris might want to assimilate preferential treatment against a patient at fault to punishment: for it would involve an historical and not an ongoing fault.

The Threat May Be Current

But historical fault may be found in self-defence. The threat may be current, but the fault may be historical [9]. Imagine the aggressor has pushed his trolley to the crest of the hill and has now tied himself in it so that he cannot jump out: you are tied to the track down which the trolley is heading and fortunately you can operate by remote control a bulldozer which, at the flick of the switch, will straddle the track, protect you but kill the aggressor when his trolley smashes into it. The fault is historical in the sense that after the trolley has crested the hill, the aggressor can do nothing more about it, and flight or effective threats are not open to the victim. This is unlike the current fault of an aggressor who is trying to strangle you and in whose power it is to desist right up to the moment of the victim's death. In this case both the threat and the fault are current. But the burden of restitution is the same in both cases. Indeed, it is not inappropriate to ask, in the present tense, 'Who *is* responsible?' in both cases of historical and current fault.

We now have a non-punitive principle of restitution. It properly belongs to rectificatory, not distributive justice, since it requires those at fault to restore those endangered or harmed to their rightful *status quo*. It is not punishment, since it is like paying damages in a civil libel suit.

Priority of Non-Smokers over Smokers in Access to Spare Organs?

What are the implications of this principle of restitution? Should medical practitioners supplement the DJC with a fault criterion that prioritises the innocent? Notoriously in ethics, as in economics and physics, there is a large gap between the enunciation of a sound principle and its practical application.

First of all, it is unclear who should apply the DJC supplemented by a rule of restitution. We have ruled out criminal courts since forfeiting priority of access to scarce resources is not a matter for punishment. But the application of the principle does introduce a dimension not covered by the DJC: assessing degrees of culpability. So expertise for assessing fault is required on any panel that is involved in the allocation: assessing fault is not a medical skill. It is to be hoped that the composition of any panel would, like juries, introduce more democracy and in some way involve consultation with those needing a transplant or with their representatives. One crucial reason for this is that if restitution is owed to another party, it does not follow that the restitution has to be made. For it is always open to the person who has the right to restitution *to waive* that right. This is not peculiar to debts of restitution, but a more general feature of obligations. After all, I do not have to pay you back the £10 I promised to repay you if you waive your right to repayment. You are morally sovereign over whether I will be held to that promise or not.

If, as law and ordinary morality suggests, it is an empirical matter whether individuals are at fault, there are undoubtedly difficulties in identifying particular cases. For example, the problem with many cases of self-inflicted heart or lung disease is that it may be caused by addiction to nicotine. Addiction as such does not rule out fault. For someone may have taken up smoking or drinking quite freely, but foreseen that he would not be able to give it up once he was addicted [10]. On the other hand, a large proportion of smokers become addicted in their early teens and so, because of immaturity, are not responsible for their addiction. Nor should we ignore the stress-related conditions that might cause much smoking in adults: unemployment, inability to keep up mortgage repayments and broken relationships are familiar examples of such causes. Fault is either negated or much reduced by such causes. But it would be a mistake to exaggerate the difficulties of assessing culpability. Let us grant that many complex cases are impossible to resolve and that many others may be resolvable only by the ratified skills of trained lawyers. Because of the constraints of time such cases would be beyond the scope of the allocation of scarce medical resources. Such cases may be contrasted with those in which the relevant histories of the parties are known and which present good, and non-conflicting, evidence of the culpability of one of them. We would insist on this if other-defence were to be justified.

We must now distinguish between being responsible for a condition and being at fault or culpable for that condition arising. For there to be a fault there must be a wrong committed as well as there being responsibility for that wrong. A miner or fireman chooses freely to subject himself to greater risk of harm or disease than is met with in most occupations. And, on the special assumption that if he were not to make that choice nobody would fill his place, it may be true that he causes a shortfall in spare healthy organs. But, because of the social value placed upon such occupations, we are not tempted to say that such a shortfall is the *fault* of the miner or the fireman. Since there is no fault there can be no case for saying that miners should have less priority than those who have no responsibility for their condition. But why should the social value of the occupations involving these risks mean that no fault occurs? The justification lies in fairness. In this case the value is one of social need: the society needs firemen and miners for its welfare. To ask people to take an extra risk (which may be rewarded by danger money) and then to give them lower medical priority than any ordinary member of the public would simply be unfair: indeed there is a case for giving them a higher medical priority in addition to danger money.

One qualification should be made here. The society asks people in dangerous occupations to take only the risks that are reasonable in the circumstances. Negligence can incur harm that was reasonably avoidable. Society did not ask the miner to harm himself in that way.

Dangerous Sports

Dangerous sports such as rock-climbing and paragliding are not pursued out of social necessity since they do not contribute to social welfare. Society does not ask people to engage in rock-climbing or paragliding. If people freely engage in these sports should they not pay all the extra costs such activities risk and so receive a lower priority in access to spare organs? The argument with smoking is that it is unfair to spread the extra risks of this self-indulgence to those who prefer not to impose an extra risk on themselves. Should not the same apply to dangerous sports? A strong case can be made here for the social value of such sports, providing they are not too dangerous, and providing they are practised non-negligently. The value does not belong to social welfare, it is not socially necessary as has been stated. But these sports do enhance lives as well as endanger them. Their value is both intrinsic and extrinsic. Intrinsically, skills of a very high order can be acquired, with an accompanying feeling of achievement; but even beginners find the activity exciting and challenging. Yet it is also a spectator sport, in the sense that it can be followed with binoculars or cameras and be read about. Extrinsically, the activity is character-forming as well as being able to provide the best exponents with a living. Activities of this kind thus become a part of our culture and their value contributes to a worthwhile life. After all, social welfare is not an end in itself: it simply enables us to choose and pursue a worthwhile life.

Moral Complicity

Do dangerous sports differ in important respects from smoking or hard drinking? I think it is easy to show that our society delivers a mixed message on this issue. On the one hand, it permits advertising and sponsorship which may target children, and which presents smoking and drinking as appendages to a glamorous life-style. And, on the whole, it does not restrict smoking very seriously in public places, even when the dangers of passive smoking are well known. Such a policy seems to countenance the sharing of risks between smokers and the general public. On the other hand, government health warnings are compulsory on packets and advertisements. I think the upshot of this is that our society may be charged with moral complicity in the tobacco companies' operations and in the smokers' self-infliction of harm. Part of the message is that there is no fault: the other part of the message is that the activity is dangerous. When combined, these messages are compatible with the claim that smoking is a valuable (chic, cool) way of living in which it would be fair that we should all, smokers and non-smokers alike, bear the costs equally in the case of access to medical care: it would be unjust if non-smokers were given priority.

The claim that smoking is socially valuable should be challenged. One familiar way of doing this is to point out that its value is an illusion created by advertisers, an illusion which can affect young people at an impressionable and vulnerable phase in their lives. We have remarked on how it can be seen as a part of stylish living: this claim might be sustainable if we could substitute a substance that had no deleterious effects on our health. But in the light of its probable effects, the illusion can be sustained only by screening off or ignoring those probable effects. Also, safer remedies are available for removing the stress that smoking can remove (for example exercise or alcohol in moderate quantities). It may be rightly claimed that smoking causes private pleasure while not harming anyone else if practised privately. But that is a reason why people's right to smoke in private should be defended, provided they are aware of the risks. It is not a reason why those risks should be shared with the general public and so reduced for the participants themselves: if the activity lacks social value then the risks should be borne by the participants alone.

So far as smoking is concerned this paper is deliberately hedged about with qualifications. A society which banned the advertising of tobacco and attached no social value to smoking would share no fault with those who smoked of their own free will. In such circumstances, it would be fair to give a lower priority to smokers in the allocation of spare organs.

The argument for this conclusion has been deontological and has been based on a principle of restitution for an historical fault. Yet deontological thinking is only part of our moral thought: we must be sensitive to the consequences of our actions. It is therefore worth remarking that it is likely that the consequences of introducing a restitutive principle would be beneficial. Now that might appear doubtful if we consider Michael Lockwood's observation about one likely consequence of adopting a rule of priority according to fault:

'... there might be good welfarist reasons for according the claims of [smokers] on health care resources a relatively low priority, if the fact were to be widely publicized and could act as an effective deterrent to such irresponsible behaviour. But I doubt whether it would. Someone who is undeterred by the prospect of seriously damaging his health is hardly likely, in my opinion, to be deterred by the prospect of less than ideal health care thereafter' [11].

Lockwood may be right about this particular consequence, at least in the vast majority of cases. Few are likely to be made *more responsible* by a rectificatory response to their fault. But he ignores the possibility that a system of equal access for all alike might induce many to become *more irresponsible* about their health. This is a phenomenon that occurs in the field of safety measures [12]. For example, if seat belts are made compulsory there is a tendency for drivers to drive faster and so restore the former accident rates.

To conclude: rectificatory but non-punitive justice has in principle a role to play in the allocation of scarce medical resources. However, this would be just only within a framework of robust preventive medicine: this would mean effective health education and the elimination of cigarette advertising and sponsorship.

References and Notes

1. For the most recent account of a sophisticated allocative criterion see Langford M J. Who should get the kidney machine? *Journal of medical ethics* 1992; 18: 12–17.
2. For the introduction of this distinction see Aristotle, *The Nicomachean ethics* bk 5: 1130a 22–1132a 27.
3. Lockwood M. Quality of life and resource allocation. In: Bell J M, Mendus S, eds. *Philosophy and medical welfare*. Royal Institute of Philosophy, Lecture Series 23. Cambridge: Cambridge University Press, 1988: 49.
4. See reference (1) 13.
5. See reference (1) 16.
6. Harris J. *The value of life*. London: Routledge and Kegan Paul, 1985: 108.
7. For a detailed account see Smart B J. Understanding and justifying self-defence. *International journal of moral and social studies* 1989; 4, 3: 231–244.
8. For such a hypothetical see Wasserman D. Justifying self-defense. *Philosophy and public affairs* 1987; 16, 4: 367, fn 29.
9. David Wasserman wrongly attempts to dissociate an aggressor from his current threat where the fault is historical and the point of no return has been passed. See reference (8) 371–372. For a fault principle characterised as distributive rather than retributive or restitutive see Montague P. The morality of self-defense. *Philosophy and public affairs* 1989; 18, 1: 88.
10. See reference (2): bk 3: 1114a 15–21.
11. See reference (3): 49.
12. See Trammell R L *et al.* Utility and survival. *Philosophy* 1977; 52: 336.

Applicants

Felicia Niume Ackerman

There were books about job interviews. There were books about college interviews. But for this interview, I was on my own. Of course, I could use some of what I had read.

LOOK YOUR BEST. I had slept with my hair braided, and now it was wavy and soft. My little mirror showed a heart-shaped face (appropriate), large light-blue eyes, skin maybe a trifle pale, but except for the bluish tinge of my lips, I thought I looked almost more like a movie invalid than the real thing. Hard to decide about makeup, though. The books said it should be effective but unobtrusive, but they weren't too specific about what that meant. Probably best to compromise: enough lipstick to give my lips a better color, but no eye shadow. I tweezed my eyebrows just enough to make the arch look natural. Yes, I liked my reflection. And I had read somewhere that attractive people were rated better on everything, even things you would think had nothing to do with looks.

BE ON TIME OR SLIGHTLY EARLY. No problem there. My interview was coming to me. Where else would that happen? Suppose I were trying to adopt a child. I'd spend hours getting the house ready: sweeping, scrubbing, vacuuming, dusting. Hiding things. My controversial books would go in boxes in a closet, my bearskin rug under my bed in case the interviewer was big on animal rights. I'd put sheet music on the piano, although I hadn't played it in years. Your home reflects you.... But I didn't have to worry about that here. This room was cleaner than I could have made it myself, even if I had been able to get out of bed. Walls, linoleum, curtains, chairs: everything was pure, dazzling white. Sterile, institutional, dehumanizing, my sister would have said. I liked it. It meant business. At the hospice where she had wanted me to go (and which took mainly cancer patients, she had added, as if I were being offered a special favor), they had wallpaper with pretty flowers, and you could even bring some of your own furniture, but they wouldn't resuscitate you if you stopped breathing. Forget it, I had told her, I'm not that stuck on my night table.

DRESS IN A WAY THAT IS BECOMING AND APPROPRIATE. I could hardly get more appropriate than a hospital gown. Over it I wore the pink-and-blue quilted bed jacket my sister had sent instead of coming. The blue was almost the shade of my eyes, and my rose quartz ring matched the pink. I pinned my circlet of pearls on the collar; no oversized Middle Eastern pendants or jangly earrings today.

REHEARSE ANSWERS TO THE QUESTIONS YOU ARE LIKELY TO BE ASKED. I had been at that for months, and last week I got Nick started, too. They would interview him separately later. It was like trying to become a corporate executive; your

---

"Applicants," by Felicia Niume Ackerman, was originally published in *Ascent* 1985; 10(2): 2–18.

family got checked out as well. You had to have a "supportive family." My sister was useless, my parents were dead, but I had Nick. My supportive family. At a price.

The gold watch that had been my mother's said nine-thirty. Half an hour to go.

***

There were two of them, and they were ten minutes late. The psychiatric screeners, keepers of the gates of life. Dr Reynolds and Dr Garner. One tall and one short, one male and one female, one black and one white. Equal opportunity.

Dr Garner was my age or maybe a few years older, 35 at most. She had blond hair cut like a helmet, gold-rimmed glasses, and wore a severely tailored charcoal gray skirt and white blouse underneath her open white coat. Nothing like how I would be dressed on the job. I favored heavily embroidered ethnic clothes, and I'd always been proud that I could get ahead without "dressing for success." But now someone who used words like "supportive" and dressed like a disciple of *The Woman's Dress for Success Book* would decide whether my personality made me fit to live.

Dr Reynolds was fortyish and heavyset, with a thick neck and broad shoulders, as though he might have played football in college. How did I feel about the prospect of having a heart transplant? he wanted to know. I looked at the two of them steadily (MAKE EYE CONTACT) and said I had never wanted anything so much in my life. Dr Garner pushed her glasses up the bridge of her nose and asked why. I thought of the woman who had interviewed me for college 15 years ago.

And why do you want to come to Wellesley, Yvonne?

I like everything I know about it. The curriculum, the campus, the high academic standards.

"It's my only chance," I said now.

Dr Garner nodded. Was I afraid of the operation?

Somewhere there was bound to be a study showing that patients who were afraid of surgery had a lower survival rate.

"No," I said firmly.

"But you realize the surgery carries a mortality risk?" Dr Reynolds asked slowly, leaning forward as if he were about to run with the ball.

I assured him that the operation was worth the risk. That I knew I couldn't last more than a few months without a transplant. That I had come here because it was the best transplant center in the world, and I had absolute confidence in the surgical team.

No, it doesn't bother me that there are no men at Wellesley, Dean Morrison. I like the idea of a women's college.

Once more with feeling. That sort of thing had never been my strong point—too hard to keep my voice from coming out singsong. But this time, I'd practiced again and again.

Dr Garner shifted her position. Now she was sitting with her legs crossed at the ankles and her hands clasped in her lap. Wasn't that how little girls sat in portraits a century ago? She wore elegant black calf shoes with stacked heels. I had not worn shoes in over a month.

Dr Reynolds was looking at his hands. Then he glanced up at me again. It struck me that he seemed more hesitant than she did. Maybe he had doubts about what he was doing. So what? I wondered if he knew what used to be said about blacks: let them earn equal rights. How did I feel about my illness? he asked finally. It must have been quite a blow to have this happen to me so young and so suddenly. At least these examiners, like the ones at my PhD oral examination six years ago, were asking nothing I had not anticipated.

"Well, at first, I could hardly believe how sick I was. I knew how sick I felt, but I kept telling myself it would go away, like mono or the flu. And then...." I let my voice trail off.

"Yes?" prompted Dr Reynolds, as sympathetically as a friend.

As sympathetically as a friend. These days, kindness affected me like music: immediately, automatically, even when I knew the kindness was professional and purposeful. Why couldn't someone invent a vaccine for it? Already I could feel myself wanting to yield, to say, Oh, Dr Reynolds, I am so scared. Please let me live. Aren't you my friend? I'll say anything you want. Do anything you want. And I'll be so grateful.

My eyes stung. Steady on. The dentist I had gone to during my year in London used to say that, and it always made me furious. Who was he to tell me how to feel? No one likes to be told to calm down.... Focus on something neutral. Dr Reynolds' tie. It was red with a design of little black puppies. Was it a present from one of his children? It didn't look like something an adult would have chosen. It looked silly. But this man would decide whether my personality made me fit to live.

"For a while, I was bitter and resentful, I have to admit," I said carefully. "And I was scared. Why did this have to happen to me? I kept wondering, as if I were the world's first person ever to become critically ill. That stage lasted about two weeks." (Psychiatrists liked stages, didn't they?) "But then..."

"Yes?" said Dr Garner. They were both nodding now—in agreement? Approval? Were they lapping it up like a pair of sleek cats? Or were they just telling me to continue? What else could I do, anyway?

"Well, resentment never accomplished anything, did it?" I said. As if it were supposed to. And anyway, it did. I never would have lost 11 pounds in junior high school if I hadn't resented how popular Kathy McKinley was.

"So after a while, something in me just got tired of using up my energy that way and started wanting to use it to combat my illness instead." (At least I hadn't said "use my energy constructively.") "And that made all the difference," I continued.

Getting my tone right was the hard part here. The trick was to make the platitudes sound both reasonable and as if I'd originated them. I plowed on through the whole growth-through-adversity speech. The interviewers looked impressed. Of course, they also looked healthy enough to fall for it, and I had all my hesitations and facial expressions down pat. Good thing I'd been so active in college dramatics. It was enough to vindicate that Wellesley dean who was always trumpeting the value of extracurricular activities.

What time was it? No way I could find out without being obvious. My hands were under the blanket. They were cold. They were always cold now. My heart was too weak to keep them warm. *How long are you going to keep this up, for Christ's sake? I'm tired. I'm deathly ill, remember? Have a heart. Have mine; let's trade.*

Dr Garner was asking whether I was afraid of death. Easy to guess the right answer. Didn't every healthy person with at least 40 years of life ahead know that a truly emotionally mature individual had worked through the fear of death? Of course, there were no right or wrong answers. The answers that could condemn me to death weren't *wrong* answers.

Did I have any questions?

I had prepared some innocuous ones just in case.

Now the interviewers were rising to leave. Would my fiancé be able to talk with them next Thursday at four?

"Yes, he will. I'll tell him. He'll be there."

***

"They want to interview you Thursday at four," I said when Nick came into my room two days later.

He kicked the door shut behind him. "I've got a choice?"

"Nick—"

"Yeah, okay." He sat down in the white plastic chair facing me, slouched forward, and started cracking his knuckles—one of his more irritating habits, I had recently decided.

"*American Historical Quarterly* turned down my paper," he said, glaring at the floor. "Did you see that pretentious Hitchens crap they published in October? Yes, if you're at Cornell. No, if you're at Tomlinson State College. What a coincidence. Almost as big a coincidence as that my mother and my father both got married on the same day. Ever occur to you that 'editor' rhymes with 'predator'?"

He transferred the glare to me as if I were one of those creatures myself. His face seemed designed for ineffectual glares. It was tired and heavy-featured, with black hair spilling across his forehead, and chronically red, puffy, irritable-looking eyes. Hardly the most prepossessing supportive family I could have chosen. If I'd had a choice.

I thought, I have got to be the world's only heart-transplant candidate who's expected to get excited about someone's rejected articles. Then again, maybe not. Who knew what went on in the other supportive families?

"You know that's the third place I sent it to? No point in my trying anywhere else now. Might as well wait until—" He cracked another knuckle. "Might as well wait."

I nodded. I knew what he had been about to say. I thought about our conversation in December, the agreement we had made.

***

I had telephoned him on a Friday evening a few weeks before Christmas. It had taken me all afternoon to get up my strength.

"Nick? It's Yvonne." I had still been at home then, propped up in bed on three pillows. I could no longer breathe lying flat. But it had been one of my better days. I could manage a long phone call.

"Yvonne? Not sure I ought to be talking to you." Over the telephone, Nick's voice had sounded harsher and duller than I'd remembered. "Think I forgot how you ditched me at the convention so you could go off with some Harvard hotshots?"

I'd had an image of Nick in his cracked old leather jacket and black chinos (he didn't dress for success, either), his face bleak and rigid as I hastily ended our conversation when the Harvard people appeared in the hotel lobby. Of course, he hadn't forgotten. But I had. I hadn't anticipated this.

"Nick, I had been corresponding with Peter for months. I explained it to you later, remember?" The following morning at the convention, I had also told Nick about the secret manuscript I was planning to spring upon the world as soon as I was done with the finishing touches. I had loved having a secret manuscript. It was so different from the way other people worked, and it had felt exquisitely private, as I supposed having a clandestine lover might feel. But, of course, Nick had accused me of picking him to hear the secret because I figured he didn't count.

"Yeah, so what's this, your winter slumming trip?" I could hear him breathing roughly into the phone. "You got the right place. Just found out I won't get tenure unless I have what they call a 'vastly improved publication record' next year. Know when my chairman's last publication was? Eight years ago. Well, what are you up to? Tell me how the other half lives."

I had told him.

"Jesus." There'd been a long pause. "Is it hard to get a transplant?"

"Harder than getting tenure. It's not just medical, anyway. It's fantastically expensive, which I can just about manage, and they have to approve of your personality and think you're stable enough. And you've got to have a family. They have some theory that what they call a supportive family is supposed to help you get through all this, so if you haven't got one, the hell with you."

"You're kidding."

"No. You've got to have a family."

"Wages of singleness is death," Nick had said, and I'd told him I had been oversimplifying. They didn't actually require relatives as long as you could prove someone cared about you enough. They had even given a transplant to a lesbian with a long-term, live-in lover, which must have made them feel very liberal.

"You're nobody till somebody loves you," Nick had said. "Yeah, very liberal. How's your family?"

"Dead. Except my sister, who believes in death with dignity. For me. She refused to help me get a transplant."

"Even though you want one?"

"That's right."

"Jesus."

My right hand had become almost numb by this point. The fingertips were startlingly blue. I'd been gripping the receiver like the edge of a raft.

"Jesus can't help me," I had said. "But you can."

"What could I do? I can't be your family."

"No, but you could fake it."

He had been bewildered. Intrigued. But most of all—I could tell—he had been afraid. Afraid of being trapped. He had his own problems; hadn't he just been telling me? And I knew perfectly well how he resented me for having tenure at UCLA and being well known in our field.

But he was practically the only unattached male friend I had, even if we hadn't seen each other much since graduate school, where I'd found his lack of the usual academic veneer refreshing. And he wouldn't actually have to marry me or live with me, I had assured him. He'd just have to say he would. Let them interview him. Come to visit me three times a week at the Center, so they would know he really cared. Lucky he lived so nearby.

"It's not so nearby. It's an hour away."

"I'll give you anything you want in return. Anything. My BMW, all my family jewelry—"

"Christ! Look, I'd like to help you, even with the crummy way you treated me. I just can't. Don't have that kind of time now, not if I want any chance to keep my lousy job. There's got to be someone else you could get."

"There isn't." He hadn't asked why. Probably he could guess that I'd been too busy being a success to get close to anyone, just as he'd been too busy resenting not being one. One thing I had to say for Nick: at least he didn't think that having no loved ones in your life was a personal defect.

"Nick, without the transplant, I'm going to—*die*, can't you see?" My voice had almost broken, and I hadn't even tried to control it. "Think it over. Please. There must be something I can give you that would make up for what I'm asking."

The next morning, Nick had called me back. "Well, I thought of something." His voice had been heavy, gritty, dragging. I'd had an image of a car being pushed uphill. "Pretty crummy, though. You'll hate it. Maybe you can guess already."

***

That had been two months ago, and now, sitting at my bedside in the white room, Nick was thinking about it again. I could tell by his expression, at once defiant and uncomfortable. He was thinking about the manuscript I'd described at the convention, the manuscript no one else knew about. No one else would ever know about it now, until it appeared under Nick's name with enough revisions to make it look as though it could be his. It would be his, if I got the transplant. Your book or your life. I had chosen my life.

"You could have said no," Nick said suddenly. "At least I gave you a choice. Would I be less of a louse if I'd been like your sister and left you to die?"

I closed my eyes. "Nick, I don't know and I don't care. It's beside the point, anyway. We made a deal." No point in telling him how horribly I minded it.

"I did try to come yesterday." Nick's voice was eerily disembodied in the dark. "They wouldn't let me in. They said you had a bad night and needed to rest."

"Yes." He didn't ask for details. I didn't give them.

"Yeah, I know you think I'm a crumb to want to get ahead off your book," Nick persisted, like a buzzing insect. "I tried it the other way. You teach at a state college, you need something special to get published anywhere decent. Yvonne?"

"What?"

"Don't you think they should have taken my paper?"

He was cracking his knuckles again. It sounded like popping corn. I opened my eyes. The air in the room seemed heavy and close, as though the window had not been opened in days.

"Nick, this is probably going to astonish you, but that isn't the main question on my mind right now." I looked at him. A muscle twitched under his left eye. I looked away. "We've been all through this sort of thing, anyhow. Your papers are good enough to be in good journals, and you're probably right about why they get turned down." I wasn't lying. But I hoped he wouldn't ask me exactly how I thought his work compared with mine.

"Will you bring me more mysteries next time?" I said.

Nick nodded. I began giving him titles to look for and some to avoid. He pulled a brown imitation-leather-covered notebook out of his back pocket and started writing with his bumpy fingers. The knuckles were misshapen and enlarged, and his fingernails were dirty. "Clean fingernails are a mark of a lady," my mother used to say, "but whether you want to be a lady is another matter."

I thought about the time Steffi Gibson in graduate school had told Nick sweetly that in addition to being offensive, cracking his knuckles would probably give him arthritis in later life. Nick had stared, then walked over to her, cracked three knuckles right in her cool Ivy League face, and slammed out of the room. "He's so crude," Steffi had said. "So what?" I had said.

The following year Steffi flunked out of the program. It was the last time I could remember Nick being really happy about anything.

Now he was finishing up my list and muttering to himself. "Anyway," he said loudly, abruptly, when I was running out of names, "I'd never have time to get anything written myself this term. Not when I've got to drive up here to see you three times a week."

***

Two days later, Nick came back with four detective novels and a Venus flytrap.

"All homey little murders, none of that spy stuff, and I checked the flaps to see that there's nothing about illness," he said, handing me the books.

"Thank you." I had read one of the Christies, and Nick had forgotten how I disliked Sayers for her cloying fascination with the British aristocracy. The other two were titles I had requested.

I had not requested a Venus flytrap. Why did he bring it? I asked.

"Better than flowers. More unusual. Impress the staff."

"Impress them how? Are they supposed to think it's a tender symbol of a beautiful relationship?" I looked at the evil little spines and began to laugh. "Really, Nick, a Venus flytrap!"

His face tightened. "Yeah, well, if you want to know, I went to three places looking for something special," he said slowly. "You don't like it? I'll take it back."

"It's okay," I said. "Are you also going to provide the flies?"

"Doesn't need them." Nick gave me a quick glance, then grinned awkwardly, as if he were out of practice. "Bring you a cactus with lots of spikes next time," he said and sat down with a small thud, slouching and rubbing his eyes with the back of his hand. "I saw one of your rivals in the corridor," he added, cracking a knuckle.

One of my rivals. My room was in a nursing home whose inmates were all candidates for transplants at the Center, but I seldom saw or heard any of the others. It was almost like living here alone. I felt a surge of curiosity as intense as hunger.

"Well?" I said.

"Man in a wheelchair, about fifty, a little overweight. Wore glasses and, you'll be happy to hear, no wedding ring. Maybe he's got no supportive family. Score one for you."

"Lots of married men that age don't wear wedding rings," I said, but I hoped Nick was right. It was like the hope I felt whenever I heard an ambulance siren: maybe that's a heart for me. A common reaction in people awaiting transplants, I had once read in a news magazine, and then, a few weeks later, someone had written in to say heart transplants should be discontinued because waiting for them was so bad for people's character.

"I hate healthy people," I said.

"I know," said Nick, as though he weren't included.

I told him about the article and the letter, and he pulled a bruised apple out of his jacket pocket and bit into it noisily. "Know what that reminds me of?" he said, his mouth full. "Feature I saw in the Tomlinson local paper about this kid who has leukemia and needs blood. It was all about how sweet and patient she was—like if she'd acted like a crabby bitch because she didn't get off on being sick all the time, she wouldn't deserve to have people donate."

Loud crunching and sucking noises were accompanying these remarks. I kept my eyes on my blanket and wished I could avert my ears as well. I had always admired Nick for not being concerned enough about social niceties to bother with polite eating habits, but I preferred to admire this without actually watching him eat. It occurred to me, though, not for the first time, that much as I hated Nick for what he was making me do, I was glad for his visits. At least with Nick, I didn't have to act like the constant epitome of mental hygiene, as if I'd washed my mind out with germicidal soap. With the staff, on the other hand, even orderlies and cleaning women, I kept myself eternally pleasant and cheerful. Nick disliked pleasantness and cheer. I wondered what he did for fun.

I pushed myself up further against the pillows and asked him.

He cracked two knuckles simultaneously. "I like to sleep."

"What?"

"You heard. I can sleep ten, twelve hours a day. Don't have much time for it now. When you sleep, you could be anyone. I have good dreams, better than being awake." He rubbed his puffy eyes longingly and glanced at his watch as if it were nearly bedtime. It was 5.15.

For a moment I felt sad. Nick had had a lot of vitality once. But then, so had I.

"Well, don't come out with that at your interview," I said. "Stick to the crossword puzzles." I had chosen crossword puzzles as the perfect hobby for an invalid's fiancé. He could do them at my bedside. I could participate. Interruptions wouldn't matter.

It also wouldn't matter that Nick in fact hated crossword puzzles and all intellectual games. If I'm thinking that hard, I want to learn something, he had told me.

"For once, give me credit for half a brain, will you?" Nick got up and tapped the top mystery on the night table. *Death Comes as the End*. "Read this one first. It looks good," he said, putting on the beat-up leather jacket I had warned him not to wear to his interview.

"Wait," I said urgently. "We have to go over the stuff for your interview again."

"We've done it a million times already. I know my lines. Don't worry; I'm not going to screw up, for Christ's sake." He turned to leave. "I've got a lot at stake, too, remember?"

***

I tried to read *Death Comes as the End*, but it annoyed me. The story was set in ancient Egypt, and I preferred mysteries where the murderer was the sort of person I could have known. Ancient Egypt was too remote and peculiar. But even my own field of history, the nineteenth-century American West, seemed remote and peculiar now. My world had shrunk to my heart and this room. Just the sort of thing invalids were always getting criticized for, but I couldn't see why. When I had no idea whether I would be alive next fall, was I supposed to be able to get excited about antebellum patterns of westward migration? My department had sent me a new book on the subject, with a note signed by everyone on the faculty. I knew the author slightly. He taught at Yale, and I'd had dinner with him twice at conventions. I liked him. Nick didn't. Nick resented everyone at Yale. But until I had gotten this illness, I had not resented anyone in all my adult life. No reason to. I had been the favored one. Yes, I'd been smug, which was maybe why I had no close friends, but I had never expected this to be a capital offense.

I put the mystery aside and opened the book from my colleagues. I was surprised to discover I could still get drawn into it. But when I came upon some flattering references to the work of Sibley, it was a few moments before I realized the author was talking about me.

***

The next two days were bad days. There was pain, I couldn't eat, and I slept a lot. I kept dreaming about wandering, thirsty and lost, alone in the Mojave desert. When I reached an oasis, there was a long line of people, like the queues I had seen in England, with everyone patiently waiting for a turn. But when it came to my turn, I was refused water. "You're too unsocial, too odd," I was told. "You weren't even in a sorority in college." "My college didn't have sororities!" I screamed silently, and woke up gasping and sweating.

God, do you have a dumb unconscious, I said to myself when I calmed down. A maladjusted and unwholesome one, too, no doubt. Good thing they couldn't monitor my dreams.

I thought about Nick, with his good dreams. He didn't deserve them.

***

On the morning of Nick's interview, I woke up refreshed and alert, but uneasy. Nick would remember his lines, I was sure, but he'd turned surlier than usual at some of my other instructions: sit up straight, speak in complete sentences, don't say "yeah" all the time, don't crack your knuckles. Don't be a slob, polish up your image, it all came down to, and I recalled how outraged he had been when his dissertation supervisor made similar suggestions when Nick was on the job market. Nick's moral code permitted plagiarism, but not the deliberate upgrading of his personal style. It had taken me 15 minutes to persuade him to go along with me on this, and I doubted he'd be much good at it, anyway.

At 5.30, Nick appeared in my room, wearing wool pants and a sports jacket, as I had insisted. The pants were too blue. The jacket was too tight. Would it matter? Who knew? But fraternities rejected people for less, much less.

"Well?" I demanded as soon as he closed the door.

Nick rubbed his eyes for a long time. He didn't sit down. "I did okay."

"What did they ask?"

"About what you expected."

"Well, sit down and tell me all about it." I gestured toward the white chair, but he just stared at it as though wondering what it was for. He hadn't looked at me once, I realized. This in itself wasn't surprising—we were hardly enough enamored of each other to spend time gazing into each other's eyes—but now he seemed almost to be avoiding me. His glance shifted to the Venus flytrap, then to the window, which faced north, away from the sun.

"Look, I—got to get home. I'm tired. I'll be back in a couple of days." He turned to leave, cracking all his knuckles at once with a sound like a little explosion. From the back he looked worse. The jacket gaped at the slit, making an inverted "V."

"Nick—is anything wrong?"

"No, I did fine. I told you. I'm just tired."

Before I could say anything else, he was gone.

***

Nothing had gone wrong, I kept telling myself, nothing could have gone wrong. Nick wouldn't lie about having done well. And he certainly wouldn't be having second thoughts at this point, not when I was counting on him. Not when he was counting on me. "I've got a lot at stake, too, remember?" he had said.

But my mind would not stop. What if something had changed? What if…he had been told he wouldn't get tenure in any case? What if he'd decided my book couldn't help him anymore? What if he'd decided no one would believe it was his?

Stop being ridiculous; he would have said something. Steady on. But when I tried to telephone Nick in the evening, there was no answer.

***

For three days there was no answer. On the morning of the fourth day, Dr Reynolds came into my room. He was smiling.

"Good morning. I have good news for you."

I had passed. Like the director of admissions at Wellesley, the director of graduate studies at Berkeley, and the chairman of the history department at UCLA, Dr Reynolds was pleased to be able to tell me that I had been weighed in the balance and found not wanting. My application had been approved. I was in.

"How long—do you think I'll have to wait a long time for the operation?"

Hard to say. But probably not a terribly long time. My blood and tissue typing had shown that I would not be difficult to match. That was one reason I had been accepted. Aside from my psychological stability and supportive family situation, of course.

I smiled. I kept on smiling. And I thanked him over and over. But there was still no sign of my supportive family situation that afternoon. No answer when I phoned. Where was Nick?

***

"Where were you?" I asked when Nick walked into my room the following afternoon as if he had never stayed away.

He grunted, sat down in the white chair, and gazed blisteringly at the floor. Even when I told him we had passed the final test, his expression did not change.

"Well, really, Nick, you'll be getting what you want, too, you know. You ought to be happy…" My voice trailed away as Nick raised his eyes and gave me a look of the most concentrated hostility I had ever seen. He *hates* me, I thought, frantically scanning my memory for all the times when, in spite of everything, we'd had a kind of momentary rapport.

"I don't want your lousy book," he said.

"*What?*" I had imagined this possibility so often during the past few days that it seemed almost as if I were still doing it. Don't be ridiculous, Yvonne; Nick would never pull out. He's got a lot at stake, too, remember. Remember? My face was growing hotter by the second, and in a moment …

"Christ! Take it easy. Jesus." Nick's voice sounded drained, disgusted, and who was he to tell me to take it easy, especially now? "Christ, I didn't say I wouldn't keep on with the supportive family crap. I'll do it. You can just keep your lousy book, like I said."

"What?" I was still faintly panicky. Disoriented.

"I said—"

"I heard what you said. Have you given up on getting tenure? Did you decide you want something else from me instead?"

"Nah."

"Then what happened?"

"I changed my mind."

"Why?"

He cracked several knuckles. "I just did. Look, do we have to talk about it?"

"I want to talk about it."

"You want to." Nick got up and started pacing the floor with tense, awkward movements. "You want to, so of course we have to. Okay, it was because of the shrinks."

"What?"

He was still pacing, not looking at me. "They made me want to puke," he muttered in a tone suggesting I had the same effect. "Especially her. She was so serene, just so goddamn sure of her right to make you bargain for your life by being the kind of person she wanted. I couldn't stand being in the same room with her. Never felt so superior to anyone, except I obviously wasn't; you don't have to tell me about it." He shot me another inflamed look. "So anyway, you don't have to bargain with me anymore."

I gaped at him. He looked about the same. (Puffy-eyed, belligerent, unappealing.) What had I expected? I said the first thing that came into my mind. "But you knew all along you were making me bargain for my life."

He sat down heavily. "You can know something all along, but it's different when you see it."

It's different when you see it. Nick had finally applied his sense of outrage to somebody's plight besides his own. I opened my mouth to speak, but what came out were small puffs of laughter, over and over with all the breath I could manage, as if I were on a roller coaster or being tickled.

"What the hell's so funny?" Nick's voice took a moment to penetrate.

"It's not funny." I stopped laughing and caught my breath. "I just think everything may turn out all right, after all."

"Sure," said Nick, "for you."

"But it was your decision."

"Christ, don't you know anything?" He began cracking his knuckles again, and maybe I only imagined that the sound was sharper than before. "I spent the whole goddamn weekend trying to make myself take your book or maybe just drop out of the whole thing. Just because I couldn't do it doesn't mean I didn't want to, for Christ's sake!"

"You actually considered leaving me to die."

"I couldn't possibly do it, so calm down." He rubbed his eyes, which were redder than usual. "Jesus, I didn't even sleep much. Drove over half the state…"

Heaven help half the state. When Nick was upset in graduate school, I suddenly remembered, he used to go off for days at a time, driving over back roads in his ancient Mustang, stopping only when he got worn out, sleeping in his car. He drove viciously but skillfully, like a teenage greaser who practically lived in his hotrod, and he returned from these journeys looking dissolute and exhausted, as if he'd been on a weeklong bender.

"I see," I said. "Well, this is very…nice of you."

"Nice?" Nick got up so roughly and abruptly that he nearly knocked over the chair. "Jesus. I'm not nice. And I wouldn't pick you to be nice to. You treat me like dirt, you know that? Do this, do that, sit the way I tell you, talk the way I say... You're the last person—"

I would ever want to be nice to, I finished in my mind. I closed my eyes and could see Nick driving furiously along the bumpiest road he could find, snarling at anyone and anything that got in his way, stuffing himself with fistfuls of French fries from the nearest McDonald's, and finally falling asleep, exhausted by the discovery that the pull to do right could be as hard to resist as the pull to do wrong, and you could feel just as terrible when you felt yourself giving in.

"Yes," I said, opening my eyes. "I think maybe I understand now. I just don't know what to say. I could say I'm grateful, only I can't stand sick people being humble and grateful, like the kids on those awful Easter Seals posters. But why don't you go get some sleep, Nick? Have some good dreams."

Nick nodded. He didn't say anything. Didn't smile. Didn't even look at me. But his face seemed to relax ever so slightly, as if maybe he hated me a tiny bit less, or maybe it was just a trick of the light.

C. International Public Health Policy and Ethics

Toward Control of Infectious Disease
Ethical Challenges for a Global Effort

MARGARET P. BATTIN, CHARLES B. SMITH,
LESLIE P. FRANCIS, AND JAY A. JACOBSON

Introduction

Despite the devastating pandemic of HIV/AIDS that erupted in the early 1980s, despite the failure to eradicate polio and the emergence of resistant forms of tuberculosis that came into focus in the 1990s, and despite newly emerging diseases like SARS in 2003 and the fearsome prospect of human-to-human avian flu, it is nevertheless a time of some excitement over prospects for effective control of much of infectious disease. Funded by national and international governmental and nongovernmental organizations, private foundations, and even popular entertainers, large-scale new efforts are

"Toward Control of Infectious Disease: Ethical Challenges for a Global Effort," by Margaret P. Battin, Charles B. Smith, Leslie P. Francis, and Jay A. Jacobson, is from Michael Boylan (ed.) (2008) *International Public Health Policy and Ethics*. Springer; pp. 191–214.

under way to address global killers like AIDS, tuberculosis, and malaria, among others. Legal standoffs over patent rights to antiretrovirals and other drugs have to some extent been resolved, and pressure is being exerted for the improvement of infrastructure issues, like clean water and improved sanitation. Research in the identification of pathogens, as well as in the prevention, diagnosis, and treatment of infectious diseases, has made very great progress in some areas, especially in vaccine development and the development of rapid tests, in pandemic forecasting, and in the establishment of globally coordinated disease outbreak surveillance networks. At last, attention is being focused on orphan infectious diseases and the so-called neglected tropical diseases. It is, we think, a moment of growing optimism. Finally, after what has seemed like a long hiatus—roughly since the late 1960s and early 1970s when the then surgeon general was apparently saying that it was time to "close the book on infectious disease," and concern over infectious disease was slipping out of public view, at least in the developed world—broad and publicly visible efforts at control are now again being made as a central part of the new concern for global health. Progress, it seems, is in the air.

A "Marvelous Momentum" for the Control of Infectious Disease

It is important to understand how very recent the new optimism is—as we write this, it is only about seven or eight years old. In 1999, the Gates Foundation announced that it would contribute $25 million to the International AIDS Vaccine Initiative (IAVI) to further the development of an AIDS vaccine, and the following year dedicated $90 million towards control of HIV/AIDS in Africa, especially to decrease the rates of new infections and maternal–child transmission, and provide resources and training in palliative care to children orphaned by AIDS (Bill and Melinda Gates Foundation 2008). The impressive size of the Gates' contributions, together with the fact that they came from a private entity rather than a governmental organization, contributed to a new optimism that at last something could be done to try to bring under control one of the world's most devastating pandemics, one that echoes the plagues of the middle ages and the 1918 influenza.

In the perception of both the public and of many professionals, this infusion of money and energy served as the turning point (Cohen 2006, 162–7) after years in which many institutions and governments, including that of the United States, had done little or nothing to try to stop the AIDS pandemic as a global phenomenon—even after effective drugs had been developed. The wealthy nations, especially the United States, had been attentive to issues of HIV treatment in their own populations and patent protections for their own pharmaceutical industries, but were seemingly oblivious to the skyrocketing death rate in the developing world and the devastation of an entire continent. HIV control on a global scale seemed impossible. However, galvanized perhaps by the infusion of both optimism and cash from the Gates Foundation, within the past decade governments, NGOs, public/private partnerships, multinational corporations, religious groups, and entertainers have rushed to contribute to a far more concerted effort to reduce the global burden of AIDS and with it other infectious diseases as well.

In fact, considerable progress toward the control of infectious disease had been being made during the decades of the 1970s and 1980s in the development of vaccines, anti-infectives, and methods for disease prevention and treatment. With the emergence of HIV/AIDS on a global scale, the public awakened as well. The World Health Organization (WHO) had been making tireless efforts over the years, culminating in the ambitious 3 by 5 program to have three million HIV patients receiving antiretroviral therapy by 2005. Other foundations as well as Gates had been concerned with global health, like the Rockefeller Foundation; so were many national and international governmental institutions. Evolving market forces and improved education also played some role. But the Gates Foundation's immense contribution of private funding to fight AIDS has served as a catalyst, giving focus to many other efforts, both those initiated beforehand and especially those introduced afterwards. Governments of affluent countries have become major donors to efforts to improve global health: the United States, France, Italy, the United Kingdom, Canada, Germany, the Netherlands, Sweden, Spain, Norway, Denmark, and Russia, ranked by size of contribution to the Global Fund as of early 2008, but less affluent countries have also been donors: Romania, Brazil, Mexico, Slovenia, Poland, and Hungary (The Global Fund, 2008). Funds have poured in from multiple sources—a total of some $35 billion, by one estimate, as of January 2006 (Cohen 2006, 162–7). Laurie Garrett, seconded by Paul Farmer, calls this "a marvelous momentum" (Garrett 2007) (Farmer and Garrett 2007) towards assistance in global health.

To be sure, this picture of progress and emerging comprehensive global efforts toward the improvement of global health, and with it the control of infectious disease, is hardly a fully coordinated or integrated one: efforts by one foundation or NGO sometimes reduplicate efforts by another, and related but not-quite-parallel research programs leave gaps where articulation of related efforts might be much closer. Competition between entities, international tensions, commercial agendas, and very different styles of research funding and priority-setting make the picture far from seamlessly smooth. Political agendas sometimes undercut research; research sometimes violates local custom or understandings of fairness; popular misunderstandings sometimes block immunization drives and other efforts to control the transmission of disease. Officials at one organization complain of dominance by another (McNeil 2008). There have been disappointments and failures: the 3 by 5 program for AIDS and Roll Back Malaria, for example, did not meet their ambitious initial goals. Only one million rather than three million people were receiving combination antiretroviral therapy for HIV/AIDS in developing countries by June 2005 (WHO/UNAIDS 2005). Roll Back Malaria's clear pledge in 1998 to cut deaths from malaria in half by 2010 was labeled a failure, its principal contributors admitting that it was "acting against a background of increasing malaria burden"—that is, that malaria deaths were going up, not down. (Yamey 2004, 1086–7).

Furthermore, attention to infectious disease has been patchwork in character, focusing on some high-profile diseases while ignoring others that cost far more lives. While AIDS, Ebola, and avian flu fuel widespread fear, some ongoing endemic killers, such as infantile diarrhea and childhood acute respiratory tract infections, receive little press and correspondingly little funding or policy attention. Indeed, Solomon Benatar laments the "siloed" character of approaches to infectious disease (Benatar 2005), one disease at a time. Laurie Garrett despairs of "stovepipe" funding: aid that is piped down narrow channels relating to a particular program or disease, ignoring broader needs and concerns: she cites as an example the case in which a government receives considerable support for an antiretroviral distribution program for mothers and children in a specific area, but nothing else. The consequence: mothers who are HIV+ receive drugs for their own infection and to prevent maternal/infant transmission at delivery, but they cannot obtain obstetric and gynecological care or infant immunizations (Garrett 2007, 22–3). Attention to specific diseases has seemed to be quite unequal: while massive research efforts have been directed towards development of a vaccine against HIV, with more than 30 candidates currently in the pipeline, no new tuberculosis vaccine has been developed since 1921, even though the TB bacillus is a technically easier target than the human immunodeficiency virus. In most developing countries the method of diagnosing TB is still the same as that used in 1847.

Yet even if not fully coordinated and sometimes seeming to undercut each other, these disease-by-disease, program-by-program efforts all focus directly or indirectly on a common goal, the reduction of the global burden of infectious disease. Thus these varied efforts can all be seen as a sort of mosaic or kaleidoscope of specific efforts that perhaps all form part of a broader one, coming incrementally into being. The many programs of research in vaccines and antimicrobials, the various water purification and public sanitation projects, the various initiatives for the control of diseases from AIDS to human papillomavirus (HPV)-caused cervical cancer to river blindness, and the multiple legal and social programs like model statutes and pandemic prioritization policies contribute to these emerging, newly coalescing global efforts towards the ultimate goal of control of infectious disease, the details of which are being continuously filled in and modified as the various individual projects are developed and become more fully integrated. We can think of it as a projection forward of current efforts and an anticipation of future ones, an ongoing, overall project under continuous development. Call this still-emerging set of efforts by a unifying name: a *Comprehensive Global Effort for the Eradication, Elimination, or Control of Infectious Disease.*

A Vision for 2020–30? A *Comprehensive Global Effort for the Control of Infectious Disease*

We want to take advantage of this forward-looking, unifying, optimistic picture of new progress and reenergized enthusiasm over the last seven or eight years to examine the ethical questions a genuinely global effort would raise. After all, practical success as the various components of this overall effort move forward does not entail ethical success, either in their mosaic diversity or as a comprehensive whole.

One way to give the notion of an emerging *Comprehensive Global Effort* concreteness and urgency is to think about what would need to happen if we were to try to bring these various efforts to fruition within a given decade—for example, to imagine implementing it fully within, say, the decade 2020–30. A clearly defined *Comprehensive Global Effort* imagined as just far enough away to give some time for coordination and preparation would nevertheless be close enough to make a real difference to the world today. This is a somewhat visionary approach, but not just fantasy—rather, it is an approach that looks ahead to a future we can reasonably foresee.

To the degree that such an approach involves extrapolating into the future from current trends, we can hardly be sure what the conditions and events even in the future will be, or whether a *Comprehensive Global Effort* could or will succeed or even partly succeed. It might work; it might not; or it might be only a partial success.

Elsewhere, we have described what we call the "patient-as-victim-and-vector view," or *PVV* for short, as a way to think about issues of policy and practice. It begins with an account of the patient—the person, indeed any person—as physically "embedded" in a web of disease, a "way-station self" who is breeding ground and launching pad for literally trillions of microorganisms, many of which are benign or crucial to human functioning but some of which are dangerous or lethal, and involves three intertwined perspectives through which to take account of the phenomenon of transmissibility of disease: self-views, population-level views, and hypothetical, Rawlsian-like views (Battin *et al.* 2008). The normative conclusion of the PVV view can be stated simply:

> *Ethical problems in infectious disease should be analyzed, and clinical practices, research agendas, and public policies developed that always take into account the possibility that a person with communicable infectious disease is both victim and vector at one and the same time.*

Using this view of the patient as both victim and vector, we can reasonably foresee something about the ethical challenges that can be expected to arise along the way as the *Comprehensive Global Effort* proceeds, and it is these challenges we wish to explore here.

A more pessimistic version of the same projection of a *Comprehensive Global Effort* despairs of the possibility of ever achieving control of infectious disease or doing so within a specific period of time. It asks instead what are the crucial features in delay—what factors are operating now or might operate in the future to make such a goal unattainable? Could the fearsome prospect of virtually total collapse of public health portrayed so effectively by Laurie Garrett in *Betrayal of Trust* (Garrett 2001) be inevitable? Could the effects of climate change and global warming destroy advances in environmental preventatives like vector control, or could the expansion of warfare and ethnic cleansing, especially that which employs deliberate tactics for spreading infectious disease, undercut any progress in disease-control programs? And what ethical failures in disease control are becoming increasingly evident, and what ethical objections might be so strong that they would be sufficient to warrant blocking of any attempt to undertake comprehensive global efforts?

Leaving these concerns aside for the moment, the optimistic picture we explore here of an emerging *Comprehensive Global Effort for the Control of Infectious Disease* is in one sense an elaboration and expansion of a comparatively simple thought-experiment about airport surveillance for infectious disease, a way of considering what constraints would be acceptable in the effort to eradicate, eliminate, or control the serious human infectious diseases. This thought experiment considered the possibility that rapid testing (and treatment) were available for all the major infectious diseases—and asked whether it would be permissible to require such testing of everyone before they boarded an airplane. The inconvenience would be limited—just a cheek swab, a short delay (perhaps 20 minutes, perhaps as short as 120 seconds), and of course a longer delay with treatment if necessary—but the possibility of reducing the global burden of infectious disease would be immense (Battin *et al.* 2008, chapter 15). In another sense, it is a projection of the overall direction we discern in the many somewhat disparate enterprises already under way, a description of an overall project on which many organizations around the globe have already embarked. And in yet another sense, casting a *Global Effort* as highly time-focused, pursued within the specific decade 2020–30, looks very much like a plan, something we are already embarked upon and should continue pursuing.

This essay's account of a *Comprehensive Global Effort* can thus be read in at least three not fully distinct ways. It lies somewhere between a sheer thought-experiment ("What if the serious human infectious diseases could be brought under control?"); a factual account of events that are now taking place ("Look at all the remarkable progress that is going on!"); and a practical proposal with a concrete, dated plan ("What would it take to bring the serious human infectious diseases under control, and to do so—this is the visionary part—*by the end of the decade 2020–30?*"). The power of a thought experiment is to help identify moral fault lines (as in our airport thought experiment), and the importance of a factual account of what is actually going on is to remind ourselves of the very substantial progress, as well as backsliding, that has been made so far. And the heuristic device of a time-pressured feature, of imagining the culmination of this *Effort* in a fast-approaching, specific, and limited period of time—the decade 2020–30—emphasizes the real-world challenges of global coordination and cooperation, if that is what would be necessary to bring the serious human communicable diseases under control. But most important for our concerns here, this chapter's broader and far more realistic exploration of what is afoot in the new "marvelous momentum" of efforts to reduce the global burden of disease also involves exploring concrete moral claims about what would be required to make this immense global effort go *ethically* well.

Some authors suggest that the moment for such a project is already past. Robert Baker, for instance, contends that humankind has "squandered" the opportunity to usher in a "Golden Age of protection from disease" (Baker 2007). But that does not preclude a renewed, reinvigorated, and better-orchestrated effort as a revitalized attempt, something we see as again under way.

Other global efforts are also beginning to attract at least some measure of global cooperation—for example, controlling global warming; rescuing endangered species; securing equitable access to water or establishing water justice; developing alternative energy sources; managing immigration; controlling drugs; and eliminating terrorism, ethnic cleansing, and war. But a common goal of the eradication, elimination, or full control of serious, human-affecting infectious disease may be, as we will consider later on, both more practicable and less controversial than these others, even though like them it may involve quite controversial policy initiatives.

In a *Comprehensive Global Effort*, coordination of effort or at least simultaneous effort on many different fronts is crucial, since many of the factors that need to be addressed are highly interrelated with others. Scientific advances accomplish little without infrastructure improvement, for example, or environmental control. Institutional cooperation and legal protections are inadequate in the face of cultural and religious attitudes that vilify carriers of infectious disease as sinful individuals, or characterize outbreaks of infectious disease as an appropriate scourge for sinful populations. To think about an emerging, overall, coordinated globe-wide project is to "think big" about all the factors across the board that affect how we might address a challenge to human well-being that had almost disappeared from ethical dialogue in the late 1960s and early 1970s, before renewed ethical debate with the emergence of HIV, even though advances like the development of new antimicrobials and the eradication of smallpox were proceeding apace. It is such an ongoing project that has now come into view again with real force, reenergized and far more publicly visible in the last seven or eight years, and that makes it imperative to "think big."

"Thinking Big," Both Practically and Ethically

A number of "think big" efforts toward reducing the global burden of infectious disease are already under way, practical efforts of a variety of sorts focusing on social realities and scientific gains. The United Nations Millennium Development Goals (MDG), for example, represent an effort to think globally about health and related problems (United Nations 2008). The Gates Foundation's Grand Challenges in Global Health Initiative is also global in scale: it seeks to achieve scientific breakthroughs against diseases that disproportionately affect the two billion poorest people on earth, though of course diseases like AIDS and tuberculosis can affect people everywhere. The Council of Science Editors has organized a global theme issue on poverty and human development involving more than 230 science and biomedical journals, focusing among other things on interventions to improve health among the poor (Flanagin and Winker 2007). These are all invaluable efforts involving the many, many parts of the overall picture, and they all "think big."

At the same time that practical efforts are converging in the effort to control infectious disease, there is an efflorescence of efforts to consider the ethical issues involved. With the exception of those directed to HIV/AIDS, most date from 1999 or later, and recent attention to the ethics issues in pandemic influenza planning has been particularly extensive. Documents like that from WHO by Coleman, Reis, and Croisier (Coleman *et al.* 2007) articulate policies; others, like the American Civil Liberties Union (ACLU) document authored by Annas, Mariner, and Parmet (Annas *et al.* 2008), vigorously critique policies already developed on the basis of ethical inadequacies. And a major effort has been mounted by the Bill & Melinda Gates Foundation to look specifically at the ethical issues in the emerging concern with global health: this is the ethical, social, and cultural program that is funded under the Grand Challenges in Global Health Initiative, designed to use bioethics considerations to assess the specific Grand Challenges projects that are planned or are currently under way (Singer *et al.* 2008). Elsewhere we document how infectious disease had been left out of bioethics during that new field's formative years (Battin *et al.* 2008, chapter 4); now it is moving back in, so to speak, with extraordinary rapidity, making up for a couple of decades of lost time.

However, much of the burgeoning new work in the ethics of infectious disease employs the conceptual categories of traditional bioethics that were developed without specific attention to the moral issues in transmissibility. To be sure, this may be perfectly adequate in addressing issues like caged field trials of genetically modified mosquitoes, as is the subject of one of the current projects under the Gates Foundation's Grand Challenges program, but the traditional approaches of bioethics' usual ethical framework within which projects are assessed needs, as we argued there, to be augmented and expanded.

Of course, many writers and theorists already instinctively appeal to both victim-related and vector-related concerns, but as far as we are aware none have done this explicitly or systematically in a way that would *guarantee* that both concerns would be addressed in any given issue. This is what we have sought to do with our PVV view. Hence, we like to think of our objective here in exploring the notion of a comprehensive global project as in concert with, and indeed admiring of, the many efforts now afoot to explore the ethical issues in infectious disease, but pushing them a good step further—a step we believe necessary for morally adequate reflection on a very broad scale.

What, then, would be involved in a *Comprehensive Global Effort for the Years 2020–30 for the Eradication, Elimination, or Control of Infectious Disease*? We point to both practical and ethical issues that would arise along at least five different though interrelated "tracks": (1) What would be desirable in the spheres of national and international policy? (2) What would we need to bring about in terms of epidemiological and health care infrastructure? (3) What are the most crucial lines of pursuit in scientific development? (4) What would need to be thought about in light of religious, social, and cultural considerations? and 5) What would need to be developed as legal and social protections for individuals? These five are all critical areas for research and policy development, most of them interdependent upon each other, and all raising substantial ethical issues we will sketch here.

This *Global Effort* is not to be imagined as starting from zero. On the contrary, many of the critical areas in Tracks 1–5 are already well known to participants in current efforts to address infectious disease across the globe, from researchers and clinical health care providers to immense organizations concerned with global health. Indeed, everyone and every organization working in infectious disease participates in some part of the global project explored here, whether aware of the emerging comprehensive effort or not. It is already in progress—indeed, in full swing.

Global Efforts: Results So Far

Can we even imagine a *Comprehensive Global Effort for the Eradication, Elimination, or Control of Infectious Disease*? Indeed, in many respects the world is already halfway there, at least in developed countries. It is important to remember as we entertain the notion of a *Global Effort* the impressive list of infectious diseases affecting humans for which effective vaccines, treatments, or preventive measures have been developed. Some of these diseases have already been eradicated, eliminated, or brought under control in the wild, though for many methods for prevention and treatment are known but not available in much of the developing world.

Here is a snapshot taken at the current moment in history of our progress so far in bringing the serious human infectious diseases under control: it is a shifting picture and highly variable from one area to another, but a picture of extraordinary achievement just the same. Some is due to the development of effective vaccines or drugs, some due to quality-of-life improvements and infrastructure development, some due to effective preventative measures, and some due to accidents of geography or environmental change, as with alterations in the ranges of animal or insect vectors.

Here is a partial list of human diseases that have been eradicated, eliminated, or can be well controlled by vaccines or effective therapies. Among these are:

- Smallpox
- Leprosy
- Plague
- Yellow fever
- Pertussis (whooping cough)
- Syphilis
- Diphtheria
- Tetanus
- Rabies
- Measles
- Mumps
- Polio
- Varicella (chickenpox)
- Rubella (German measles)
- Invasive pneumococcal disease
- *Hemophilus influenzae* type B
- Hepatitis A and B
- Meningococcal meningitis
- Japanese encephalitis
- Seasonal influenza

Other infectious diseases, particularly those common in developing countries, have effective therapies or methods for control, but these controls have not been widely implemented. They include:

- Tuberculosis
- Malaria
- Trypanosomiasis (sleeping sickness, Chagas disease)
- Cholera
- The "neglected tropical diseases" for which effective oral treatments are already known (Reddy *et al.* 2008, 1911–24):
  - Roundworm
  - Whipworm
  - Hookworm
  - Schistosomiasis (snail fever or bilharzias)
  - Elephantiasis
  - Trachoma
  - River blindness

Still other infectious diseases remain essentially uncontrolled or currently lack any effective vaccines or therapies, among them:

- Ebola
- Marburg

- HIV
- Dengue fever and dengue hemorrhagic fever
- West Nile virus
- Hantavirus
- SARS viruses
- Leishmaniasis (sandfly fever)
- Creuztfelt-Jakob Disease and variant Creutzfeldt-Jakob Disease
- Food-borne toxigenic *E. coli*
- Evolving highly antimicrobial-resistant strains of tuberculosis
- Influenza type A

So far, successes in reducing the burden of disease in the developed world have been remarkable. In the United States, the death rates for smallpox, diphtheria, and polio have declined by 100% since vaccines were approved; for another nine diseases, they have declined by 90% (McNeil 2007). To be sure, there have been major setbacks (like the reemergence of tuberculosis, polio, yellow fever, even plague), but in general progress towards the full control of infectious disease is astonishing—at least where it is fully implemented, as in the wealthy parts of the world. In contemplating the possibility of eradication, elimination, or control of the serious human infectious diseases, it might be said, we are halfway there, at least in the developed world.

Human Health in Epidemiological Perspective

The already impressive successes of an emerging *Comprehensive Global Effort*, if we can think of them as part of a long-term effort, are after all evident in the history of demographic shifts in causes of human mortality. Up through the middle of the 19th century, everywhere in the world, parasitic and infectious diseases were the principal cause of human mortality (Olshansky and Ault 1987, 207–17). With the development of clean water, public sanitation, immunization, the germ theory of disease, hand washing by physicians, antibiotics, and many other factors, infectious disease (with the single exception of pneumonia) is not even on the standard list of the top ten causes of death in the developed world. At the same time, infectious diseases remain a major factor in the developing world, where death rates particularly for children remain high. Just a century or two ago, infectious and parasitic diseases were the way most people everywhere in the world died; in the developed world, they are a much reduced threat, and where they do kill, kill mainly the old. Infectious disease mortality in the United States has declined remarkably in the past century, and now represents a small percentage (<5%) of disability-adjusted life-years lost (Armstrong *et al.* 1999). The stark differences in life expectancy around the world, ranging roughly from a high of between 75 and 86 years for both sexes in Japan, Australia, Iceland, Canada, the Netherlands, Cuba, and the United Kingdom at the top end of the range, downward to 40–60 years in the poorer, developing nations, and in some countries, like Malawi, Mozambique, Zimbabwe, Zambia, still lower, to Sierra Leone, with a low of 37–40 years, is not just a matter of disparate human development indices but differential death rates from infectious disease (WorldHealth Organization, data for 2005). A *Comprehensive Global*

Effort, it is painfully obvious, has already been very largely successful in the developed world—this may be part of what has allowed the developed world to become developed—but has a long, long way to go in those countries left behind.

Is a *Comprehensive Global Effort* Realistic? On Eradication, Elimination, and Control

It is crucial in understanding any *Global Effort* to recognize the differences between eradication, elimination, and control. Complete eradication by eliminating entirely the pathogen which causes disease is realistic in only a small proportion of cases, those which involve human vectors only and no intermediate stages: e.g., smallpox, polio, measles, and tuberculosis. The eradication of all human infectious disease—that is, completely ridding the world of all disease-causing pathogens in the wild—is not a realistic goal, since many human-affecting infectious diseases also have nonhuman vectors or reservoirs. Tetanus, for example, lives in the soil; so do the spores of coccidioidomycosis, a fungal infection responsible for valley fever (McKinley 2008). Malaria involves a transmission stage in mosquitoes; so do yellow fever, dengue fever, and many other arthropod-borne infectious diseases. Other common infections—such as staphylococcal skin infections, or peritonitis due to ruptured bowel—are due to organisms that we normally carry on our skin or in our gastrointestinal tracts, and attempts to eliminate one pathogen would be foiled by the rapid appearance of other potential pathogens to refill the microbial niche in the skin or gastrointestinal (GI) tract.

Furthermore, many pathogenic organisms do not require humans for their perpetuation and are not acquired from other humans. Elimination of these organisms in humans, for instance by means of universal immunization or effective treatment, would still not eliminate these organisms, and the diseases they cause will remain a continuing threat. Some human-affecting diseases also affect animals and are carried by animals—Rift Valley fever, for example—and unless contact between these animals and humans were completely interrupted, control of these diseases in humans could not be complete without achieving control in the animal population as well. Some pathogens affect both people and plants, like the bacterium *Burkholderia cepacia* (people and onions), which can be lethal for people with cystic fibrosis, or *Serratia marcescens* (people and squash plants), which reaches immunocompromised hospital patients through floral arrangements, salads, and intravenous tubes (Milius 2007, 251); it is hard to see how these pathogens could be entirely eradicated. And some infectious diseases, such as influenza and HIV, reappear in modified form and potentially require ongoing prevention or treatment in generation after generation. At this point in the human history of infectious disease, there is just one extant example of complete eradication: smallpox. But there are many examples of elimination, that is, reduction to a very low level, like leprosy, plague, and polio, the latter on the verge of eradication despite recent outbreaks. And there are many examples of full or nearly full control, at least in the developed world, where disease is preventable, treatable, or curable by means of immunization, antimicrobials, sanitation measures (e.g., clean water), or other effective prevention or treatment.

Of course, there is an immense gap between diseases which can be eliminated and diseases which are in fact eliminated. Leprosy, for example, falls in this category, as do many of the so-called neglected tropical diseases for which effective treatment is known but not widely available: here the gulf between the developed world and the developing world is at its greatest. It is already possible in principle, despite enormous practical obstacles, to reduce dramatically much of the huge burden of disease suffered by those in poorest parts of the globe, and as new diagnostic technologies, vaccines, and treatment modalities are developed, so does the likelihood of elimination or full control for many additional diseases.

Obviously, even in the developed world control of infectious disease will never be complete. There will always be newly emerging diseases: in recent years, some 39 new communicable diseases with the potential to become pandemic have jumped species, including SARS, monkeypox, and bird flu (Rubin 2008). The prospect of newly designed or already known pathogens used as bioweapons cannot be ruled out (Selgelid 2007; Zilinskas 2007). Climate change, settlement of newly cleared land, and warfare and its dislocations can also play a role in the emergence or evolution of disease.

Some theorists might argue that certain serious diseases should not be eliminated because they are useful in other respects, as when pneumonia serves as the "old man's friend," a bringer of death more easeful than that from other human maladies. Others might point to research suggesting that exposure to infectious disease has played a major role in mammalian evolution, resulting among other things in the development of the amniotic sac and other adaptive advantages (Zuk 2007), and thus argue that continuing exposure should not be eliminated, lest further evolutionary gains be lost. Still others claim that the overuse of antibacterial soaps and other "germ-proofing" methods results in higher rates of asthma and allergies. A *Comprehensive Global Effort* certainly would not seek to exterminate all parasites, fungi, bacteria, viruses, and prions (the microorganisms that affect human beings), since many are essential for human health, but only the pathogenic ones that do not have beneficial functions and are responsible for extensive human morbidity and mortality. It is this process of overcoming *disease* that we see as already well under way in any long-term *Comprehensive Global Effort*.

We may ask, then, phrasing the question in three ways that correspond to seeing a *Comprehensive Global Effort*—as a thought experiment, as a report of current activity, or as a plan—what would it be like if, what is happening that, or what do we need to do to try to achieve the eradication, elimination, or full control of serious human affecting infectious disease, say within the decade 2020–30, around the globe? The question, in each of these forms, is not just about what practical projects of research, policy development, or implementation would be most urgent, but also about what ethical issues most urgently require attention as a *Global Effort* proceeds.

We suggest five tracks along which to consider these questions.

Track 1: National and international organizations and the development of collective will

If a *Comprehensive Global Effort* is to succeed fully, it would be important to foster the cooperation of institutions and players of all sorts, public and private. Many are already committed—but not all. Thus a first part is to consider what sorts of institutions are critical to infectious disease control, which are helpful, which are problematic—and how the support of such institutions could be enlisted and maintained, or modified where it has been counterproductive. This is to seek to establish and maintain the collective, global will to try to reduce the global burden of infectious disease as low a level as possible. The practical challenge is to develop the global political will to try to work together to bring infectious disease under control in the first place, and it is a substantial challenge. If the many sorts of institutions are all to cooperate, it would require laying aside infighting, reducing political competition, avoiding distraction by shifting from one to another "short-term numerical target" (Farmer and Garrett 2007), avoiding turf wars, and other things that could derail progress (Cohen 2006, 162–7). Could all these institutions contribute cooperatively in their myriad ways to a common project, even for just a decade? How such matters should be addressed is a crucial issue for reflection in the development of this track of a *Global Effort to Close the Book on Infectious Disease*. After all, the *Effort* cannot succeed, or succeed quickly, if some institutions undercut the efforts of the whole.

Track 2: Epidemiologic and health care infrastructure

Track 2, epidemiologic and health care infrastructure, is widely recognized as indispensable in the control of infectious disease. The absence of adequate health care infrastructure, including the absence of adequate diagnostic and surveillance measures as well as adequate immunization and treatment measures, can contribute dramatically to the unchecked spread of infectious disease. An outbreak unnoticed (or ignored) can have an immense amplification effect down the road; the "stitch in time" approach to infectious disease is key to prevention, in that it is almost always easier to stop one case now than ten cases down the road—or a hundred, or a hundred thousand. Poverty and war have crucial amplifying effects: diseases that might be mild or resisted altogether by individuals who are healthy and well nourished may spread rapidly in disrupted conditions where people endure malnourishment, parasites, and chronic illness. Natural disasters can also produce similar effects, if populations are cut off from care, and if the conditions of the disaster—standing water after a flood, for instance—create risks of disease. Economic practices can also affect disease transmission: for example, the practice common in many developing countries that physicians see private patients rather than poor, charity ones, exacerbates disease transmission, since it is poor, charity patients who are most likely to be afflicted because of their crowded living conditions and lack of access to clean water and adequate sanitation.

Poverty, war, and natural disaster are also typically associated with inadequate infrastructure: for those who do become ill, health care is hardly available; clinics, if there are any, are overcrowded; personnel are inadequately trained and hopelessly stressed; medications are outmoded or unavailable. Poverty and war are often closely intertwined: northeast Kenya, for example, has a million refugees from Somalia, people for whom the risks of infectious disease are compounded over the already difficult lives they had previously led. Another 300,000 have been internally displaced following the postelection violence in early 2008, and the chief among the many health risks they face is cholera (Harvard World Health News 2008). Life in refugee camps or urban slums, often without adequate sanitation facilities, is, as our PVV view might describe it, life most fully "enmeshed in the web of disease," life in which people are most obviously "way-station selves" as microorganisms travel unchecked among them. Thus, in seeking greater control of infectious disease, attention to social and sanitary infrastructure issues is crucial:

- Clean water
- Sanitation
- Waste disposal
- Control of insect and animal vectors (mosquitoes, fleas, rats, etc.)
- Control of environmental toxins
- Health-related transportation, including roads or airlifts and other ways of bring health care to people in remote or disrupted communities
- Enhancement of health care delivery systems, especially vaccine delivery systems, treatment facilities, and easy-access clinics
- Encouragement of use of low-tech, low-cost modalities for infectious-disease prevention: bed nets (Bradley 2007), water filters, "drinking straws," and pond attendants, etc.
- Development of novel health care delivery modalities, e.g., *accompagnateurs* (Farmer and Garrett 2007) as Partners in Health has utilized in HIV/TB treatment in Haiti
- Attention to the causes of poverty associated with infectious disease, particularly those associated with the neglected tropical diseases and with disease outbreaks among dislocated populations like refugees
- Attention to the causes of war, civil conflict, guerilla actions, and related hostilities that exacerbate the risks of infectious disease
- Rapid response to natural disasters, with particular attention to special characteristics of a disaster that might encourage the spread of disease

Ethical questions associated with this enormous variety of concerns might range from consideration of who should receive how many bed nets and what they may or may not do with them, to requiring contributions or labor for the installation of sanitary systems, to the very substantial privacy and confidentiality issues that arise with local and global surveillance systems. Modeling methods used in planning, whether for endemic disease in poverty and war or for outbreaks associated with pandemics of newly emerging diseases or in natural disasters, are of particular ethical significance under the PVV view, since they often incorporate assumptions about what levels of disease can be tolerated; the PVV view warns against cavalier acceptance of leaving a significant proportion—indeed, any proportion—of a population still subject to preventable or treatable disease, since that is to ignore the fact that those who suffer disease are indeed victims.

Particularly important under the PVV view is attention to how large-scale programs are formulated. Classic epidemiology tracks disease movement through populations. Research agendas focus on issues of particular salience in specific populations but leave aside others. Treatment programs often target just those populations or population subgroups at highest risk of contracting and transmitting disease. There are obvious advantages of design and efficiency here, but at some moral cost. Our PVV view insists that those left outside these categories—people not in high-risk groups who nevertheless contract disease, people whose groups are not the focus of research efforts, and sufferers from "orphan diseases"—be recognized too, both in their own roles as vectors but especially as victims.

Track 3: Scientific development

Effective control of human infectious disease cannot be possible without continuing scientific development. Examples of scientific efforts—many already well under way—that would be essential to achieving any measure of success involve better diagnosis, better treatment, better mechanisms for prevention, and better background science in the understanding microbial pathogenesis, defense mechanisms in humans, and evolutionary, genetic and other factors relevant to human vulnerability to infectious disease. The Gates Foundation's handsomely funded Grand Challenges in Global Health program already includes some 14 research incentives which serve seven long-term goals in global health: improving childhood vaccines, creating new vaccines, controlling insects that transmit agents of disease, improving nutrition to promote health, improving drug treatment of infectious diseases, curing latent and chronic infection, and measuring health status accurately and economically in developing countries (Singer *et al.* 2007). These are immense important goals; many others are in progress or remain to be developed. A group of comparatively realistic research goals would include:

- Improvement or development of rapid, reliable tests for all infectious diseases, based on PCR, proteomic, or nanotechnology methods:
  - Goal: 100% specificity, 100% sensitivity: 0 false positives, 0 false negatives, including field-usable tests available at point-of-care
  - Goal: rapid speed of identification, in minutes or seconds
  - Goal: low cost, easy use
- Improvement of genetic identification methods for pathogens and other means for transmission tracking:
  - In humans
  - In animal vectors
- Development of improved methods of rapid identification of emerging diseases

Pathogen identification and disease diagnosis are crucial in prevention, and central to a *Global Effort* already under way. Particularly challenging scientific goals include treatment as well, especially since treatment possibilities change with the rapid replication rate of many infectious organisms, with the development of drug resistance, and other factors. A drug that may have worked in one context, like chloroquine for malaria, for example, may not work in other contexts or with the same disease in other regions (Bradley 2007); developing effective prevention and treatment is an ongoing challenge. Other obviously crucial scientific goals include:

- Development of improved vaccines and vaccine administration and storage methods
- Development of improved antimicrobials and other treatment methods
- Development of safer insecticides and vector controls

The PVV view also urges that governments and entities recognize the hypothetical as well as actual reasons for support of scientific research and cooperation in a

Comprehensive Global Effort: although epidemics may at the current historical moment seem particularly likely to afflict some countries or continents rather than others, when it comes to globally transmissible disease, it could be otherwise. After all, dengue may be spreading to areas that, it is claimed, are warming with global climate change, but influenza flourishes in colder weather, and we may be quite unable to predict the ranges of future, not-as-yet emerging diseases.

Track 4: Religious, social, and cultural considerations

Track 1's concern with developing cooperation among the various major institutions of the world—governmental, corporate, private, intergovernmental, and so on—also included religious institutions. Inasmuch as religious traditions and their institutions influence much of what people in every part of the globe think about disease and also govern their disease-transmission behavior, from hand washing before meals to sexual contact, the participation of religious institutions is crucial to the success of a *Global Effort*. However, some religious traditions preserve scriptural or traditional characterizations of infectious disease as "scourge," as "punishment" that is divinely ordained, or as the product of wrong behavior in this or previous lives. Addressing these often archaic characterizations of infectious disease is of consummate importance in securing the cooperation of people and their religious institutions, often enormously powerful, around the globe.

Consider the various portrayals of leprosy or plague or other infectious diseases in the scriptures of religious traditions. In the Hebrew/Christian Bible, for example, God allows Satan to test the loyal Job with any hardship that is short of fatal, and Satan begins with infectious disease (perhaps leprosy or a staph infection?): Satan "smote Job with running sores from head to foot, so that he took a piece of broken pot to scratch himself as he sat among the ashes" (Job 2:7–9, *New English Bible* translation). In the Muslim *Hadith*, plague is described as "a means of torture which Allah used to send upon whomsoever He wished, but He made it a source of mercy for the believers, for anyone who is residing in a town in which this disease is present, and remains there and does not leave that town, but has patience and hopes for Allah's reward, and knows that nothing will befall him except what Allah has written for him, then he will get such reward as that of a martyr"—in other words, plague is a punishment, though it can also become a blessing for those who believe (al-Bukhari 1959). In many religious traditions, the implication is that people or groups afflicted by disease deserve it in one way or another, and that such illnesses are a product of divine wrath visited upon them or perhaps an opportunity for spiritual growth.

Attitudes about HIV/AIDS or other STDs expressed in some contemporary religious groups sometimes construe contracting the disease as punishment for homosexuality, infidelity, promiscuity, or other sinful behavior, either of individuals or of groups. Fatalism may also be associated with religious views, as when it is held that the visitation of infectious disease is God's will and hence that nothing can be done about it. Both religious and cultural attitudes may be involved in ancient practices like belling lepers or shunning victims with pocks, boils, open sores, or other visible evidence of disease. In some traditions, such attitudes may include views that the afflicted not only deserve it but are "not our problem," that justice is being done and others have either no obligation to intervene, or no intervention is appropriate. Some religious groups appear to fear that attempts to reduce infectious disease transmission, especially of sexually transmitted diseases like HIV, might interfere with teachings prohibiting homosexuality or encouraging chastity. And some religious traditions value the contingency of human life *per se*, appearing to hold that efforts to forestall illness or delay death are contrary to divine plan.

Religious beliefs and attitudes can of course play a strongly positive role in encouraging cooperation with a societal project to protect the life and health of human beings. Religious commandments like "do not kill" and "respect life" speak in favor of bringing potential lethal infectious disease under control. Traditions which stress compassion and the relief of suffering would presumably also support the underlying concern of a *Global Effort*, to extricate humankind from the web of disease within which it is enmeshed. Some religious traditions stress the unity of human beings in divine creation; some stress stewardship of the environment and with it, concern for human health; some emphasize attitudes of caring, concern, and compassion for those who are ill. And many stress the value of sacrifice and dedicated work for the good of the community, a commitment believed to be viewed favorably by the divine or rewarded well in the next life. These are all attitudes that suggest that religious institutions might play a powerful role in engendering cooperation with a *Global Effort* by the world's faithful who subscribe to these views.

But not all religious views concerning infectious disease favor constructive cooperation. To challenge entrenched social or religious beliefs is never easy, and rarely fully successful. This is the issue our PVV view expects us to put on the table: that entrenched beliefs and practices may fail to regard people, both as individuals and in groups or populations, as both victim and vector at one and the same time, in ways that work to the detriment of all.

Track 5: Legal and social protections for individuals and groups

Our PVV view here also recognizes that a *Global Effort* for the control of infectious disease cannot satisfy the conditions of this view unless it attends to legal and social protections for individuals and groups, to ensure that neither individuals nor groups are victimized by institutional measures, scientific research programs, infrastructure changes, or other matters that are part of the *Global Effort*. This is to recognize that, under our PVV view, "victimhood" can have a dual sense: a person or group, or entire population, may be the victim of a disease—this is the primary sense of "victim" in the PVV view—but may also be the victim, so to speak, of policies, programs, prejudices, and other matters associated with disease, or both.

Legal and social protections for individuals, groups, and populations, under our PVV view, should include at least:

- Development of rigorous local, national, and international protections for privacy and confidentiality of individual information in surveillance systems:
  - In reporting of data
  - In contact tracing and transmission tracking
  - In follow-up for health care

- Development of policies concerning rights to privacy and/or confidentiality for information that poses a risk to other people, or a right to privacy in a public place
- Development of protections and systems for maximum communication among families and social groups during isolation, quarantine, home quarantine, or other restrictions in epidemics
- Development of protections for things that matter to people, e.g., pets and property
- Attention to animal rights and animal-welfare issues
- Erection of special protections for the least well-off (and most likely to be affected by infectious disease):
  - Refugees
  - Prisoners
  - The institutionalized, including those in mental institutions
  - The homeless
  - The elderly
  - Infants and children
  - People with disabilities, poor health, or compromised immune systems

As Michael Parker puts it, echoing the British pandemic plan, "Everyone matters" (Parker 2007). This notion is essential to our PVV view: while it recognizes that trade-offs between concerns like privacy and surveillance or confidentiality and interruption of transmission must sometimes be made, it still insists that policies not victimize or exempt those whom they affect.

A further area of concern about legal and social protections for individuals and groups involves attention to micro- and macroeconomic issues. What will be the impact of a *Global Effort* on all parties? Some concerns might involve those whose current income depends on treatment of infectious disease. After all, if a *Global Effort* were to succeed and the global burden of infectious disease dramatically reduced, this income would be eliminated. Who will be out of a job? Larger economic concerns might focus for instance on the impact of higher rates of infant and child survival on domestic and social situations where poverty is severe, or on changed patterns of survival—reflecting the success of a *Global Effort* in reducing death rates—on economies around the world. There would presumably be relatively little effect on economies in the advanced industrial nations where infectious disease is already largely under control, but there could be dramatic effect in the worst-off nations of the world. Like everything else associated with it, a *Comprehensive Global Effort* should be subjected to adequate scrutiny in the decades prior to and during the culminating phase itself, with of course an eye to mitigating economic damage where it threatens to occur and but reaping the economic benefits of effective disease control as well.

A *Comprehensive Global Effort*: From Thought Experiment to Plan

Attempts to control infectious disease are already going on in many areas—indeed, in all five practical and policy tracks considered above—and they all raise important ethical issues. A *Comprehensive Global Effort for the Control of Infectious Disease*, incompletely developed as it is, is already well under way, whether we see it as a thought experiment, a description of current events, or a plan. Whichever way we interpret it, it requires us to consider the importance of not only global coordination and cooperation, but also the importance of coordinated, across-the-board *ethical* reflection. This ranges from reflection on comparatively focused issues like how to balance considerations of confidentiality versus public interest, how to weigh the impact of mandated treatment, or how to prioritize access to prevention and care in epidemics, to the deeper but at the moment more diffuse sorts of philosophical issues, such as whether attempts to control infectious disease should be given priority over attempts to control cancer or whether bioweaponry is intrinsically worse than conventional arms. In part because attention to the full control of infectious disease on a global scale has not so far been unified, the ethical issues each distinct effort raises have not been unified either, and have to a considerable extent been treated in comparatively isolated, discrete, "siloed" ways, even now that they are finally coming to be discussed at all in bioethics and other fields. This is not to say that ethical issues are to be viewed in a monolithic way, but rather that reflection on them must include understanding them in the larger context of a world in which we are "all in this together," all potentially victims and vectors of transmissible infectious disease.

No writer, as far as we are aware, is currently advocating the kind of universal surveillance or mandated treatment imagined in our airport thought-experiment, and no writer is advocating a decade of intense dedication to infectious disease control. But part of the point of a thought experiment like that is to test the ethical challenges to be faced in the real world, not just in a fictional one, and hence the challenges that would and do arise in what we see as an already-emerging *Comprehensive Global Effort*. Ethical reflection in the context of infectious disease, we have been arguing all along, must be far broader than it has been, even during the efflorescence of the last seven or eight years—that is why we appeal not only to a limited thought-experiment about airport surveillance but to the much broader constellation of developments we have called an emerging *Comprehensive Global Effort for the Control of Infectious Disease*.

If a *Global Effort* as imagined here seems too grand—an overly far-fetched thought experiment, a misdescription of current reality, or an unworkable concrete plan—imagine what is involved in trying to extricate the globe from any *one* of the particularly serious diseases that are currently widespread—say, HIV/AIDS, or tuberculosis, or malaria. These are all recognized as devastating. AIDS has already killed 19 million people and, as of 2007, another 33.2 million are infected with the HIV virus. Tuberculosis infects or has infected an estimated 30% of the global population and kills about 2 million people a year. Worldwide, malaria infects between 350 and 500 million people every year, and between 2 to 3 million die from it—90% in Africa, where it is estimated that one child dies from malaria every 30 seconds (Packard 2007, xvi). The new movement for global health, building on the steady work of the WHO and others over many years and galvanized less than a decade ago by the remarkable private contribution of the Gates Foundation, is already committed to the elimination of these diseases; it has become a top global priority. Yet—here is the key to our project in this "think big" essay—eliminating any one of these diseases will raise virtually *all* the issues we have posed in the five tracks outlined above. So would eliminating all three. Indeed, for any disease or group of diseases for which we might consider trying to achieve global or even local eradication, elimination, or control, issues about institutional cooperation, infrastructure improvement, scientific development, religious and cultural attitudes, and social and legal protections are all relevant. Comprehensive ethical reflection is crucial in such an enterprise as well: while it is important to be sensitive to the specific, factual features of any given case, we cannot do ethics piecemeal, as an iterated effort one disease after another for the indefinite future, or in response to one new technology, or one political challenge, or one scientific development at a time, without a larger picture of human embeddedness in webs of mutual disease transmission, within which they occur.

"Think Big" thought experiments are unlimited in scope, in this case fueled by an elective optimism and bounded only by the limits of plausibility in assembling the resources of the world to confront one of its most pervasive problems. We can imagine, as we have said, other *Global Efforts* directed towards other global problems—climate change and global warming, endangered species rescue, water justice, immigration management, global drug control, and so on. But the vision of a *Comprehensive Global Effort for the Years 2020–30 for the Eradication, Elimination, or Control of Infectious Disease* may be, in contrast, simpler: its overall purpose of reducing the burden of infectious disease may be less controversial; its methods are not technically impossible; its science is reasonably well understood; and it does not require the change of institutions, only coordination and cooperation. Imagining such a project is of course to "think big," but we can certainly imagine what this project would take, as the culmination of the efforts of several centuries, to achieve within a single decade a goal with which the fate of humankind might be dramatically improved. There is no way to guarantee that it would succeed. But it is a project already well under way, since the time of Jenner and with the best efforts of dedicated researchers, clinicians, and workers in public health. There is no practical or moral reason not to undertake this project, though plenty of reason to be cautious about how to do so—that is what we have tried to explore.

There is another, darker reason for exploring the practical and ethical issues in the *Global Effort* in this comprehensive way. A *Global Effort*, or even just continuing ordinary efforts to control infectious disease, might contain repressive, biased, insensitive, or otherwise morally indefensible elements, particularly if it were pursued under a tight time schedule by zealous institutions or highly competitive players. That there is a current efflorescence of ethical reflection does not entail that the various components of the overall global effort will go ethically well, and ethical reflection by itself will not prevent abuse. It is important to understand how even an admirable project with a highly desirable goal—extricating humankind from the web of infectious disease—could go wrong, that is, how it could be done, but not done well. It remains to look at a variety of policies of the sort that might be involved in a *Global Effort* to see what can go wrong with them as well as right, using our PVV view as a tool for examining actual, real-world policies as a way of thinking about larger aims.

We would like to thank a number of people who helped us "think big" at a conference in July 2007 at the Uehiro Center for Ethics, Oxford University: David Bradley, Nim Pathy, Angela McLean, Helen Fletcher, Paul Kelly, Anders Sandberg, Carl H. Coleman, Michael Parker, Harold Jaffe, Angus Dawson, Michael J. Selgelid, Marcel Verweij, Dan Brock, Søren Holm, Ray Zilinskas, and Matthew Liao. This chapter is an earlier, abridged and differently titled version of chapter 20 from: Margaret P. Battin, Leslie P. Francis, Jay A. Jacobson, and Charles B. Smith, *The Patient as Victim and Vector: Ethics and Infectious Disease* (New York: Oxford University Press, forthcoming 2009).

References

al-Bukhari Sahih (1959), *Hadith*, vol. 8, book 77, n. 616, tr. Muhammad Mushin Khan, "The Translation of the Meanings of Sahih al-Bukhari" in *Fath al-Bari*. Cairo: Egyptian Press of Mustafa al-Babi, al-Halab.

Annas, George J., Wendy K. Mariner, and Wendy E. Parmet. 2008. "Pandemic Preparedness: The Need for a Public Health—Not a Law Enforcement/National Security—Approach," *American Civil Liberties Union: Technology and Liberty Project*, available at http://www.aclu.org/privacy/medical/33642pub20080114.html (accessed January 20, 2008).

Armstrong, Gregory L., Laura A. Conn, and Robert W. Pinner. 1999. "Trends in Infectious Disease Mortality in the United States During the 20th Century," *Journal of the American Medical Association* 281(1): 61–6.

Battin, Margaret P., Leslie P. Francis, Jay A. Jacobson, and Charles B. Smith. 2009. *The Patient as Victim and Vector: Ethics and Infectious Disease*. New York: Oxford University Press.

Benatar, Solomon R. 2005. "Moral Imagination: The Missing Component in Global Health," *PLoS Medicine* 2(12): e400.

Bill and Melinda Gates Foundation. 2008. "The Bill & Melinda Gates Foundation Announces New HIV/AIDS Grants at World AIDS Conference," available at http://www.gatesfoundation.org/GlobalHealth/Pri_Diseases/HIVAIDS/Announcements/Announce-245.htm (accessed February 16, 2008).

Bradley, David. 2007. "Ethical Barriers to Malaria Control." *Lecture, Uehiro Center, Oxford University, Oxford, England, July 4, 2007*.

Cohen, Jon. 2006. "The New World of Global Health," *Science* 311(5758): 162–7.

Coleman, Carl, Andreas Reis, and Alice Croisier. 2007. "Ethical Considerations in Developing a Public Health Response to Pandemic Influenza," World Health Organization, available at www.who.int/csr/resources/publications (accessed February 16, 2008).

Farmer, Paul, and Laurie Garrett. 2007. "From 'Marvelous Momentum' to Health Care for All: Success Is Possible With the Right Programs," *Foreign Affairs* 86(2). http://www.foreignaffairs.org/20070301faresponse86213/paul-farmer-laurie-garrett/from-marvelous-momentum-to-health-care-for-all-success-is-possible-with-the-right-programs.html.

Flanagin, Annette, and Margaret A. Winker. 2007. "Global Theme Issue on Poverty and Human Development," *Journal of the American Medical Association* 298(16): 1942; Council of Science Editors, *Global Theme Issue on Poverty and Human Development* (October 22, 2007), available at http://www.councilscienceeditors.org/globalthemeissue.cfm (accessed February 16, 2008).

Garrett, Laurie. 2007. "The Challenge of Global Health," *Foreign Affairs* 86(1): 22–23.

The Global Fund. 2008. *Donors' Pledges and Contributions* (February 2008), www.theglobal-fund.org/ (accessed February 14, 2008).

Harvard World Health News. 2008. "Kenya: Homeless Face Myriad Risks," whn@hsh.harvard.edu, January 17, 2008, quoting *The Standard, Nairobi*.

McKinley, Jesse. 2008. "Infection Hits a California Prison Hard, and Experts Ask Why," *New York Times*, December 30, 2007, available at http://query.nytimes.com/gst/fullpage.html?res = 9A0 6E6D81130F933A05 751C1A9619C8B63&scp = 2&sq = Valley + Fever&st = nyt (accessed January 21, 2008).

McNeil, Donald G., Jr. 2007. "Sharp Drop Seen in Deaths From Ills fought by Vaccine," *New York Times*, Health Section, National Edition, November 14, 2007.

McNeil, Donald G. Jr., 2008. "WHO Official Complains of Gates Foundation Dominance in Malaria Research," *New York Times*, February 16, 2008.

Milius, Susan. 2007. "Not Just Hitchhikers: Human Pathogens Make Homes on Plants," *Science News*, October 20, 2007, 251.

Olshansky, S. Jay, and A. Brian Ault. 1987. "The Fourth Stage of the Epidemiologic Transition: The Age of Delayed Degenerative Disease," in Timothy M. Smeeding *et al.*, eds., *Should Medical Care Be Rationed by Age?* Totowa, NJ: Rowman & Littlefield; 11–43.

Packard, Randall, M. 2007. *The Making of a Tropical Disease: A Short History of Malaria*. Baltimore, MD: Johns Hopkins University Press; xvi.

Parker, Michael. 2007. "Methods of Pandemic Planning: The UK Task Force," lecture, Uehiro Center, Oxford University, Oxford, England, July 4, 2007.

Reddy, Madhuri, *et al.* (2008). "Oral Drug Therapy for Multiple Neglected Tropical Diseases: A Systematic Review," *Journal of the American Medical Association* 298(16): 1911–24, table 1.

Rubin, Harriet. 2008. "Google's Searches Now Include Ways to Make a Better World," *New York Times*, sec. C1, January 18, 2008.

Selgelid, Michael J. 2007. "Dual Use Discoveries: Censorship Policy Making," lecture, Uehiro Center, Oxford University, Oxford, England, July 4, 2007.

Singer, Peter A. *et al.* 2007. "Grand Challenges in Global Health: The Ethical, Social and Cultural Program" *PLoS Medicine* 4(9): 1440–4.

United Nations. 2008. UN Millennium Development Goals, available at http://www.un.org/millennium goals (accessed February 16, 2008).

World Health Organizations/UNAIDS. 2005. Report, 3 by 5 Initiative (June 29, 2005), available at: http://www. who.int/3by5/progressreportJune2005/en/ (accessed February 16, 2008).

World Health Organization. 2008. Life Expectancy Data, available at http://www.who.int/countries/en/ (accessed February 16, 2008).

Shaping Ethical Guidelines for an Influenza Pandemic

ROSEMARIE TONG

Introduction

When the North Carolina Institute of Medicine (NC IOM) and the North Carolina Department of Public Health (NCDPH) asked me to join a 37-member statewide North Carolina Institute of Medicine/Department of Public Health Task Force to develop ethical guidelines for an influenza pandemic, I thought they had dialed the wrong number mistakenly. I told the NC IOM administrator who contacted me I knew next to nothing about influenza pandemics, including the Avian Flu. She said that my infectious-disease ignorance was of little concern to her; the NC IOM/DPH Task Force would have among its members many public health and safety experts. In addition, there would be representatives from government agencies, health care organizations, businesses, industries, faith communities, and advocacy groups. What the Task Force lacked were ethicists. Specifically, it needed an ethicist to serve as co-Chair together with the Director of the North Carolina Department of Public Health, and I had been identified as a likely candidate for this role.

Intrigued by the NC IOM administrator's request, I asked her to be honest. Would the NC IOM/DPH Task Force really be serious about ethics? Or would it simply want to use ethics as a sweet frosting to lather over a cake of political deals made between special-interests' lobbies? She responded: "Come to the first meeting. If you do not like the way it goes, you never have to come to another meeting." I went to the first meeting of the Task Force; I was very impressed by the sincerity and genuine ethical concern of its members. After that meeting, I agreed to co-Chair the Task Force.

"Shaping Ethical Guidelines for an Influenza Pandemic," by Rosemarie Tong, is from Michael Boylan (ed.) (2008) *International Public Health Policy and Ethics*. Springer; pp. 215–32.

During the months that followed, I learned how alternately heartening and disheartening the process of producing a set of guidelines that merit the descriptor "ethical" can be. It is not easy to get 37 diverse people to develop and endorse a set of ethical guidelines. On the contrary, it is very hard work!

The Threat of an Influenza Pandemic in the Twenty-First Century

Influenza pandemics constitute a public health threat of global proportions. Although people in the United States may think that such disease outbreaks are confined mainly to their television screens and disaster films, history teaches that influenza pandemics typically occur three times in a century. In the twentieth century, the three influenza pandemics were the 1918 Spanish Flu, the 1957 Asian Flu, and the 1968 Hong Kong Flu (NC IOM/DPH Task Force 2007, 21). All were of avian (bird) origin, and the worst of them was the Spanish Flu; worldwide, 50 million people died. In the United States the death toll was 675 000 (Berlinger 2006). A particularly vexing feature of the Spanish Flu was that it did not strike the populations that annual flus generally hit hardest: the very young and the very old. Instead it targeted people in their twenties and thirties (Engel 2007, 32). The other two twentieth-century influenza pandemics (the Asian Flu and the Hong Kong Flu), though not as devastating, were no small matter. The Asian Flu killed 2 million people worldwide, 70 000 of them in the United States; and the Hong Kong Flu killed 700 000 people worldwide, 34 000 of them in the United States (Garloch 2006, A1).

Because the Avian Flu has yet to reach US shores, the US population has moved on to worrying about other problems, the war in Iraq and the economy to name two. But just because the Avian Flu has not visited the United States during the first eight years of the twenty-first century, does not mean it will not. The first human cases were reported in China and Vietnam in 2003. They were four in number, and all were fatal. In 2004, 46 cases were reported in Vietnam and Thailand; of these, 32 were fatal. In 2005, 97 cases were reported in Vietnam, Thailand, China, Cambodia, and Indonesia; 42 were fatal. In 2006, 116 cases were reported in a large range of countries: Azerbaijan, Cambodia, China, Djibouti, Egypt, Indonesia, Iraq, Thailand, and Turkey. Of these, 80 were fatal (Engel 2007, 34). To be sure, the Avian Flu has not killed many people to date, and no US citizen has succumbed to its horrors. Yet, according to public health authorities, we are closer now to an influenza pandemic than at anytime since the Asian Flu outbreak in 1968–9 (World Health Organization 2007). When the first influenza pandemic of the 2000s hits it will kill somewhere between 209 000 to 1 903 000 members of the US population (Department of Health and Human Services 2006).

Although both pandemic flu and regular seasonal flu are similar in that they spread easily between people by coughs and sneezes, they are quite different in several other ways. With respect to regular seasonal flu, outbreaks typically occur in the wintertime; the same type of flu virus occurs each year; and vaccine is generally available, with shortages being the exception rather than the rule. The situation is quite different with respect to an influenza pandemic, however. Outbreaks can occur any time; the type of flu virus is novel; and an *effective* vaccine takes months to identify, develop, and get to market in large enough supplies to meet the demand (Adler 2005, 44).

More than likely, an influenza pandemic will begin in a developing nation where animal-to-human contact is close and public health systems are either nonexistent or very fragile. An international traveler probably will bring the disease to US shores, having exposed at least some of his or her traveling companions to the virus. Infected patients will start trickling in to primary care offices, urgent care clinics, and hospital emergency rooms. Regrettably, health care personnel may not have much in their medical arsenal, over and beyond the antiviral Tamiflu, to treat the initial wave of infected patients. Worse, before too long, health care personnel may find themselves drowning in a sea of infected patients, unable to assist but a small fraction of them.

In North Carolina, public health officials know there is no way to be totally prepared for a severe influenza pandemic. As they see it, even a *mild* or *moderate* influenza pandemic would probably last eight weeks and result in 1.6 million physician visits, 35 000 hospital admissions, and 7900 deaths statewide (McGorty *et al.* 2007, 39). Nonetheless, despite their realization that their best preparedness efforts may not be enough to meet North Carolinians' needs during an influenza pandemic, NC public health officials are determined to prepare as much as they can.

Laying the Foundation for an Ethical Preparedness Plan for an Influenza Pandemic

To their credit, NC public health officials think North Carolinians need to be *ethically* as well as medically prepared for an Avian Flu attack. As difficult as it is to get medical systems of command and control, surveillance, vaccine and antiviral production, and health care delivery prepared for a deadly pandemic, it is even more difficult to get ethical codes and guidelines prepared for it. Experience teaches that once an influenza pandemic hits full force, it is too late to formulate ethical codes and guidelines to help citizens meet its distinctive ethical challenges. Accustomed to using ethical guidelines that work well enough in the clinical context, people may discover that the principles of autonomy, beneficence, nonmaleficence, and justice need to be interpreted and/or prioritized differently in the public health context. In addition, they may discover that these principles need to be supplemented by ethical principles they rarely, if ever, invoke in the clinical context. For example, individual freedom may have to give way to the public good.

Interestingly, the prime movers behind the NC IOM/DPH Task Force on which I served were very much influenced by the work of the University of Toronto Joint Center for Bioethics. In the aftermath of the 2003 Severe Acute Respiratory Syndrome (SARS) outbreak in Canada and several Asian nations, members of Toronto's Joint Center for Bioethics drafted a document entitled "Stand on Guard for Thee: Ethical Considerations for Pandemic Preparedness Planning" (University of Toronto Joint Centre for Bioethics Pandemic Influenza Working Group 2005). The phrase "stand on guard for thee" occurs in the Canadian national anthem. It signals to Canadians their obligation to be on the lookout for each other's best interests. Whatever befalls one Canadian potentially affects all Canadians. Although Canadians behaved well enough during the SARS crisis, manifesting their traditional communitarian spirit, the drafters of the Stand-on-Guard-for-Thee document felt Canadians would have acted even better had they been *ethically* as well as medically prepared for SARS. Among the things that went wrong ethically during Canada's SARS experience were: (1) some health care personnel refused to care for people infected with SARS and were subsequently dismissed for failing to report for duty; (2) other health care personnel were socially ostracized or stigmatized because they willingly cared for infected patients (Rhyne 2007, 51); (3) some physicians and nurses left their respective professions voluntarily because they did not want to continue in what they had come to regard as a truly life-threatening job (Rhyne 2007, 51); (4) some Canadians infected by or exposed to SARS did not comply or fully comply with quarantine restrictions (University of Toronto Joint Centre for Bioethics 2005, 12–13); and (5) some Canadians boycotted all Chinese businesses everywhere in Toronto just because the initial case of SARS was linked to an international traveler from China (Yount 2005, 21).

Wanting to avoid SARS-like mistakes in the event that an influenza pandemic hit the United States, the leaders of the NC IOM/DPH Task Force invited Alison Thompson, PhD, to discuss the reasoning process behind Toronto's Joint Center for Bioethics document. The Task Force wanted to explore with her whether the ethical values guiding the Canadian document were exportable to the United States. Dr Thompson stressed that two interrelated but nonetheless distinct sets of values, one *procedural* and the other *substantive*, were embedded in the Stand-on-Guard-for-Thee document. She then identified the procedural values as: (1) reasonability, (2) openness, (3) inclusiveness, (4) responsiveness, and (5) accountability; and the substantive values as: (1) individual liberty, (2) protection of the public from harm, (3) proportionality, (4) privacy, (5) equity, (6) duty to provide care, (7) reciprocity, (8) trust, (9) solidarity, and (10) stewardship (University of Toronto Joint Centre for Bioethics 2005, 6–7).

No one on the NC IOM/DPH Task Force had a problem with the Toronto team's procedural values, but several members of the Task Force questioned Dr Thompson about the Toronto team's definitions for the substantive values of solidarity, steward-ship, and reciprocity, respectively. In addition, they interrogated her about the Toronto team's views on the duty to care as it applied to licensed health care professionals in particular, but to others as well. Did licensed health care professionals really have a duty to risk their own lives in order to serve infected patients? Was this duty professional, contractual, legal, or moral? Did nonlicensed health care professionals have the same or different duties as licensed health care professionals? Did other professionals have the same or different duties as health care professionals? Did families have either a legal or a moral duty to take care of their infected relatives? Was a duty the same as an obligation? A responsibility? Was there a difference between a *moral* duty/obligation/responsibility and an *ethical* duty/obligation/responsibility?

After Dr Thompson's visit and nearly two months of sometimes heated, but always careful, discussions the NC IOM/DPH Task Force decided not to embrace the substantive values of solidarity and stewardship. Because some Task Force members associated the substantive value of solidarity with unions and/or socialism/commu-nism, the Task Force as a whole decided to forsake this value as too politically charged. Solidarity does not play as well on North Carolina soil as on Canadian ground. Americans are, on the average, more individualistic and less communal than Canadians; and solidarity with fellow citizens is not as important to Americans as being able to chart the course of their own individual destinies.

NC IOM/DPH Task Force members' reasons for rejecting the substantive value of stewardship ranged from very serious ones to fairly comical ones. One Task Force member objected to the substantive value of stewardship because he feared it connoted heavy fiduciary burdens. Another Task Force member stated the term "stewardship" had too many religious connotations. Yet another Task Force member could not disassociate the term "stewardship" from memories of the stewards who had served him on a recent ocean cruise. Realizing that stewardship was a substantive value without which the Task Force could still accomplish its mission, I suggested that, on balance, it was one we need not embrace.

Thinking that the IOM/DPH Task Force also would dismiss the substantive value of reciprocity as yet another unpalatable Canadian import, I was surprised when the entire Task Force embraced the value of reciprocity as one of its premier substantive values. Apparently, most Task Force members reasoned it was only fair that those who performed their usual duties and/or accepted heavier/riskier new duties during an influenza epidemic should be reciprocated in some way during and/or after the outbreak. Although some Task Force members interpreted reciprocity in a way that suggested they had not progressed beyond Stage Two ("I'll scratch your back, if you scratch mine") on Lawrence Kohlberg's well-known six-stage trajectory for moral development (Kohlberg 1971, 164–5), other Task Force members interpreted the substantive value of reciprocity in quite demanding ways, such as requiring those who receive services in an influenza pandemic to feel duty-bound to give back something of at least equal value to those who rendered the services to them.

Health Care Personnel and the Duty/Obligation/Responsibility to Work During an Influenza Pandemic

As I indicated above, one of the most prolonged and uncomfortable NC IOM/DPH Task Force meetings centered on health care personnel's purported duty to care for infected patients during an influenza pandemic. Several Task Force members asserted the term "duty" was too strong. To them, the term implied that health care personnel had an *ethical* duty to care for infected patients. I responded that, as I saw it, at least *licensed* health care personnel (e.g., physicians and nurses) did indeed have an ethical duty to care for infected patients for three reasons. First, licensed health care professionals have a greater ability than any other segment of the public to provide medical care, a fact that increases their obligation to provide it. Second, licensed health care professionals have a contract with society, resulting from the privilege of self-regulation and self-licensure, that calls on them to be available in times of emergency. Third, licensed health care professionals, by freely choosing a profession devoted to caring for the ill, prima facie accept an ethical obligation to act in the best interests of the ill and to assume a proportional share of the risks to which their profession exposes them (NC IOM/DPH Task Force 2007, 28).

Within nanoseconds of my response, several vociferous objections were made to it. Some Task Force members claimed that individuals' professional ethics were separate from their personal ethics. As they saw it, a professional duty was less ethically binding than a personal duty. When I asked them why, they had no definite answer. However,

I did find plausible the suggestion that because professional duties *typically* are less linked to one's central self-identity than to personal duties, they may be less ethically binding. Yet even though this suggestion made sense to me, it also made me want to run for cover. Suddenly, I realized the extent to which ethical theory has failed to clearly specify whether professional duties are "perfect" or "imperfect" in the Kantian sense of these terms. For Kant, a perfect duty is one "which admits of no exception in the interests of inclination" (Kant 1964, 96). In contrast, an imperfect duty is one that must be performed at least sometimes when the opportunity arises. Did licensed health care professionals always have a duty to treat infected patients during an influenza pandemic or could they, with clear conscience, balance their duty to care for infected patients against their duty not to infect others, including themselves under certain circumstances? In answer to my question, one Task Force member noted that the American Medical Association (AMA) Policy E-9.067 Physician Obligation in Disaster Preparedness and Response states:

> The physician workforce … is not an unlimited resource; therefore, when participating in disaster responses, physicians should balance immediate benefits to individual patients with ability to care for patients in the future. (Rhyne 2007, 52)

He then claimed that, at most, health care professionals had an imperfect duty to care for infected patients. Other members of the Task Force disagreed. They worried that unless health care professionals were exhorted to think they have a perfect duty to care for infected patients, they would always find a reason not to discharge their "imperfect" duty to care for infected patients.

The perfect/imperfect duty debate was never resolved. Rather it was shelved for future consideration. But not every uncomfortable debate was shelved. Sometimes the Task Force had the fortitude to resolve a moral disagreement relatively quickly. For example, when two Task Force members referred to Ayn Rand's *The Virtue of Selfishness* (Rand 1964), claiming that the only moral duty individuals had was the duty to maximize their own self-interest, they were immediately challenged by the majority of Task Force members who claimed either that individuals had moral duties to others or that it was in individuals' self-interest to serve the interests of others. Realizing there was major opposition on the Task Force to Ayn Rand's brand of ethical egoism, her two followers quickly decided it was probably in their own self-interest to soft-pedal their point of view. However, one of them suggested the Task Force reserve the term "duty" or "obligation" for (1) licensed health care personnel's *professional* obligation to care for infected patients; and (2) unlicensed as well as licensed health care personnel's *contractual* obligation to meet the terms of their respective employment agreements. He further suggested that a weaker term like "responsibility" be used to refer to everyone else's purported duty/obligation to assist each other in times of need. Although I was not certain I agreed with these two suggestions, I ultimately voted with the rest of the Task Force to accept them as verbal distinctions that probably would not make much of a substantive difference in the Task Force's final report.

Relieved to have the duty/obligation/responsibility "wordsmithing" session behind it, the NC IOM/DPH moved on to a matter more easy for it to understand and discuss; namely, what society "owed" to health care personnel willing to put their lives on the line for the sake of the common good. As it considered society's debt to those who serve it in times of crisis, the NC IOM/DPH Task Force repeatedly invoked the value of reciprocity. To its credit, the Task Force was alert to the fact that if health care personnel and other critical workers were asked to fulfill their duties/obligations/responsibilities to society, it was only fair that society express its gratitude to them. Thus, the Task Force insisted that frontline health care personnel and others at increased risk of infection should have priority for protective equipment, antiviral medications, vaccinations, counseling services, and adequate on-the-job training if necessary (NC IOM/DPH 2007, 29–32). In addition, most, if not all, of the Task Force members insisted that families of frontline health care personnel be given priority for preventive measures and/or curative treatments, so as to increase the likelihood of health care personnel reporting for duty. Finally, the Task Force urged government authorities to take measures such as the following three:

1. Establish liability immunity for good faith medical treatment and triage judgments.
2. Suspend Health Insurance Portability and Accountability ACT (HIPAA) regulations enforcement in cases of necessary and/or inadvertent violations in a crisis situation.
3. Provide a compensatory program modeled on workman's compensation for physicians who die or become disabled as a consequence of providing care in a pandemic (Rhyne 2007, 52).

Interestingly, the NC IOM/DPH Task Force considered, but ultimately rejected, the suggestion that health care personnel, nonlicensed as well as licensed, be paid extra for working during an influenza pandemic. Several Task Force members feared that extra pay might entice infected health care personnel to report for work. They had in mind relatively low-paid health care personnel such as nurse aides.

As much as I wanted to believe that most health care personnel would continue to work during an influenza pandemic, reciprocated or not, my inner skeptic chipped away at my inner optimist. My unease increased when several Task Force members recommended that we rely on *volunteers* during an influenza pandemic. The idea of relying on volunteers is, in the Southeast region of the United States, still enormously popular. The region is characterized by a particularly large number of charitable organizations, many of them church based. A remarkably high number of physicians and other health care personnel volunteer to work at free clinics, respond to medical crises whenever and wherever they occur, and serve desperately ill people in developing nations. Yet, in time of an influenza pandemic, there may be something wrong about relying on volunteers. I asked the Task Force if risk of death should not be distributed equally among all health care personnel, particularly the licensed ones. I noted that during the height of the HIV AIDS crisis, when a sizeable number of physicians and nurses refused to treat infected patients, Abigail Zuger, MD, argued that the American Medical Association (AMA) code of 1847 had it right when it stated: "When pestilence prevails, it is their duty to face the danger and to continue their labors for the alleviation of suffering, even at the jeopardy of their own lives" (Zuger 1987). The 1847 code imposed on *all* licensed health care professionals, and not merely the volunteers among them, the duty to care for infected patients during an influenza pandemic.

To be sure, there are times when a health care professional justifiably may refuse to treat an infected patient on the grounds that his or her attempt to do so would most probably (or nearly certainly) result in more harm than good for the patient. For example, the Task Force imagined the following scenario as one which might constitute a justification for a licensed health care professional, in this case a psychiatrist, not to treat an infected patient:

> A psychiatrist has been called in to help hospital personnel cope with the stresses of the influenza pandemic. Suddenly, while waiting to speak with emergency department physicians, a patient on a gurney begins to turn blue and struggle to breathe. All of the other physicians and healthcare personnel are busy with equally ill patients. The psychiatrist knows that she must intubate the patient (e.g., insert a breathing tube into the patient's airway) to help him breathe but has concerns because she has not intubated a patient since she was an intern 10 years ago. Should she intubate the patient? Is the risk of him dying greater than the risk of her injuring him while attempting to intubate him? What if something goes wrong? (NC IOM/DPH 2007, 32)

Still, even in this scenario, from a patient's point of view, he or she might reasonably prefer the help of a psychiatrist with rusty intubation skills to no help at all. If not the psychiatrist, then who? The health care ethicist on call? A food service employee?

Although the Task Force seemed particularly worried that not enough health care personnel would be willing to risk their lives for infected patients, the health care personnel on the Task Force all expressed the sentiment that if an influenza pandemic did hit US shores, *they* intended to report for duty. They felt personally, as well as professionally and contractually, bound to do so. However, one physician in this group, who described himself as a realist, said his and other health care personnel's good intentions might weaken or even disappear if a sizeable number of health care personnel died as a result of serving infected patients. He noted that during the three-century long pandemic of bubonic plague in Europe, each new outbreak provoked physicians to reconsider their duty to treat infected patients. I added that during this plague many physicians ultimately followed the advice they gave patients: namely "leave fast, go far and return slowly" (Jonsen 2000, 45).

Other Critical Workers and Duty/Obligation/Responsibility to Work During an Influenza Pandemic

Although the NC IOM/DPH Task Force spent considerable time addressing the concerns of health care personnel, throughout its deliberations it always was aware that health care personnel were only one among many types of workers *critical* to maintaining society during an influenza pandemic. Although there are significant differences between a medical crisis like an influenza pandemic on the one hand and a natural disaster like a hurricane, earthquake, or tsunami on the other, there are certain similarities. When the situation gets dire—and people find themselves in a survivor scenario, scrambling for water, food, shelter, and other necessities—morality's grip on people's minds and hearts is severely tested. To be sure, such disastrous states of affair often bring out the best in people; but sometimes they also bring out the worst. Therefore, the Task Force reasoned it would be incumbent upon government officials to get not only health care personnel but also other socially essential personnel to do their jobs.

In its deliberations about the degree to which workers in critical, nonhealth-related industries would have duties, obligations, and/or responsibilities to work during an influenza pandemic, the NC IOM/DPH Task Force struggled to draft a complete list of industries "critical" for social functioning. It found some helpful leads in the US Department of Homeland Security's (DHS) list of 17 critical industries that comprise the national infrastructure and would require protection in the event of a terrorist attack or other hazard: agriculture and food; energy; public health and health care; banking and finance; drinking waters and water treatment systems; information technology and telecommunications; postal and shipping; transportation systems including mass transit, aviation, maritime, ground or surface, and rail and pipelines systems; chemical; commercial facilities; government facilities, emergency services; dams; nuclear reactors, materials and waste; the defense industrial base; and national monuments and icons (NC IOM/DPH 2007, 35). Absent from this list (and rightly so because it is a list of *industries*) were two sets of critical workers whom the Task Force thought would be essential during an influenza pandemic: the police and the military.

No doubt, it was largely the memory of the aftermath of Hurricane Katrina in New Orleans that prompted the NC IOM/DPH Task Force to realize how much social order depends on a disciplined, fair, and humane police force and military to stay the course during times of civil unrest or even panic. In a *Newsweek* article written shortly after Katrina hit New Orleans, the reporter noted that within the space of days, the city was "on the verge of anarchy" and "policemen [sic], many of whom had lost their homes, were turning in their badges rather than face … looters for another day" (Thomas 2005, 47–48). The National Guard had to be called in. Eventually order was restored, in large measure because so many people had left New Orleans voluntarily or involuntarily. There were other places to go—safer places. But in a full-scale influenza pandemic there will be no safe places to which to flee. The Task Force theorized that although most workers in critical industries probably did not have the same degree of duties/obligations/responsibilities to work as, for example, licensed health care personnel had, the police and military probably did.

To the Task Force's relief, the police personnel Task Force members on it stated they viewed themselves (as well as the military) as having a professional as well as contractual duty/obligation/responsibility to do their job during an influenza pandemic. Police personnel had some concerns, however, about how to maintain order at pressure points such as grocery stores and pharmacies. They also were worried about the role they might be required to play in enforcing isolation, quarantine, and social-distancing regulations. Significantly, none of the Task Force members were official representatives of the military sector, a fact that concerned me. Given the role the National Guard had played in trying to restore and keep order in the aftermath of Katrina, for example, I thought it would be important for the Task Force to at least be informed about the NC National Guard's influenza pandemic plans. Do they exist? I felt we were largely avoiding discussions about a worse-case influenza pandemic during which police personnel and military personnel might need to resort to force (even deadly force) to maintain order.

Significantly, the police personnel on the NC IOM/DPH Task Force were not the only group of nonhealth critical workers who voiced more than a contractual obligation to work during times of crisis. The Task Force was most impressed by the influenza pandemic preparedness plans of North Carolina's energy industry. One representative of this industry spoke with particular eloquence about the *ethos* behind his company's preparedness plan. He said, "We know folks will need light and heat and we are determined not to leave them in a lurch during a crisis situation even if we take a major financial hit." The Task Force noted how sensitive the company in question was not only to its customers' needs but also to its employees' needs (Kerin 2007, 62–4). Indeed, the company put many health care institutions' preparedness plans to shame.

In contrast to the NC police force and the NC energy industry, the food industry seemed to be significantly unprepared for an influenza pandemic. No one was quite sure whether the food industry included only farms and groceries, or whether it also included restaurants; and Task Force members from the food industry confessed their companies had no explicit ethos about their duty/obligation/responsibility to feed the public in time of crisis. Most people who work in the grocery stores at which the public shops and the restaurants at which it eats are paid fairly minimal wages. During an influenza pandemic, food-industry employees may respond in dramatically different ways to "come-to-work" summons. Some may refuse to work for fear of being infected by customers or coworkers; others may insist on working for fear of having no income or being fired.

The more the NC IOM/DPH Task Force focused on the food industry, the more it realized that during an influenza pandemic, food might become a scarcer resource than medical treatment. How would food be delivered to isolated, quarantined, or socially distanced people? Who would deliver it? Who would pay for it? And so forth. I thought to myself: Does any ethicist I know have good answers to such everyday, but crucial, questions? What, if anything, do workers in the food industry owe the public; and what, if anything, does the public owe them? I was relieved when the Task Force decided to move on to another topic, largely because I realized that as much as ethicists like to talk about applied ethics, they rarely address issues such as whose obligation it is to feed the grumpy old man down the street who has a hard time walking and communicating and who seems to have no visitors.

Social Distancing, Isolation, and Quarantine

Unfortunately, the next major topic of discussion also proved to be a difficult one for the Task Force to address. During an influenza pandemic, some individuals' rights would need to be temporarily suspended to protect the public from harm. For example, during a mild influenza pandemic (1 on a scale of 1 to 5), public health officials may require isolation of actually infected persons at home or in a secure environment. They may also require quarantine of individuals exposed to the virus, once again in their own homes or in a secure environment. The rest of the public could go about its usual business. In contrast, in a severe influenza pandemic (4 or 5 on the 1–5 scale), not only would isolation and quarantine measures be implemented, so too would social-distancing measures be implemented. Schools and day care centers might be asked or required to close (NC IOM/DPH Task Force 2007, 41–42). Large social gatherings including church services as well as sports and entertainment events might be discouraged or even prohibited. Moreover, in a worst-case scenario all nonessential businesses might be asked or required to close and/or all nonessential workers might be asked or required to stay at home (ibid.).

Although most of the Task Force wanted to believe that North Carolinians would *voluntarily* isolate, quarantine, and/or socially distance themselves in order to protect the public from harm, some members of the Task Force were more skeptical about North Carolinians' behavior in an influenza pandemic. They noted that at each of the four public meetings the Task Force held, in the cities of Asheville, Charlotte, Greenville, and Raleigh, respectively, those assembled said most people's economic situations would determine whether they stayed home from work voluntarily. If their workplace was open and they needed the money to pay their bills, people would drag themselves to work. Many members of the public suggested that the only sure ways to prevent this state of affairs would be to force workplaces to close or to pay workers to stay home. Of course, the wisdom of the state actually implementing either of these suggestions is highly questionable. The former suggestion might be financially devastating for many businesses, and the latter only marginally less so. Businesses could ask the government to provide them with funds to mitigate their major financial hits, but whether the government could do this without jeopardizing the economy as a whole is an open question. During the SARS pandemic in Canada—a very mild pandemic—about $2 billion was lost (Jha 2004). The bulk of these dollars was confined to the Toronto area, sparing the vast majority of Canada. In the case of an influenza pandemic, however, the economic impact would likely not respect any borders nor be limited to a single metropolitan area.

On the whole, the people who came to one of the Task Force's public meetings stated they were willing to forgo church services and other events, including entertainment and sports events, which sometimes seem as sacred to North Carolinians as church events. They also expressed willingness to keep their children home from school and to tend the sick in their own homes, provided their families' basic needs were met and they received adequate instructions and supplies for tending their infected loved ones and themselves. Once again, the NC IOM/DPH Task Force was sobered by the fact that during an influenza pandemic, so much would depend on society having well-developed systems to meet people's basic needs and on having adequate reservoirs of community goodwill and public service at hand. But did North Carolina have such systems and reservoirs? Was it realistic, for example, to expect family members to care for their infected relatives? Maybe. But studies indicate that many people would prefer their families not take care of them if they fall victim to an influenza pandemic. Should such studies prove to be true, who would take care of these people and where? Health care facilities would be without enough beds, and thoughts of housing infected people in Superdome-type quarters are frightening. Should people be housed in schools? In churches? In fitness centers? Who should staff these facilities? What about people for whom no one seems to care? As usual, I asked myself why is it that society creates task forces to meet all people's, but especially vulnerable people's, needs during an influenza pandemic or subsequent to a major natural disaster, when that same society ignores and/or neglects meeting vulnerable people's needs in relatively good times? Why is *care* reserved for moments of crisis? As much as I wanted to pose these fundamental questions to the Task Force, I knew they would serve only to sidetrack it. I held my tongue and focused on the Band-Aid at hand.

Allocation of Scarce Health Care Resources

The last major issue the NC IOM/DPH Task Force discussed was the allocation of scarce health care resources during an influenza pandemic. In an effort to avoid wasting time, the Task Force read the results of the Center for Disease Control's (CDC) 2005 Public Engagement Pilot Program on Pandemic Influenza (PEPPPI) project. The leaders of this project wanted to ascertain the general public's views on distributing scarce vaccine during an influenza pandemic. They asked citizens to rank order the following ethical guidelines for distributing scarce vaccine fairly: (1) Save those most at risk; (2) put children and younger people first; (3) limit the larger effects in society; (4) use a lottery system; and (5) use the principle of "first come, first served." After much discussion, the consulted citizens concluded:

> [W]ith a very high level of agreement—that *assuring the functioning of society* should be the first immunization goal followed in importance by *reducing the individual deaths and hospitalizations due to influenza* (i.e. protecting those who are most at risk). Because of the still high importance of the second goal, the groups added that the first goal should be achieved using the minimum number of vaccine doses required to assure that function. This would allow the remaining doses to be used as soon as possible for those at highest risk of death or hospitalization. There was little support for other suggested goals to vaccinate young people first, to use a lottery system, or a first come first served approach as top priorities. (Public Engagement Pilot Program on Pandemic Influenza 2005, 7)

Although the NC IOM/DPH Task Force learned much from the PEPPI report, it felt it had not learned enough. The Task Force wanted to establish ethical guidelines for a wide range of scarce medical resources. Vaccines would not be the only scarce medical resource in an influenza pandemic. So too would be antiviral medicines, ventilators, hospital and nursing home beds, masks, and health care professionals' time. Complicating the Task Force's allocation deliberations was the empirical fact that during an influenza pandemic priorities inevitably shift depending on whether prevention of disease (early stages) or treatment of disease (later stages) is central. Thus, the Task Force would need at least two sets of allocation guidelines: one for healthy people who needed vaccines and other preventive measures in order not to get sick; and another for sick people who needed treatment.

The NC IOM/DPH Task Force's list of possible allocation criteria included:

1. Priority should be given to assure the functioning of society.
2. Priority should be given to reduce the incidence or spread of disease.
3. Priority should be given to reduce illness, hospitalizations, and death due to the influenza.

4. Priority should be given to protect people with the most years of life ahead of them.
5. There should be no priority given for the distribution of limited health care resources to ensure that everyone has an equal chance of being protected. (NC IOM/DPH Task Force 2007, 49–50)

Although most of the Task Force wanted to limit its deliberations to the five possible allocation criteria listed above, at least one member of the Task Force wanted to add Ezekiel J. Emanuel's allocation criterion of "quality of life years left or the life cycle principle" (Emanuel and Wertheimer 2006, 854). The idea behind this criterion is that "each person should have an opportunity to live through all the stages of life," with priority given to young adults over young children (around one year old, say). Emanuel's reasoning for favoring young adults over young children is that young adults *supposedly* have more developed interests, hopes, and plans than young children, but like young children have not had an opportunity to realize them (ibid.). In other words, young adults have consciously articulated to themselves their school, career, marriage, and family plans, whereas young children have not. Thus, dying during an influenza pandemic would entail more suffering for a young adult than a young child.

For all the merits of Emanuel's criterion, the objection can be raised that if a young child survives an influenza pandemic, he/she will probably live to be a young adult with the kind of plans noted above. Moreover, given the fact that people are living ever longer and healthier lives, who is to say that a 40, 50, 60, 70, or even 80-year-old has had a chance to realize their hopes and interests? What if someone wasted the first 40 years of his or her life and wanted to use the next 40 years or so to make up for their wasted years? Why should his or her plans count less than a young adult's plans? If it adopted Emanuel's criterion, would the Task Force be perceived as ageist? To be sure, Task Force members thought that during an influenza pandemic many grandparents would willingly sacrifice their lives for the lives of their grandchildren, but this sentiment was captured in the less controversial principle that priority should be given to protect people with the most years of life ahead of them. Without the Emanuel principle ever coming to a vote, it gradually disappeared from the Task Force's radar screen, resurfacing as a "mention-only" in the Task Force's final report (NC IOM/ DPH 2007, 50, footnote c).

In addition to largely ignoring the Emanuel criterion, the Task Force loudly rejected the first-come, first-serve criterion. It made no sense to Task Force members to give vaccines to people who could not benefit from them just because they got first in line for them. Therefore, said the Task Force, many sorts of unfairnesses built into the "first-come, first-served" criterion, beginning with the fact that not everyone has the means to get to a vaccine-delivery location. During the aftermath of Hurricane Katrina, for example, it became clear that many of the people left behind did not have the transportation or help to flee. Should people be penalized an influenza pandemic simply because they have no access to transportation?

In the end, the NC IOM/DPH Task Force recommended a relatively nuanced list of ethical guidelines for a fair allocation of scarce medical resources during an influenza pandemic. The intent behind the Task Force's allocation guidelines was three-fold: (1) to preserve lives of workers critical for the functioning of society; (2) to prevent the spread of the disease; and (3) to treat people who could benefit from the treatment. Having previously been advised that its ethical allocation priorities would need to shift, depending on the state and severity of an influenza pandemic, and on whether preventive resources (both nonpharmaceutical and pharmaceutical) or treatment resources (both nonpharmaceutical and pharmaceutical) were under consideration, the Task Force issued the following ethical guidelines for distributing scarce medical resources:

a.   Allocation of vaccines (pharmaceutical prevention resources) should be made with the primary goal of assuring the functioning of society and the secondary goal of minimizing the spread of the disease.
b.   Allocation of nonpharmaceutical prevention resources (such as personal protective equipment) should be made with the goal of assuring the functioning of society and preventing the spread of the disease.
c.   Allocation of antivirals (pharmaceutical treatment resources) should be made with the primary goal of minimizing illness, hospitalization, and death and the secondary goal of assuring the functioning of society.
d.   Allocation of non-pharmaceutical treatment resources (e.g., ventilators and hospital beds) should be made with the goal of reducing illness, hospitalization, and deaths (NC IOM/DPH Task Force 2007, 53).

In addition to providing these four basic ethical guidelines, the Task Force stressed that within priority groups, decisions should be based on clinical and epidemiological factors only. They should not be based on socioeconomic status, gender, race, ethnicity, or, more controversially, immigration/legal-documentation status. (North Carolina has a large number of Hispanic immigrants, many with proper documentation, but an increasingly large number without proper documents).

Conclusion

After a unanimous vote, the Task Force's final ethical guidelines were published with the title "Stockpiling Solutions: North Carolina's Ethical Guidelines for an Influenza Pandemic." I came away from the experience convinced that Stephen Toulmin had it right in his now quarter-century old article, "The Tyranny of Principles" (Toulmin, 1981). Neither absolute adherence to principles, nor relativistic acceptance of all "moral" views, is likely to result in a set of ethical guidelines that most people in a highly-diverse society can accept as substantially their own. Rather, any such set of ethical guidelines is likely to be built "taxonomically, taking one difficult class of cases at a time and comparing it in detail with other clearer and easier classes of cases" (Toulmin 1981, 31). The NC IOM/DPH Task Force stalled when it tried to agree on abstract definitions of terms like "duty," "obligation," and "responsibility," but it made substantial progress as soon as Task Force members began to share cases in which it was clear to them, for example, that a physician had a duty/obligation/responsibility to work and cases in which it was not clear. By comparing and contrasting clear and unclear cases, the Task Force was able to write ethical guidelines that, in its collective estimation, would help decision-makers handle, fairly and compassionately, all but the hardest cases—the kind of cases which tragically result in someone or some group being harmed despite everyone's best intensions and efforts to avoid this state of affairs.

I left my role as co-Chair of the NC IOM/DPH Task Force convinced that when an influenza pandemic arrives, the kind of ethics most likely to persuade people to do their duty and more is not a rights-based, duties-based, or utility-based ethics, but a care-based ethics. We human beings are a very vulnerable lot. We are radically dependent on each other for survival and we need to view ourselves as folks in a life-boat in the middle or the ocean with no visible sign of rescue. If there aren't enough supplies to go around until help arrives, we can do several things: we can ask for volunteers to jump off the boat; we can start drawing straws for who gets pushed off the boat; we can have a majority vote about which lives are most dispensable; or we can look in each other's eyes and see ourselves—fearful, hopeful, and in need of compassion. Then start paddling together to get to shore, knowing that although we might not all make it, we didn't turn on each other in our panic. What we need most to weather a pandemic is an ethics of trust, reciprocity, and solidarity. If we have that, we will have the most precious health care resource of all.

References

Adler, J. 2005. "The fight against the flu." *Newsweek* (October 31, 2005): 44.

Berlinger, N. 2006. "Influenza pandemic and the fair allocation of scarce life-saving resources: how can we make the hardest of choices?" *The Hasting Center Bioethics Backgrounder*, berlinger@thehastingscenter.org.

Department of Health and Human Services. 2006. "Pandemic planning assumptions." Available at http://www.pandemicflu.gov/plan/pandplan.html. Accessed December 11, 2006.

Emanuel, E. J. and Wertheimer, A. 2006. "Who should get influenza vaccine when not all can?" *Science* 312(5775): 854–5.

Engel, J. P., MD. 2007. "Pandemic influenza: the critical issues and North Carolina's preparedness plan." *North Carolina Medical Journal: A Journal of Health Policy Analysis and Debate* 68(1): 32.

Garloch, K. 2006. "Avian flu: are we ready?" *The Charlotte Observer* (Sunday, April 9, 2006): A1.

Jha, P. 2004. "Doing good on a global scale." *University of Toronto Bulletin*. November 8, 2004. Accessed May 25, 2007 from www.news.utoronto.ca/bin6/thoughts/041108–665.asp.

Jonsen, A. 2000. *A Short History of Medical Ethics*. New York: Oxford University Press.

Kant, I. 1964. *Groundwork of the Metaphysic of Morals*, translated and analyzed by H.J. Paton, New York: Harper & Row; p. 96.

Kerin, J. 2007. "Business preparation for an influenza pandemic." *North Carolina Medical Journal* 68(1): 62–4.

Kohlberg, L. 1971. "From is to ought: how to commit the naturalistic fallacy and get away with it in the study of moral development." In *Cognitive Development and Epistemology*, ed. T. Mischel, 164–5. New York: Academic Press.

McGorty, E. K., JD, MA; Devlin, L. DDS, MPH; Tong, R. PhD; Harrison, N.; Holmes, M., PhD; and Silberman, P., JD, PhD. 2007. "Ethical guidelines for an influenza pandemic." *North Carolina Medical Journal: A Journal of Health Policy Analysis and Debate* 68(1): 39.

NC IOM/DPH Task Force (North Carolina Institute of Medicine and Division of Public Health Task Force on Ethics and Pandemic Influenza Planning). 2007. "Ethical guidelines for an influenza pandemic." DRAFT. North Carolina Department of Health and Human Services, 23.

PEPPPI (Public Engagement Pilot Program on Pandemic Influenza). 2005. "Citizen voices on pandemic flu choices: a report of the public engagement pilot program on pandemic influenza." The Keystone Center: Denver, 7.

Rand, A. 1964. *The Virtue of Selfishness*. New York: Signet.

Rhyne, J. A. MD. 2007. "Likely ethical, legal, and professional challenges physicians will face during an influenza pandemic." *North Carolina Medical Journal: A Journal of Health Policy Analysis and Debate* 68(1): 51.

Thomas, E. 2005. "The lost city—special report: after Katrina." *Newsweek* (September 12, 2005): pp. 47–8.

Toulmin, S. 1981. "The tyranny of principles." *The Hastings Center* 11(6): 31–9.

University of Toronto Joint Centre for Bioethics Pandemic Influenza Working Group. 2005. "Stand on guard for thee: ethical considerations in preparedness planning for pandemic influenza." University of Toronto Joint Centre for Bioethics.

World Health Organization. 2007. Current WHO phase of pandemic alert. Available at http://www.who.int/csr/disease/avian_influenza/phase/en/index.html. Accessed February 14, 2007.

Yount, K. 2005. "Man vs. virus: why we're worried about 'bird flu.'" *UAB Magazine* (Fall 2005): 21.

Zuger, A., and Miles, S. H. 1987. "Physicians, AIDS and occupational risk: historic traditions and ethical obligations." *JAMA* 258: 1924–8.

TB Matters More

Michael J. Selgelid, Paul M. Kelly, and Adrian Sleigh

Bioethics and Infectious Disease

Medical research resources are poorly distributed. This is illustrated by the 10/90 divide, a phenomenon whereby less than 10% of medical research resources focus on diseases responsible for 90% of the global burden of disease (Resnik 2004). While medical research focuses on development of profitable products, research and development (R&D) on infectious diseases remains largely neglected. This is because infectious diseases primarily affect poor people who cannot afford even inexpensive medications. The world's most urgent health care needs remain largely neglected as a result.

An analogous misdistribution of research resources applies to bioethics. Though infectious disease should be recognized as a topic of primary importance for bioethics, it has historically been neglected by this discipline (Selgelid 2005; Francis *et al.* 2005). There are numerous reasons why infectious disease warrants the central attention of bioethics. First, the historical and likely future consequences of infectious diseases are almost unrivalled. Throughout history, infectious diseases have caused more morbidity and mortality than any other cause, including war (Price-Smith 2001); and they are currently the biggest killers of children and young adults. The continuing threat of infectious disease is revealed by the extent of AIDS, TB, and malaria; the increasing number of newly emerging infectious diseases (such as Ebola, SARS, West Nile Virus, and avian influenza); the growing problem of drug resistance (which may imply return to a situation analogous to the pre-antibiotic era); and the specter of bioterrorism. Second, because they can be contagious and cause acute illness and death, infectious

"TB Matters More," by Michael J. Selgelid, Paul M. Kelly, and Adrian Sleigh, is from Michael Boylan (ed.) (2008) *International Public Health Policy and Ethics*. Springer; pp. 233–48.

diseases raise difficult ethical questions of their own (Smith *et al.* 2004; Selgelid 2005). Public health measures for controlling epidemics may include surveillance, mandatory treatment or vaccination, and coercive social distancing measures such as isolation and quarantine. Because measures such as these may conflict with human rights to privacy, consent to medical treatment, and freedom of movement, an ethical dilemma arises. How should the social aim to promote public health be balanced against the aim to protect human rights and liberties in the context of diseases that are to varying degrees contagious, dangerous or deadly? Third, because infectious diseases primarily affect the poor and disempowered, the topic of infectious disease is closely connected to the topic of justice, a central concern of ethics.

Bioethics has not entirely ignored the topic of infectious disease. AIDS, in particular, has received a great deal of discussion in the bioethics literature. In a related development, public health ethics has become a rapidly growing subdiscipline of bioethics as is evidenced by a number of recent books (Coughlin *et al.* 1998; Beauchamp and Steinbock 1999; Gostin 2002; Boylan 2004; Anand *et al.* 2004; Selgelid *et al.* 2006; Balint *et al.* 2006; Dawson and Verweij 2007) and (as of 2008) a new journal—*Public Health Ethics* (Oxford University Press). At least some of this literature has emphasized infectious disease in particular. With the exception of AIDS, however, bioethics discussion of infectious disease remains in its infancy, and coverage of topics has been patchy at best (Tausig *et al.* 2006). Much of the emerging literature has focused on SARS, pandemic influenza, and bioterrorism in particular. There has also been an increase in relevant debate about intellectual property rights in pharmaceuticals—and the barriers patents pose to medication access in poor countries (Schüklenk and Ashcroft 2002; Cohen and Illingworth 2003; Sterckx 2004; Pogge 2005; Cohen *et al.* 2006).

Neglected Disease

Tuberculosis (TB) is a bacterial infectious disease that is usually spread by coughing. TB illness is debilitating in the short term; and it is associated with high mortality if untreated, and with significant disability even if successfully cured. Whilst pulmonary TB (disease affecting the lungs) is the most common and most infectious form of the disease, TB can affect any part of the body. TB is strongly associated with poverty and is common in less-developed countries, particularly in Asia, Africa, and South America. There has been a resurgence of TB in relation to the HIV/AIDS pandemic, particularly in sub-Saharan Africa (Dye *et al.* 2007). The public health implications of TB are enormous. Until recently TB was the world's leading infectious cause of mortality, and it is now second only to AIDS.

It is surprising and unfortunate that there has not been much focused discussion of ethical issues associated with TB,[1] which is arguably the most important neglected topic in bioethics. Because TB kills nearly as many people as AIDS each year, one would expect TB to receive a proportionate amount of discussion in health ethics literature. There are, furthermore, good reasons for thinking that the problem of TB is even more ethically important than AIDS. In the vast majority of cases TB drugs can provide cure, and they are much less expensive than AIDS medications. While

1.6 million people die from TB each year (WHO 2007a) and 2.1 million die from AIDS (UNAIDS 2007), the former deaths are, economically speaking, much easier to prevent. A standard course of TB medication can cost as little as US$10 or US$20, and TB therapy is considered to be one of the most cost-effective health care interventions. In best case scenarios, AIDS medication costs as little as $100 for a year of treatment in developing countries, but it often costs much more. In the case of AIDS, furthermore, lifelong treatment is required because no cure exists. Given cost considerations, the case for increasing access to TB medication appears stronger than the case for increasing access to AIDS medication (which is not to say that the case for increasing access to AIDS medication is not itself enormously powerful). In 1998, only 56% of those in need had access to TB therapy recommended by World Health Organization (WHO), and the rate was only 23% just a few years earlier in 1995 (Lienhardt *et al.* 2003). There have been impressive gains in access to TB services in many countries in recent years, and approximately 62% of those in need were receiving treatment in 2007 (Floyd 2007). Significant gaps remain, however, in many of the countries where TB is most prevalent (Dye *et al.* 2007).

A final reason for thinking that TB is ethically more important than AIDS is that the former, being airborne, is both contractible via casual contact and much more contagious. While behavior modification (with respect to IV drug use and sexual practice) can essentially eliminate the risk of infection with AIDS, TB can be passed from one individual to another via coughing, sneezing, and even talking. In many ways, then, the threat to "innocent individuals"—and public health in general—is greater in the case of TB.

Though the ethical importance of TB at least rivals, if it does not surpass, the ethical importance of AIDS; the former has received comparatively little attention from bioethicists. The lack of attention to ethical issues associated with TB is revealed via searches on the Internet. A *PubMed* search of titles and abstracts (conducted in October 2007) for the terms "ethics" and "AIDS" yielded 2998 entries; while a similar search for the terms "ethics" and "tuberculosis" yielded only 179. Rather than reflecting difference in ethical importance, the disproportionate amount of bioethics attention to AIDS in comparison with TB reflects the fact that the former disease has affected an economically powerful and articulate community and has been much more highly politicized.

The global TB status quo, meanwhile, is alarming. The World Health Organization (WHO) declared TB a global health emergency in 1993. One third of the world population is currently infected with latent TB. Approximately nine million people develop active illness each year, and "there are between 16 million and 20 million persons with active tuberculosis at any one time" (Gandy and Zumla 2002, 385). Though a cure for TB has existed for over 50 years, and though in the 1950s TB was believed to be eradicable, TB "is now more prevalent than in any previous period of human history" (Gandy and Zumla 2002, 385). The TB burden is highest in Asia, which accounts for two thirds of the global burden of TB (WHO 2006b). The Southeast Asia Region has the *largest number* of new incident cases, accounting for 34% of incident cases globally. The *incidence rate* in sub-Saharan Africa, however, is nearly twice as high—"at nearly 350 cases per 100 000 population" (WHO 2007b). Like most other infectious diseases, the burden of TB is most heavily shouldered by the poor: 95% of TB cases and 98% of TB deaths occur in developing countries (Gandy and Zumla

2002). This is because the poor lack good nutrition, and this weakens their immune systems. It is also because crowded living and working conditions, and lack of sanitation and hygiene, increase chances of exposure and infection. Because the poor so often lack access to (even inexpensive) medical care, they are more likely to suffer adverse outcomes when infection occurs. Direct and indirect costs of illness can have a catastrophic effect on TB sufferers and their families (Bates *et al.* 2004; Jackson *et al.* 2006). Matters have been made worse by the growing HIV/AIDS epidemic. Those living with HIV/AIDS are much more likely to contract TB, and more likely to develop severe illness when they do (Harries and Dye 2006).

Though the impact of TB is most heavily felt in developing countries, the emergence and spread of multidrug-resistant TB (MDRTB) poses serious threats to developed nations as well. A primary cause of drug resistance is the failure of patients to always complete a full course of TB medication. This often occurs in developing countries when patients cannot afford to continue therapy, cannot afford time off work to visit health providers, or cannot afford travel to clinics. Another cause of drug resistance is the weakness of health care infrastructures in poor countries. Patients often fail to complete therapy because hospitals and clinics in poor countries fail to maintain a steady supply of standard TB medications (Farmer 1999; Farmer 2003). Drug resistance is also driven by the market presence of drugs that are low quality, old, or often counterfeit.

Like ordinary TB, drug-resistant TB is contagious. With increased global trade and travel, drug-resistant TB spreads frequently from country to country. Though it is usually curable, MDRTB requires longer and more expensive treatment. Ordinary TB can be treated with a six month course of medication costing US$10–20. MDRTB takes two years to treat, and treatment can be up to 100 times more expensive. The "second-line" medications used to treat MDRTB are, furthermore, both more toxic and less effective than the "first-line" drugs used to treat ordinary TB.

The problem of untreatable TB is suddenly on the rise. In 2006, the US Centers for Disease Control and Prevention (CDC) and WHO announced the emergence and spread of "extreme" or "extensively" drug-resistant TB (XDR-TB). MDRTB is defined as TB resistant to at least two (namely isoniazid and rifampicin) of the four first-line TB medications. XDR-TB is defined as TB resistant to at least two of the four first-line TB medications and at least two of the six second-line medications (a fluoroquinolone and an injectable agent; CDC 2006; WHO 2006a). A recent study showed that 20% of TB isolates from around the world were MDRTB and that 10% of these were XDR-TB. XDR-TB was found in every region, and the study showed that isolates of MDRTB obtained from the USA, Latvia, and South Korea were, respectively, 4%, 19%, and 15% XDR-TB (CDC 2006). The most dramatic epidemic of XDR-TB is currently underway in South Africa. A study in March 2006 showed that 41% of suspected patients in Tugela Ferry were infected with MDRTB and that 24% of these had XDR-TB. Of the 53 patients with the latter, 52 died within 25 days (MSF 2006). Many are worried that XDR-TB may "swiftly put an end to all hope of containing the [AIDS] pandemic [in Africa] through treatment". According to one expert: "There is no point investing hugely in ARV [anti-retro viral] programmes if patients are going to die a few weeks later from extreme drug-resistant tuberculosis" (Boseley 2006). Implications of XDR-TB for the international community are starkly revealed by the CDC's conclusion that XDR-TB "has emerged worldwide as a threat to public health and TB control, raising concerns of a future epidemic of virtually untreatable TB" (CDC 2006).

Mapping the Terrain of Ethical Issues Associated with TB: A Research Agenda

Bioethics research in the context of TB should address the following issues.

Duty to treat

A common topic in bioethics discussion of infectious disease has been the question of health workers' duty to treat patients infected with diseases that pose risks to health workers themselves. A related question concerns the duty of society, or the health care system, to provide safe conditions for health workers through provision of masks, room ventilation, and other infection control measures in hospitals and clinics. Most of the debate has thus far focused on AIDS, SARS, and avian influenza. The existing literature reveals that there are no simple answers to these kinds of questions and that different issues arise in the context of different diseases (Reid 2005). Though these questions are pertinent to TB, given that it is highly contagious—and increasingly dangerous in the context of MDRTB and XDR-TB, and/or when health workers are living with HIV (Cobelens 2007)—they have in the specific context of TB received little if any dedicated discussion in mainstream bioethics literature. Bioethics should examine the extent of risk involved with treating TB patients; the nature and extent of health care workers' "duties" to face such risks; possible means (and ethical justification) for reducing such risks through improvement of infection control in health care settings; and the propriety of rewarding health workers willing to face greater risks (Savulescu, in discussion) and/or the propriety of compensating those who actually become infected on the job (University of Toronto Joint Centre for Bioethics 2005).

Clinical research

A major topic of debate in the context of HIV/AIDS research has been the question of what should count as an ethically acceptable control arm in studies involving human subjects. Most of the attention has focused on placebo controlled studies of mother-to-child transmission of HIV in Africa. Critics argued that these studies conflicted with the Declaration of Helsinki requirement that patients in the control arm of a study should receive the "best proven" or "best current" therapy for the condition in question (Lurie and Wolfe 1997). Others argued that it would have been too expensive to provide such treatment in developing world contexts—and that no harm was done because patients were denied no treatment they would have received if they had not participated in the studies (because the standard of care in poor countries was *no treatment* to prevent vertical transmission of HIV). Given that the WHO has recently declared that the standard of care for MDRTB requires provision of second-line drugs, it will not be surprising, given what commonly occurred in the context of HIV, if there are proposals for studies where control arm subjects would not receive this expensive, high level of care (apparently) still required by the Declaration of Helsinki. Would it be wrong to deprive control arm subjects of second-line drugs if they would not receive them if they did not participate in the study in question—given the poverty situation in the local context? How are the ethical issues in the context of TB similar to, or different from, those that arose in the context of HIV/AIDS?

Another issue arising in clinical research involves the management of third-party risks. A study of a new drug for resistant strains of TB, for example, may pose risks to third parties. If the investigational drug is not effective, then a patient-subject who receives it may remain infectious and thus endanger family members and other close contacts. Isolation of the patient-subject or informed consent of third parties might thus be called for. This general issue has been neglected by research ethics guidelines (Francis et al. 2006).

Treatment exclusion

There have been reports of prescription practices in poor countries where health workers decide to exclude TB patients from treatment in cases where it is believed that the patient is unlikely to complete therapy (Singh et al. 2002). While withholding treatment from unreliable patients may serve the aim to avoid promotion of drug resistance, a practice like this may be inappropriately discriminatory. Such a practice may also have counterproductive results if infectious patients remain at large in the community. Because the ability of health workers to make sound judgments about such matters is suspect, the extent and quality of institutional policy calling for patient exclusion warrants further analysis. In addition to concerns about unjust discrimination, a major question is whether or not, or why, it is reasonable to think that the harm to excluded individuals would be outweighed by greater goods to society in the way of public health. These are partly, though not entirely, empirical questions—i.e., about what the actual harms and benefits are (to individuals and society, respectively). The more ethico-philosophical question is how benefits to society should be weighed against harms to individuals.

Obligation to avoid infecting others

If there is a duty to do no harm, then infected—or potentially infected—persons have duties to avoid infecting others (Harris and Holm 1995; Verweij 2005). This interesting and important topic has received surprisingly little attention in general, and discussion to date has primarily focused on AIDS and influenza. Bioethics should examine the extent to which a duty like this applies in the context of TB in particular. Because it would be unreasonable to expect potentially infected persons to take all possible measures to avoid infecting others, appropriate limitations to the duty must be considered. Because TB is transmissible via casual contact, anyone who has been breathed or coughed on by someone who *might* (for all one knows) be infected with TB should, epistemologically speaking, consider herself to be "potentially-infected". But that means almost all of us! (This is just one of the ways in which the case of TB is different from AIDS.) Even those who actually have been in (limited) contact with someone sick with active TB, however, will usually not themselves become infected as a result.

Though potentially deadly and considered highly contagious, TB is not nearly so contagious as the flu. (This is just one of the ways in which the case of TB is different from flu.) To what extent should someone who knows she has been exposed to TB limit her interactions with others afterwards? The answer will partly depend on whether we are talking about ordinary TB, MDRTB or XDR-TB—*if these details are known*.

Third-party notification

In cases where a contagious patient fails to take adequate precautions to avoid infecting others—and fails to warn close contacts about his infectious status—then the question of whether or not the health worker should inform identifiable third parties at risk arises. On the one hand, notification of third parties about a patient's health status would breach the widely acknowledged patient right to confidentiality. On the other hand, failure to warn could (especially in the context of XDR-TB) conflict with the innocent third party's right to life—which many would say is more important than the incautious patient's right to confidentiality. This matter is complicated because a routine practice of breaching confidentiality may decrease trust in the health care system, reduce health-seeking behavior, and thus drive the epidemic underground. What the actual public health implications of third-party notification would be is an empirical question that warrants further study.

Domestic surveillance

Mandatory TB testing in schools, the workplace, or elsewhere in the community may potentially conflict with the right to privacy. If information concerning the health status of individuals is not well protected, then stigma and discrimination will result. Surveillance measures, on the other hand, are sometimes important to the protection of public health. Bioethics should consider the extent to which current surveillance measures are—or the extent to which more wide-reaching surveillance measures would be—justified in the context of TB, especially now that MDRTB and XDR-TB are growing threats to global public health.

Migrant screening

It is common for countries to screen migrants for TB before granting entry visas. Some have questioned the public health efficacy and/or cost-effectiveness of a practice like this in comparison with other means of TB control (Coker 2003). Whilst identification of active disease offshore is a commonly used method for TB control in countries with a low prevalence of TB (and sometimes countries with high prevalence), it is not always possible to perform due to the lack of resources or a lack of time prior to arrival (Coker 2003). Additionally, one-off screening for TB with x-ray does not completely eliminate the risk of TB transmission to the public in the receiving nation due to the lifetime latency of the disease (MacIntyre *et al.* 1997). The offshore TB screening policy relies on a "user pays" philosophy, where visa applicants are responsible for the costs incurred. Aside from questions of equity, where the poor who are most likely to have TB are also least likely to be able to pay for the screening tests, this model works well when a private sector health system is in operation. The International Organization for Migration (IOM) has called for a "paradigm shift from exclusion to inclusion" to address this, amongst other unintended effects of premigration screening for the benefit of the migrant and the host nation (Maloney 2004). In many countries from which refugees are resettled, there are no private for-profit radiological or microbiological facilities and government clinics are stretched to capacity. Is it appropriate for developed countries to shift costs for their public health onto the overburdened health systems of other, less well-resourced, countries? Additional ethical issues arise in the context of asylum seekers. This form of migration has posed enormous problems in the northern hemisphere. In situations like this, host countries' duties of beneficence potentially conflict with duties to protect public health. Ethical issues associated with migrant screening in the context of infectious disease are a generally neglected area of discussion that is becoming increasingly important in the contemporary era of "globalisation" and "emerging infectious diseases". These issues are especially pertinent in the context of TB.

Social distancing

In the past, patients with infectious TB were isolated in sanatoria for prolonged periods—and sometimes even for life. This was done to protect others from infection. Even today, in many countries, it is common to isolate patients with pulmonary symptoms (i.e., "active TB") until they are deemed uninfectious— usually about two weeks after therapy is started. Such detention is usually brief and voluntary. It is common, however, to coercively confine patients with active TB, and sometimes patients with inactive TB, when they refuse to take their medicine or when it is believed they are unlikely to adhere to treatment regimens (Coker 2000).

Bioethics should consider the extent to which (coercive) restriction of movement is ethically justified in the name of public health protection against TB. Of particular importance is the question of what should be done with XDR-TB patients, who pose threats of infection with an especially dangerous form of TB whether they take their medicines or not. Defenders of confinement in the context of treatable TB sometimes suggest that confinement is justified when patients are at least given a choice between confinement and treatment—the idea being that this respects their autonomy (Bayer and Dupuis 1995). If XDR-TB patients are confined because they are untreatable, then no autonomous choice would remain. Though this does not go to show that mandatory confinement is therefore inappropriate, the point is that the question of what to do with XDR-TB patients is not automatically settled by conclusions about what to do with noncompliant patients with treatable TB. Additional new questions are whether or not, the extent to which, or the conditions under which, it would be ethical to quarantine the large number of people exposed to, though not known to be infected with, XDR-TB—or those suspected, though not known, to be infected with XDR-TB (Singh et al. 2007)—while diagnostic confirmation is awaited.

Coercive long-term confinement may again become common in the case of patients actually diagnosed with (untreatable) XDR-TB. In a widely reported case in Arizona, for example, an XDR-TB patient has been detained in a prison hospital for over a year (Democracy Now 2007). And there are already calls in Africa for a return to compulsory sanatoria for such patients (Sakoane 2007). If the spread of untreatable XDR-TB becomes sufficiently alarming, we may be faced with quarantine and confinement at a scale not seen for decades. In 2007 a patient suspected of infection with XDR-TB was subjected to the first US federal isolation order since 1963.

Among other questions, the following should be further considered: (1) the extent to which coercive social distancing measures are justified in light of the available evidence (or lack thereof) regarding their efficacy and (2) arguments calling for compensation provision to those whose liberties are coercively restricted.

It is true that untreatable TB was the norm prior to development of cures in the middle of the 20th century, and we should examine historical debates regarding the social acceptability of confinement and so on that took place in public health circles in the pre-antibiotic era. No developed discipline of bioethics existed at that time, however, and so it remains to be seen how policy decisions made then will be viewed under the lens of rigorous ethical analysis. More importantly, given population growth and globalization, the contemporary world is different from that when untreatable TB previously existed. Because population dynamics have changed, there is no reason to assume that public health solutions to untreatable TB in the past (even if it is determined that such policies were ethically and epidemiologically sound at the time) will be appropriate to the contemporary world.

Mandatory treatment and ethical issues associated with DOTS

As indicated above, it is commonly the case that (treatable) patients are required to either undergo therapy or be held in confinement. Insofar as the threat or actual use of force is involved, TB treatment involves coercion and thus conflicts with individual autonomy (despite the fact that patients are usually given at least some choice in the matter). The worldwide standard of care for TB treatment is known as Directly Observed Therapy, Short Course (DOTS). Among other things, DOTS involves health or social workers' observation of patients' medication-taking; and patient cooperation is (often) part of what is required to avoid detention. Though DOTS has (arguably rightly) been hailed as a great success in global TB control (partly because it promotes patient "compliance" and thus helps prevent drug resistance) ethical issues are raised by the coercion involved. It is generally thought that informed consent to medical treatment is important—and that it must be voluntary. Autonomy, however, may be outweighed by societal benefits if the stakes are sufficiently high. Additional issues involve threats to privacy and dangers of stigmatization in contexts where DOTS practices are visible to the community; and the costs/inconvenience of DOTS in comparison with unmonitored treatment (especially when we are talking about reliable patients). Though issues associated with mandatory treatment and DOTS have perhaps received more bioethics attention than others considered in this chapter, much of the debate to date has focused on the limited context of New York City in the 1980s and 1990s (see Bayer and Dupuis 1995 and references therein).

Coercive in the prevention of Zoonosis

Coercion is also involved in attempts to remove *Mycobacterium bovis* ("bovine TB") from the food supply in rich countries by culling infected herds and pasteurizing milk. In part this is done to increase the safety and value of bovine (or ovine and other herbivore) products, especially milk and cheese. In poor areas of the world with ongoing high rates of TB among cattle or buffalo and use of raw milk products, bovine TB still causes much disease among humans, usually as an extrapulmonary infection of the throat (scrofula), stomach, abdomen or bones. Although control of animal TB may seem to be of obvious benefit to a community, the affected farmers may object to testing and culling of their infected animals, even when paid compensation, if herds cannot easily be replaced with disease-free equivalents. Also, farmers may be emotionally attached to the animals, especially dairy cattle, the main target for control of bovine TB. Another issue arises with compulsory pasteurization of milk. Some people even break the law to exercise their "right to consume natural products". How important are these liberties—and are they outweighed by public health benefits requiring coercion? Again these are, but only partly, empirical issues.

Justice and the distribution of health resources

As a disease of poverty, TB raises issues of international distributive justice. Though sufficient resources for health improvement are lacking in poor countries, there are numerous powerful moral (egalitarian, utilitarian, and libertarian) and self-interested reasons for wealthy nations to do more to help improve health care in poor countries (Selgelid OnlineEarly 2007). These issues are complex and intertwined with the above questions regarding liberty violating public health measures. If health care provision and thus global health were better to begin with, for example, then the occasions upon which liberty infringing public health measures are called for would arise less often.

In addition to improving access to existing medications, increased R&D for drugs and diagnostics is sorely needed in the fight against TB. At present, "[w]orldwide only $20 million is spent annually for clinical trials for TB drug[s] compared to around $300 million for HIV drugs in the US alone" (MSF 2007). Bioethicists should debate recent proposals (Pogge 2005; Kremer and Glennerster 2004) and current activities (Moran *et al.* 2005) aimed at stimulating R&D on neglected diseases—and the extent to which they are apt for TB in particular. They should also examine the extent to which *targeted* funding for TB control is warranted in comparison with other infectious diseases. Because it has been argued that donor aid should aim to improve developing countries' general health care infrastructures—and improvement of general health indicators—rather than targeting particular diseases such as AIDS and TB (Garrett 2007), the propriety of targeted TB funding should be evaluated. Because infectious diseases, including drug-resistant infectious diseases such as XDR-TB, fail to respect international borders, bad health in poor countries threatens global public health in general. The strength of associated self-interested reasons for wealthy nations to help reduce TB in poor countries (through targeted or untargeted funding) should therefore, finally, be a major focus of analysis.

A "Moderate Pluralist" Ethical Approach to TB Control

Our recommended approach to ethics and infectious disease may be characterized as "moderate pluralism". This approach aims to identify the plurality of (intrinsic) values at stake in the context under study and strike a balance between potentially conflicting values without giving absolute priority to any one value in particular. In the context of XDR-TB, for example, the utilitarian aim to promote public health *might* best be promoted through coercive confinement of infected patients. Such a policy, however, would conflict with apparent rights and liberties of infected individuals; and it is not generally believed that individual rights and liberties should be sacrificed whenever this would promote the greater good of society. Resolving a conflict like this requires assessment of the overall threat to society, assessment of the centrality/importance of the rights under threat, and consideration of features that might make one value (i.e., utility) or the other (i.e., liberty) especially important in the context in question. Most ethicists, policymakers, and ordinary citizens would, upon reflection anyway, deny that either of these two social values should always be given absolute priority over the other. The ideal solution to conflict between values is to bypass the conflict to begin with. We should thus, whenever possible, aim for a policy that promotes both utility and liberty—and also equality, another legitimate social value—at the same time. TB reduction via increased health care provision would reduce the frequency of occasions where we are faced with the conflict between utility and liberty under consideration; and it would likely also promote equality (given that TB reduction would generally involve improving the situation of those who are worst off).

This is not to say that the initially considered conflict would never eventuate if TB reduction occurs. Difficult decisions will need to be made in cases where conflict is unavoidable; and a principled rationale for favoring one value over another is needed in cases of conflict. One idea is that the aim to promote utility should be weighted more heavily as a function of the extent to which utility is threatened. Another idea is that the weight of a right/liberty should be weighted as a function of its centrality. More basic rights/liberties deserve more protection than others. When catastrophe would result from protection of the most basic rights, however, then even these must be compromised. We sometimes think it is appropriate to violate the most basic right of all—i.e., the right to life in time of war.

When rights violations are found to be necessary in the context of TB, amends can be made by compensating individuals whose rights are compromised (Ly *et al.* 2007). The living conditions of those confined should be made as comfortable as possible—and those who succumb to liberty restrictions should perhaps receive additional (e.g., financial) rewards. It would be unfair to expect coerced individuals to shoulder the entire cost of societal benefit. If a net social dividend results from liberty infringement, then part of this should be returned to the victims of coercive social policy. This is a matter for reciprocity (University of Toronto Joint Centre for Bioethics 2005).

Note

1   A recent exception was the workshop organized by Anne Fogot-Largeault—with participation of Mary Edginton, Lourdes Garcia-Garcia, and Brigitte Gicquel—on "TB Ethics" at the 8th World Congress of the International Association Bioethics (2006) in Beijing. We also admit that the New York epidemic of the 1980s and 1990s received some important coverage.

References

Anand, S., Peter, F., and Sen, A. (eds) 2004. *Public health, ethics, and equity.* New York: Oxford University Press.

Balint, J., Philpott, S., Baker, R., and Strosberg, M. (eds) 2006. *Ethics and epidemics.* Amsterdam: JAI.

Bates, I., Fenton, C., Gruber, J., Lalloo, D., Medina Lara, A., Squire, S.B., Theobald, S., Thomson, R., and Tolhurst, R. 2004. Vulnerability to malaria, tuberculosis, and HIV/AIDS infection and disease. Part 1: determinants operating at individual and household level. *Lancet Infectious Diseases* 4(5): 267-77.

Bayer, R. and Dupuis, L. 1995. Tuberculosis, public health, and civil liberties. *Annual Review of Public Health* 16: 307-26.

Beauchamp, D.E. and Steinbock, B.S. (eds) 1999. *New ethics for the public's health.* New York: Oxford University Press.

Boseley, S. 2006. Global alert over deadly new TB strains. *Guardian.* Available at: http://www.guardian.co.uk/print/0,329569751-110418,00.html (Accessed 15 May 2007).

Boylan, M. (ed.) 2004. *Public health policy and ethics.* Dordrecht: Kluwer.

CDC 2006. Emergence of *Mycobacterium tuberculosis* with extensive resistance to second-line drugs—worldwide, 2000-2004, *Morbidity and Mortality Weekly Report* 55(11): 301-5.

Cobelens, F.G. 2007. Tuberculosis risks for health care workers in Africa. Available at: http://www.journals.uchicago.edu/CID/journal/issues/v44n3/41151/41151.text.html - fn1#fn1 *Clinical Infectious Diseases* 44: 324-6.

Cohen, J.C. and Illingworth, P. 2003. The dilemma of intellectual property rights for pharmaceuticals: the tension between ensuring access of the poor to medicines and committing to international agreements. *Developing World Bioethics* 3(1): 27-48.

Cohen, J.C., Illingworth, P., and Schüklenk, U. (eds) 2006. *The power of pills: social, ethical, and legal issues in drug development, marketing and pricing.* London: Pluto.

Coker, R. 2000. Tuberculosis, non-compliance and detention for the public health. *Journal of Medical Ethics* 26: 157-9.

Coker, R. 2003. Asylum and migration working paper 1: migration, public health and compulsory screening for TB and HIV. London: Institute for Public Policy Research.

Coughlin, S.S., Soskolne, C.L., and Goodman, K.W. (eds) 1998. *Case studies in public health ethics.* Washington, DC: American Public Health Association.

Dawson, A. and Verweij, M. (eds) 2007. *Ethics, prevention, and public health.* Oxford: Oxford University Press.

Democracy Now. 2007. Is sickness a crime? Arizona man with TB locked up indefinitely in solitary confinement. Available at: http://www.democracynow.org/article.pl?sid=07/04/06/142246 (Accessed 10 May 2007).

Dye, C., Hosseini, M., and Watt, C. 2007. Did we reach the 2005 targets for tuberculosis control. *Bulletin of the World Health Organization,* 85: 364-9.

Farmer, P. 1999. *Infections and inequalities: the modern plagues.* Berkeley, CA: University of California Press.

Farmer, P. 2003. *Pathologies of power: health, human rights, and the new war on the poor.* Berkeley, CA: University of California Press.

Floyd, K. 2007. Global progress towards the TB control targets (with a special attention to TB/HIV and MDR-TB). Presentation at the Stop TB Symposium, 38th World Conference on Lung Health, 8 November, Cape Town, South Africa.

Francis, L.P., Battin, M.P., Jacobson, J.A., Smith, C.B., and Botkin, J. 2005. How infectious disease got left out—and what this omission might have meant for bioethics. *Bioethics* 19(4): 207-322.

Francis, L.P., Battin, M.P., Botkin, J., Jacobson, J., and Smith, C. 2006. Infectious disease and the ethics of research: the moral significance of communicability. In *Ethics in biomedical research: international perspectives* ed. by Hayry, M., Takala, T., and Herissone-Kelly, P. New York: Rodopi.

Gandy, M. and Zumla, A. 2002. The resurgence of disease: social and historical perspectives on the 'new' tuberculosis. *Social Science and Medicine* 55: 385–96.

Garrett, L. 2007. The challenge of global health. *Foreign Affairs*, January/February 2007. Available at: http://www.foreignaffairs.org/20070101faessay86103/laurie-garrett/the-challenge-of-global-health.html?mode=print (Accessed 20 February 2007).

Gostin, L.O. (ed.) 2002, *Public health law and ethics*. Berkeley, CA: University of California Press.

Harris, A. and Dye C. 2006. Tuberculosis. *Annals of Tropical Medicine and Parasitology* 100(5–6): 415–31.

Harris J. and Holm S. 1995. Is there a duty not to infect others? *British Medical Journal* 311: 1215–17.

Jackson, S., Sleigh, A.C., Wang, G.J., and Liu, X.L. 2006. Poverty and the economic effects of TB in rural China. *International Journal of Tuberculosis and Lung Disease* 10(10): 1104–10.

Kremer, M. and Glennerster, R. 2004. *Strong medicine*. Princeton, NJ: Princeton University Press.

Lienhardt, C., Ogden, J., and Sow, S. 2003. Rethinking the social context of illness: interdisciplinary approaches to tuberculosis control. In *The return of the white plague: global poverty and the 'new' tuberculosis* ed. by Gandy, M., and Zumla, A. London: Verso.

Lurie, P., and Wolfe, S. 1997. Unethical trials of interventions to reduce perinatal transmission of the Human Immunodeficiency Virus in developing countries. *The New England Journal of Medicine* 337: 853–6.

Ly, T., Selgelid, M.J., and Kerridge, I. 2007. Pandemic and public health controls: toward an equitable compensation system. *Journal of Law and Medicine* 15(2): 296–302.

MacIntyre, C.R., Plant, A.J., Yung, A., and Streeton, J.A. 1997. Missed opportunities for prevention of tuberculosis in Victoria, Australia. *International Journal of Tuberculosis and Lung Disease* 1(2): 135–41.

Maloney, S. 2004. National migration health policies: shifting the paradigm from exclusion to inclusion. IOM's International Dialogue on Migration, seminar on health and migration, Geneva, 9–11 June 2004. Available at: http://www.iom.int/en/know/idm/smh_200406.shtml (Accessed 11 May 2007).

Moran, M., Ropars, A.L., Guzman, J., Diaz, J., and Garrison, C. 2005. The new landscape of neglected disease drug development. London: The Wellcome Trust.

MSF, Extensive drug resistant tuberculosis (XDR-TB). 2006. Available at: http://www.accessmed-msf.org/prod/publications.asp?scntid=271020061722542&contenttype=PARA& (Accessed 12 February 2007).

MSF. 2007. No time to wait. Available at: http://doctorswithoutborders.org/news/tuberculosis/tb_statement.cfm (Accessed 10 February 2007).

Pogge, T. 2005. Human rights and global health: a research program. *Metaphilosophy* 36(1/2): 182–209.

Price-Smith, A.T. 2001. *The health of nations: infectious disease, environmental change, and their effects on national security and development*. Cambridge, MA: MIT Press.

Reid, L. 2005. Diminishing returns? Risk and the duty to care in the SARS epidemic. *Bioethics* 19(4): 348–61.

Resnik, D.A. 2004. The distribution of biomedical research resources and international justice. *Developing World Bioethics* 4(1): 42–57.

Sakoane, R. 2007. XDR-TB in South Africa: back to TB sanatoria perhaps? *PLoS Medicine* 4(4): e160.

Schüklenk, U. and Ashcroft, R.E. 2002. Affordable access to essential medication in developing countries: conflicts between ethical and economic imperatives. *Journal of Medicine and Philosophy* 27(2): 179–95.

Selgelid, M.J. 2005. Ethics and infectious disease. *Bioethics* 19(3): 272–89.

Selgelid, M.J. OnlineEarly 2007. Improving global health: counting reasons why. *Developing World Bioethics*. Forthcoming in print, doi:10.1111/j.1471-8847.2007.00185.x.

Selgelid, M.J., Battin, M.P., and Smith, C.B. (eds) 2006. *Ethics and infectious disease*. Oxford: Blackwell.

Singh, J.A., Upshur, R., and Padayatchi, N. 2007. XDR-TB in South Africa: no time for denial or complacency. *PLoS Medicine* 4(1): e50.doi:101371/journal.pmed.0040050.

Singh, V., Jaiswal, A., Porter, J.D.H., Ogden, J.A., Sarin, R., Sharma, P.P., Arora, V.K., and Jain, R.C. 2002. TB control, poverty, and vulnerability in Delhi, India. *Tropical Medicine and International Health* 7: 693–700.

Smith, C.B., Battin, M.P., Jacobson, J.A., Francis, L.P., Botkin, J.R., Asplund, E.P., Domek, G.J., and Hawkins, B. 2004. Are there characteristics of infectious disease that raise special ethical issues? *Developing World Bioethics* 4(1): 1–16.

Sterckx, S. 2004. Patents and access to drugs in developing countries: An ethical analysis. *Developing World Bioethics* 4(1): 58–75.

Tausig, M., Selgelid, M.J., Subedi, S., and Subedi, J. 2006. Taking sociology seriously: A new approach to the bioethical problems of infectious disease. *Sociology of Health and Illness* 28(6): 839–49.

UNAIDS. 2007. *AIDS epidemic update: December 2007*. Available at: www.unaids.org (Accessed 4 March 2008).

University of Toronto Joint Centre for Bioethics, Pandemic Influenza Working Group. 2005. Stand on guard for thee: ethical considerations in preparedness planning for pandemic influenza. Available at: http://www.utoronto.ca/jcb/home/documents/pandemic.pdf (Accessed 15 May 2007).

Verweij, M. 2005. Obligatory precautions against infection. *Bioethics* 19(4): 323–35.

WHO. 2006a. Weekly epidemiological record, September 2006. Available at: http://www.who.int/wer (Accessed 10 February 2007).

WHO. 2006b. *The stop TB strategy*. Geneva, World Health Organization.

WHO. 2007a. Fact sheet no. 104: tuberculosis (revised March 2007). Available at: http://www.who.int/mediacentre/factsheets/fsl04/en/index.html (Accessed 8 December 2008).

WHO. 2007b. *Global tuberculosis control: surveillance, planning, financing*. WHO Report. Geneva, World Health Organization. WHO/HTM/TB/2007.376.

Evaluating a Case Study
Structuring the Essay

In previous sections, you have moved from adopting an ethical theory to weighing and assessing the merits of deeply imbedded cost issues and ethical issues conflicts. The process involves (a) choosing an ethical theory (whose point of view you will adopt), (b) determining your professional practice issues and ethical issues lists, (c) annotating the issues lists by examining how imbedded each issue is to the essential nature of the case at hand, (d) creating a brainstorming list that includes both key thoughts on the subject and arguments for and against the possible courses of action, (e) comparing pivotal premises in those arguments using ethical considerations as part of the decision-making matrix, (f) making a judgment on which course to take (given the conflicts expressed in d and e, (g) presenting your ideas in an essay. The essay is your recommendation to a professional review board about what to do in a specific situation.

This section represents stage (g) in this process. If we continue with the IUD case, your essay might be something like the following.

Sample Essay

Executive Summary. Although my profession would advocate my continuing to distribute IUDs to women in less-developed countries, it is my opinion that to do so would be immoral. Human life is too precious to put anyone at risk for population control. If IUDs are too dangerous to be sold in the United States, then they are too dangerous for women in poor countries as well. People do not give up their right to adequate health protection just because they are poor. For this reason, I am ordering a halt to the distribution of IUDs until such a time that they can be considered safe again. Furthermore, I will step up efforts to distribute alternate forms of birth control (such as the birth control pill) with better packaging that might encourage regular use.

The Introduction. In this case study, I have chosen the point of view of the regional director. This means that I must decide whether to continue distributing IUDs in less-developed countries despite a health hazard to 5 percent of the women who use this form of birth control. I will argue against continuing the distribution based on an argument that examines: (a) the imperatives of my profession, public health; (b) the imperatives of ethics; and (c) the rights of the women involved. I will contend that after examining these issues, the conclusion must be to cease IUD distribution in less-developed countries until IUDs no longer pose a significant problem to women's health.

The Body of the Essay. Develop paragraphs along the lines indicated in the introduction and executive summary.

The Conclusion. Although the dictates of the normal practice of public health would seem to suggest that IUD distribution continue, the ethical imperatives that human life is individually precious and that each woman has a right to safe medical attention over-rule the normal practice of the profession. For these reasons, my office will suspend distribution of IUDs until they no longer pose a health risk to the general population.

Comments on the Sample. The sample provides an essay structure that contains a brief epitome and the essay itself. I often encourage my students to come in with their epitome, key issues, arguments for and against, and brainstorming sheets before writing the essay itself. This way I can get an "inprogress" view of the process of composition.

Obviously, the preceding sample represents the briefest skeleton of an essay proposing a recommendation. The length can vary as can any supporting data (charts, etc.) for your position. Your instructor may ask you to present your outcomes recommendation to the entire class. When this is the assignment, remember that the same principles of any group presentation also apply here including any visual aid that will engage your audience. It is essential to include your audience in your argument as it develops.

Whether it is a written report or a group presentation, the methodology presented here should give you a chance to logically assess and respond to problems that contain moral dimensions.

The following are some general questions that some of my students have raised about writing the essay, that is, the ethical outcomes recommendation.

What if I cannot see the other side? This is a common question from students. They see everything as black or white, true or false, but truth is never advanced by prejudice. It is important as rational humans to take every argument at its face value and to determine what it says, determine the objections to the key premises, determine the strongest form of the thesis, and assess the best arguments *for* and *against* the thesis.

What is the best way to reach my assessment of the best alternative? The basic strategy of the essay is to take the best two arguments that you have selected to support the conflicting alternatives and then to focus on that single premise that seems to be at odds with the other argument. At this point, you must ask yourself, Why would someone believe in either argument 1 or argument 2?" If you do not know, you cannot offer an opinion—yet.

The rational person seeks to inform herself by getting into the skin of each party. You must understand why a thinking person might think in a particular way. If you deprecate either side, you lessen yourself because you decrease your chances to make your best judgment.

The rational individual seeks the truth. You have no need to burden your psyche with illogical beliefs. Therefore, you will go to great lengths to find the truth of the key premises that you wish to examine.

In the your final essay, you will focus on one of the argument's premises and find the following:

A. The demonstrated truth of the conclusion depends on the premises that support it.
B. If those supporting premises are false, then the conclusion is not proven.
C. Since we have assumed that the premises are all necessary to get us to the conclusion, if we refute one premise, we have refuted the conclusion.

What if I place professional practice issues or ethical issues too highly in my assessment of the outcome? The purpose of preparing an imbedded issues analysis is to force you to see that not all ethical issues are central to the problem. Some issues can be solved rather easily. If this is the case, then you should do so. When it is possible to let professional practice issues determine the outcome without sacrificing ethical standards, it is your responsibility to do so. Clearly, some ethical principles cannot be sacrificed no matter what the cost. It is *your* responsibility to determine just what these cases are and just which moral principles are "show stoppers."

Are ethical values the only values an individual should consider? Each person holds a number of personally important values that are a part of his or her worldview. These must be taken into account in real situations. Often they mean that although you cannot perform such and such an act, it is not requisite that the organization forgo doing whatever the professional practice issues dictate in that situation. For example, you may be asked to perform a task on an important religious holy day. Since your religion is important to you, you cannot work on that day, but that does not mean that you will recommend the company abandon the task that another person who does not share your value could perform.

What happens when you confuse professional practice issues and ethical issues? This happens often among managers at all levels. The problem is that one set of issues is neglected or is too quickly considered to be surface imbeddedness. Stop. Go through the method again step-by-step. It may restore your perspective.

Macro and Micro Cases[1]

Macro Case 1. You are a powerful member of the United States Senate. You have decided not to run for reelection and want to leave a piece of legislation on U.S. health care policy that will be the highlight of a distinguished career in public service. You sense that there is an interest in legislation that will set the health care landscape for the next fifty years. You want to mark that terrain.

Your staff has four alternatives before you. The first is universal health care financed by industry (existing voluntary program) with the government creating a pool of last resort that will provide basic coverage for those who cannot afford to purchase health insurance (although the coverage is not as extensive as many privately funded programs). On a scale of 1 to 10, this plan has a cost of 7.5. The second alternative is a universal health care program that is a single payer system similar to the one in Canada. This alternative has a cost of 6. The third option is a patient's bill of rights plan that only refines our present system by fixing annoying glitches that bother us all. This alternative has a cost of 0.5. The final alternative is government-run universal health care similar to the British system. This alternative has a cost of 8.5 (including the creation of basic benefits, which are not as extensive as many privately funded plans as is true for the first alternative).

Your job is to create a policy statement to share with your staff advocating any of these four plans for another plan that you create. Since this is the crowning point of your career, be sure to justify your decision in both practical and ethical terms.

Macro Case 2. You are the chief administrator of a hospital in a major U.S. city. This hospital must review its procedures for accepting charity patients who arrive at the hospital via ambulance. According to accepted professional practice, many hospitals send these patients to the nearest charity hospital designated to receive such patients. That hospital receives special funds to make its charity mission possible. Your hospital receives no such money, yet in the past it has treated any patient whose condition might be worsened by a move to another hospital. You can treat such patients only by charging *all* patients with insurance more.

If you let this practice continue without restraint, the private physicians who use your hospital might leave because various managed care companies that would find your hospital costs too high would not approve a procedure scheduled there.

This is a real problem. You would like to continue your hospital's practice of seeing these charity cases because you know that sending these emergency admissions elsewhere can often mean that they could be harmed medically. (In one study, moving such patients increased mortality by 27 percent.) But you also know that hospitals cannot act in a vacuum. All the good intentions in the world will be of no avail if your hospital closes its doors.

Tomorrow you will address the hospital's governing board. You must prepare an argument that will combine practical and ethical arguments to convince the board to pursue a course of action.

Macro Case 3. You are a powerful adviser to the president of the United States and have been chosen to head a commission on the allocation of transplant organs (and other related policies). Your committee is deadlocked as to which option to choose. The first is to allocate according to need (the sickest person gets the organ). The second option is to allocate according to an ordered pair (desert, need). In the ordered pair formula, people who have abused their bodies will be considered only after others who have not abused their bodies have received their transplants. The third proposal suggests that those who have not agreed to be organ donors (usually by a declaration on their driver's license) should be put at the end of the list.

Your vote is key for the majority. As chairperson, you will write the majority's recommendation. What will you recommend? Why?

Macro Case 4. You are the chief administrator at a major hospital. A famous person has been admitted to your hospital in need of a liver transplant. The average waiting time for a liver in your section of the country is 385 days. This person's name is a "household word." Your board of governors knows that this hospital depends on contributions from famous people who organize various charity drives and events. In fact, this particular person organized a charity auction that raised $12 million for the hospital only two years ago.

You have some discretion in allocating vital organs, especially ones that originate from deaths in the hospital. Allocation according to need is somewhat subjective, and you could put this celebrity at the top of the list above seven others who have been waiting for a liver transplant. All things being equal, the rules say that the celebrity should not receive the liver. But you, as chief administrator can tip the balance. What do you do? Why?

Macro Case 5. You are a public health specialist who has just been appointed to head the President of the United States' task force on public health. Your job is to effectively plan a strategy for countering an anticipated H5N1 influenza pandemic that has shown signs of breaking out in China. Outline what you feel would be an effective strategy to minimize our losses using the tools of public health. Try to minimize the mistakes of the SARS outbreak.

Micro Case 1. You work at a major health insurance company in its public relations department. The president of the United States has proposed legislation for universal health insurance that will severely hurt your company. Your own personal values support universal health insurance. Your company is launching a campaign to sabotage this piece of legislation by promoting half-truths and outright lies about the president's plan. You are to play a major part in this campaign. Your company is asking you to do your best to promote these half-truths and lies to defeat a policy initiative that you believe in. What should you do? Good jobs are not easy to obtain, and this is a well-paying job with numerous benefits. You are confused and decide to list the reasons you should and should not promote the company's campaign. Once you decide, how do you justify your decision?

Micro Case 2. You are a recently graduated physician from a poor rural region of the United States. Where you come from, the region's doctor has no set fee schedule and charges people what they can afford (even if it is barter, such as a chicken or a good car wash). This model of serving everyone and the community feelings that it generated were what made you first want to become a doctor. However, when you did your residency, your work was so outstanding that a prominent clinic that caters to the affluent has offered you a high-paying job. This facility is also on the cutting edge of many new medical techniques. This offer would certainly make your life more comfortable, yet you think about all of those folk from where you came and who inspired you to go into medicine.

When you talk this over with others, however, they think you are crazy even to consider the needs of these rural people. "You should take account of your own needs," they say, "both your financial and intellectual requirements." You hear what they are saying, but you are unsure about what to do. It is time to write a letter to your mother to tell her of your decision and to justify it.

Micro Case 3. You are a woman who works for Mr. Alvarez, who is a very fine boss and one of the kindest people you have ever met. He is a widower with one child. You are happily married with two children. There is no romantic relationship between you and Mr. Alvarez; however, you do consider him to be your closest friend (aside from your husband), and he has helped your career and has given you time off when your children were born and when one of them was severely ill.

Mr. Alvarez's kidneys are failing. He has been on dialysis, but even that is failing him. Nothing short of a kidney transplant will save his life. A coworker distributed a description of the criteria for a prospective donor to everyone in the building. Privately, you decided to be tested to see whether you could be a match for him and found that you could be a match. Now you must decide whether you should offer your kidney to him. To rationally discuss this with your husband, you must list the competing interests at stake and then determine what to do. What will be your choice? Why?

Micro Case 4. You are a nurse at a regional transplant center. In your care are patients who are very ill and awaiting transplant organs. One day you discover that the patient in bed 4 has cheated the system to get ahead on the list. You discovered this information by listening behind a drawn curtain around the bed when the patient had a visitor. The patient was discussing with the visitor how he had "jumped the list."

You are uncertain about what to do. On the one hand, you feel a duty to the other patients awaiting donor organs who have played by the rules. If you follow this line of thinking, you would report the patient's behavior to the hospital's organ allocation review board. The consequences for the patient in bed 4 might be severe. On the other hand, revealing what you heard might be construed as violating the patient's privacy and your oath of confidentiality. Write an essay detailing the issues involved and then recommend a course of action.

Micro Case 5. You are a fieldworker for the World Health Organization (WHO) with a master's degree in public health. You have data that show that an outbreak of tuberculosis in India is not responding to the strongest antibiotics that we have. This concerns you because of the highly contagious nature of this disease. You need to create a strategy for combatting the disease using the tools of public health: quarantine, travel restrictions, and continued research. Create a five-year plan that you will submit to your supervisor at WHO.

Note

1 For more on macro and micro cases see the overview on p. 58.

Further Reading

Chapter 2 Health: The Aim of Medicine

Ereshefsky, M. (2009) Defining "health" and "disease." *Studies in History and Philosophy of Biological and Biomedical Sciences* 40 C: 221–7.

Hamilton, R.P. (2010) The concept of health: beyond normativism and naturalism. *Journal of Evaluation in Clinical Practice* 16: 323–9.

Messer, N. (2011) Toward a theological understanding of health and disease. *Journal of the Society of Christian Ethics* 31: 161–78.

Tengland, P. (2007) A two-dimensional theory of health. *Theoretical Medicine and Bioethics: Philosophy of Medical Research and Practice* 28: 257–84.

Weinstock, D.M. (2011) How should political philosophers think of health? *Journal of Medicine & Philosophy* 36: 424–35.

Chapter 3 Physician, Nurse, and Patient: The Practice of Medicine

A. Paternalism and autonomy

Annas, G.J. (1982) The emerging stowaway: patient's rights in the 1980's. In: B. Gruzalski and C. Nelson (eds), *Value Conflict in Health Care Delivery*. Cambridge, MA: Ballinger; pp. 89–100.

Bassford, H.A. (1982) The justification of medical paternalism. *Social Science and Medicine* 16: 731–9.

Beauchamp, T.L. 1990) The promise of the beneficence model for medical ethics. *Journal of Contemporary Health Law and Policy* 6 (Spring): 145–55.

Berger, J. (2009) Paternalistic assumptions and a purported duty to deceive. *American Journal of Bioethics* 9: 20–1.

Buchanan, D.R. (2008) Autonomy, paternalism, and justice: ethical priorities in public health. *American Journal of Public Health* 98: 15–21.

Childress, J.F. (1982) *Who Should Decide? Paternalism in Health Care*. Oxford: Oxford University Press.

Childress, J.F. and Siegler, M. (1984) Metaphors and models of doctor-patient relationships: their implications for autonomy. *Theoretical Medicine* 5: 17–30.

Medical Ethics, Second Edition. Edited by Michael Boylan.

Coleman, L. (1984) *The Reign of Error*. Boston: Beacon Press.

Dworkin, G. (1988) *The Theory and Practice of Autonomy*. Cambridge: Cambridge University Press.

Hope, T., Springings, D., and Crisp, R. (1993) Not clinically indicated: patients' interests or resource allocations. *British Medical Journal* 306: 379–81.

Jansen, L.A. and Wall, S. (2009) Paternalism and fairness in clinical research. *Bioethics* 23: 172–82.

Kon, A.A. (2007) Silent decisions or veiled paternalism? Physicians are not experts in judging character. *American Journal of Bioethics* 7: 40–2.

Luna, F. (1995) Paternalism and the argument from illiteracy. *Bioethics* 9 (July): 283–90.

Mahowald, M.B. (1980) Against paternalism: a developmental view. *Philosophical Research Archives* 6: 1386.

Pinkus, R. (1996) The evolution of moral reasoning. *Medical Humanities Review* 10 (Fall): 20–44.

Sulmasy, D. (1995) Managed care and the new paternalism. *Journal of Clinical Ethics* 6 (Winter): 324–26.

Wicclair, M.R. (1991) Patient decision-making capacity and risk. *Bioethics* 5 (April): 91–104.

Wulff, H. (1995) The inherent paternalism in clinical practice. *Journal of Medicine and Philosophy* 20: 299–311.

Zomorodi, M. and Foley, B.J. (2009) The nature of advocacy vs. paternalism in nursing: clarifying the 'thin line'. *Journal of Advanced Nursing* 65: 1746–52.

B. Privacy and confidentiality

Appelbaum, P.S., Kapen, G., Walters, B., Lidz, C.W. and Roth, L.H. (1984) Confidentiality: an empirical test of the utilitarian perspective. *Bulletin of the American Academy of Psychiatry Law* 12: 109–16.

Beech, M. (2007) Confidentiality in health care: conflicting legal and ethical issues. *Nursing Standard* 21: 42–6.

Bok, S. (1984) *Secrets: On the Ethics of Concealment and Revelation*. Oxford: Oxford University Press.

Cohen, E.D. (1990) Confidentiality, counseling, and clients who have AIDS. *Journal of Counseling and Development* 68 (Jan/Feb): 282–6.

Curtin, L. (2007) When patient privacy endangers staff. *American Nurse Today* 2: 16–18.

Dewitt, D.E., *et al.* (2009) Patient privacy versus protecting the patient and the health system from harm: a case study. *Medical Journal of Australia* 191: 213–16.

Dowd, S. (1996) Maintaining confidentiality: health care's ongoing dilemma. *Health Care Supervisor* 15: 24–31.

Edgar, A. (1994) Confidentiality and personal integrity. *Nursing Ethics* 1: 86–95.

Farber, N. (1997) Confidentiality and health insurance fraud. *Archives of Internal Medicine* 157: 501–4.

Frawley, K. (1997) Secretary of HHS's recommendations regarding confidentiality of individually identifiable information. *Journal of AHIMA* 68: 14, 16, 18.

Furlong, M. (1996) Reconciling the patient's right to confidentiality with the family's need to know. *Australian and New Zealand Journal of Psychiatry* 30: 614–22.

Glen, S. (1997) Confidentiality: a critique of the traditional view. *Nursing Ethics* 4 (September): 403–6.

Harrington, C. (1998) Disclosure of child sexual abuse. *British Medical Journal* 317: 208–9.

Maclin, R. (1991) HIV-infected psychiatric patients: beyond confidentiality. *Ethics and Behavior* 1: 3–20.

Martin, D.A. (1990) Effects of ethical dilemmas on stress felt by nurses providing care to AIDS patients. *Critical Care Nursing Quarterly* 12: 53–62.

Mitchell, P. (1997) Confidentiality as risk in the electronic age. *Lancet* 349: 1608.

Sobel, R. (2007) The privacy rule that's not. *Hastings Center Report* 37: 40–50.

Sperry, L. and Pies, R. (2010) Writing about clients: ethical considerations and options. *Counseling & Values* 54: 88–102.

C. Informed consent

Capron, A. (1974) Informed consent in catastrophic disease research. *University of Pennsylvania Law Review* 123: 340–438.

Cohen, S. (2011) The Gettier problem of informed consent. *Journal of Medical Ethics: The Journal of the Institute of Medical Ethics* 37: 642–5.

Cowles, J. (1976) *Informed Consent*. New York: Coward, McCann & Geoghegan.

DeVille, K. (1998) Treating a silent stranger. *Healthcare Ethics Committee Forum* 10 (March): 55–70.

Drane, J.F. (1984) Competence to give informed consent: a model for making clinical assessments. *Journal of the American Medical Association* 252: 925–7.

Faden, R.R. and Beauchamp, T.L. (1986) *A History and Theory of Informed Consent*. New York: Oxford University Press.

Flax, R. (1997) Silicone implants: two stories. *Biolaw* 2: 311–30.

Furrow, B.R. (1984) Informed consent: A thorn in medicine's side? An arrow in law's quiver? *Law, Medicine and Health Care* 12 (December): 268–73.

Gaylin, W. and Macklin, R. (eds) (1982) *Who Speaks for the Child: The Problems of Proxy Consent*. New York: Plenum Press.

Geller, G. (1997) Informed consent regarding breast cancer. *Hastings Center Report* 27: 28–33.

Gupta, M. (2011) Improved health or improved decision making? The ethical goals of EBM. *Journal of Evaluation in Clinical Practice* 17: 957–63.

Kihlbom, U. (2008) Autonomy and negatively informed consent. *Journal of Medical Ethics: The Journal of the Institute of Medical Ethics* 34: 146–9.

Kotva, J. (1997) Was this consent informed? *American Journal of Nursing* 97 (May): 23.

Lidz, C.W., Appelbaum, P.S., and Meisel, A. (1988) Two models of implementing informed consent. *Archives of Internal Medicine* 148: 1385–9.

Marwick, C. (1997) Exceptions to informed consent. *Journal of the American Medical Association* 278: 1392–3.

Morrissey, M.M., Hoffmann, A.D., and Thrope, J.C. (1986) *Consent and Confidentiality in the Health Care of Children and Adolescents: A Legal Guide*. New York: Free Press.

Rosoff, A.J. (1981) *Informed Consent: A Guide for Health Care Providers*. Rockville, MD: Aspen.

Stoljar, N. (2011) Informed consent and relational conceptions of autonomy. *Journal of Medicine and Philosophy* 36: 375–84.

Waller, B.N. and Repko, R.A. (2000) Informed consent: good medicine, dangerous side effects. *Cambridge Quarterly of Healthcare Ethics* 17: 66–74.

D. Gender, culture, and race

Baier, Annette C. (1985) *Postures of the Mind: Essays on Mind and Morals*. Minneapolis, MN: University of Minnesota Press.

Blacksher, E. (2008) Healthcare disparities: the salience of social class. *Cambridge Quarterly of Healthcare Ethics* 17: 143–53.

Card, C. (1990) Gender and moral luck. In: O. Flanagan and A. Rorty (eds), *Identity, Character, and Morality: Essays in Moral Psychology*. Cambridge, MA: MIT Press; pp. 199–218.

Collins, P.H. (1991) *Black Feminist Thought: Knowledge, Consciousness, and the Politics of Empowerment*. NY: Routledge, Chapman & Hall, Inc.

Friedman, M. (1987) Beyond caring: the de-moralization of gender. In: M. Hanen and K.Nielsen (eds), *Science, Morality and Feminist Theory*. Calgary: University of Calgary Press; pp. 87–110.

Friedman, M. (1991) The social self and the partiality debates. In: C. Card (ed.), *Feminist Ethics*. Lawrence, KS: University of Kansas Press; pp. 161–79.

Gilligan, C. (1982) *In a Different Voice: Psychological Theory and Women's Development*. Cambridge, MA: Harvard University Press.

Gilligan, C. (1987) Moral orientation and moral development. In: E.F. Kittay and D.T. Meyers (eds), *Women and Moral Theory*. Totowa, NJ: Rowman & Littlefield; pp. 111–28.

Held, V. (1993) *Feminist Morality: Transforming Culture, Society, and Politics*. Chicago: University of Chicago Press.

Held, V. (ed.) (1995) *Justice and Care: Essential Readings in Feminist Ethics*. Boulder, CO: Westview Press.

Holmes, H.B. and Purdy, L.M. (eds) (1992) *Feminist Perspectives in Medical Ethics*. Bloomington, IN: Indiana University Press.

Hunt, L.M. and Megyesu, M.S. (2008) Genes, race and research ethics: who's minding the store? *Journal of Medical Ethics* 34: 495–500.

Jaggar, A. (1983) *Feminist Politics and Human Nature*. Totowa, NJ: Rowman & Allanheld.

Neal, K.C. (2008) Use and misuse of race in biomedical research. *Online Journal of Health Ethics* 5: 1–14.

Noddings, N. (1984) *Caring: A Feminine Approach to Ethics and Moral Education*. Berkeley, CA: University of California Press.

O'Brien, M. (1983) *The Politics of Reproduction*. London: Routledge.

O'Connor, D. (2010) This is what happens when you forget about gender. *American Journal of Bioethics* 10: 27–9.

Rogers, W. and Ballantyne, A. (2008) Gender and trust in medicine: vulnerabilities, abuses, and remedies. *IJFAB: International Journal of Feminist Approaches to Bioethics* 1: 48–66.

Rorty, A. (ed.) (1980) *Explaining Emotions*. Berkeley, CA: University of California Press.

Ruddick, S. (1989) *Moral Thinking Toward a Politics of Peace*. Boston: Beacon Press.

Tannen, D. (1991) *You Just Don't Understand: Women and Men in Conversation*. New York: Ballantine Press.

Thomas, L. (1980) Sexism and racism: some conceptual differences. *Ethics* 90: 239–50.

Thomas, L. (1989) *Living Morally: A Psychology of Moral Character*. Philadelphia: Temple University Press.

Williams, P.J. (1991) *The Alchemy of Race and Rights*. Cambridge, MA: Harvard University Press.

Wolf, S. (1996) *Feminism and Bioethics: Beyond Reproduction*. New York: Oxford University Press, 1996.

Chapter 4 Issues of Life and Death

A. Euthanasia

Angell, M. (1990) Euthanasia. *New England Journal of Medicine* 263: 1348–9.

Annas, G.J. (1991) At law—killing machines. *Hastings Center Report* 21(2): 33–5.

Anonymous (1988) It's over, Debbie. *Journal of the American Medical Association* 259: 272. "It's over, Debbie" [Letters]. *Journal of the American Medical Association* 259: 2094–8.

Begley, A.M. (2008) Guilty but good: defending voluntary active euthanasia from a virtue perspective. *Nursing Ethics* 15: 434–45.

Callahan, D. (1983) On feeding the dying. *Hastings Center Report*. 13(5): 30–2.

Callahan, D. (1987) *Setting Limits: Medical Goals in an Aging Society*. New York: Simon & Schuster.

Callahan, D. (1991) Aid-in-dying: the social dimensions. *Commonweal* 118(14 Suppl.): 476–80.

Dessaur, C.I. and Rutenfrans, C.J. (1988) The present day practice of euthanasia. *Issues in Law and Medicine* 3: 399–405.

Engelhardt, H.T. Jr (1989) Death by free choice: modern variations on an antique theme. In: B.A. Brody (ed.), *Suicide and Euthanasia: Historical and Contemporary Themes*. Philosophy and Medicine, vol. 35. Dordrecht, The Netherlands: Kluwer Academic Publishers; pp. 251–80.

Fairman, R.P. (1992) Withdrawing life-sustaining treatment: lessons from Nancy Cruzan. *Archives of Internal Medicine* 152: 25–7.

Fletcher, J. (1974) Attitudes toward defective newborns. *Hastings Center Studies* 2(1): 21–32.

Fletcher, J. (1975) Abortion, euthanasia, and care of defective newborns. *New England Journal of Medicine* 292: 75–8.

Fletcher, J. (1987/88) The courts and euthanasia. *Law, Medicine and Health Care* 15: 223–30.

Garcia, J.L.A. (2007) Health versus harm: euthanasia and physicians' duties. *Journal of Medicine and Philosophy* 32: 7–24.

Gillet, G. (1988) Euthanasia, letting die and the pause. *Journal of Medical Ethics* 14: 61–8.

Gomez, C. (1991) Consider the Dutch. *Commonweal* 118: 5–8.

Grisez, G. (1990) Should nutrition and hydration be provided to permanently unconscious and other mentally disabled persons? *Linacre Quarterly* 57: 30–43.

Husebo, S. (1998) Is euthanasia a caring thing to do? *Journal of Palliative Care* 4: 111–14.

Jecker, N.S. (1991) Giving death a hand: when the dying and the doctor stand in a special relationship. *Journal of the American Geriatrics Society* 39: 831–5.

Kamisar, Y. (2012) Are the distinctions drawn in the debate about end-of-life decision making 'principled'? If not, how much does it matter? *Journal of Law, Medicine & Ethics* 40: 66–84.

Lynn, J. (1988) The health care professional's role when active euthanasia is sought. *Journal of Palliative Care* 4: 100–2.

Mclachlan, H. (2008) The ethics of killing and letting die: active and passive euthanasia. *Journal of Medical Ethics: The Journal of the Institute of Medical Ethics* 34: 636–8.

Mclachlan, H. (2011) Moral duties and euthanasia: why to kill is not necessarily the same as to let die. *Journal of Medical Ethics: The Journal of the Institute of Medical Ethics* 37: 766–7.

Musgrave, C.F. (1990) Terminal dehydration: to give or not to give intravenous fluids. *Cancer Nursing* 13: 62–6.

Schepens, Ph. (1988) Euthanasia: our own future?" *Issues in Law and Medicine* 3: 371–84.

Thomasma, D.C. (1988) The range of euthanasia. *Bulletin of the American College of Surgeons* 73: 4–13.

B. Abortion

Bolton, M.B. (1979) Responsible women and abortion decisions. In: O. O'Neill and W. Ruddick (eds), *Having Children: Philosophical and Legal Reflections on Personhood*. New York: Oxford University Press; pp. 40–51.

Brody, B. (1974) On the humanity of the foetus. In: R.L. Perkins (ed.) *Abortions: Pro and Con*. Cambridge, MA: Schenkman; pp. 69–90.

Chervenak, F.A. and McCullough, L.B. (2009) An ethically justified practical approach to offering, recommending, performing, and referring for induced abortion and feticide. *American Journal of Obstetrics & Gynecology* 201: 560.e1–6.

Dworkin, R. (1985) *A Matter of Principle*. Cambridge, MA: Harvard University Press.

Dworkin, R. (1993) *Life's Dominion: An Argument about Abortion, Euthanasia, and Individual Freedom*. New York: Knopf.

Englehardt, H.T. Jr (1974) The ontology of abortion. *Ethics* 84: 217–34.

English, J. (1975) Abortion and the concept of a person. *Canadian Journal of Philosophy* 5: 233–43.

Finnis, J.M. (1994) 'Shameless acts' in Colorado: abuse of scholarship in constitutional cases. *Academic Questions* 10 (Fall): 10–41.

Giubilini, A. (2012) Abortion and the argument from potential: what we owe to the ones who might exist. *Journal of Medicine & Philosophy* 37: 49–59.

King, P. (1989) Should Mom be constrained in the best interests of the fetus? *Nova Law Review* Spring; pp. 393–404.

Maltz, E.M. (1992) Abortion, precedent, and the constitution: A comment on Planned Parenthood of Southeastern Pennsylvania v. Casey. *Notre Dame Law Review* 68: 11–32.

Marquis, D. (2008) Abortion and human nature. *Journal of Medical Ethics* 34: 422–6.

McClimans, L. (2010) Elective twin reductions: evidence and ethics. *Bioethics* 24: 295–303.

Noonan, J. (ed.) (1970) *The Morality of Abortion: Legal and Historical Perspectives.* Cambridge, MA: Harvard University Press.

Pojman, L.P. and Beckwith F.J. (1994) *The Abortion Controversy: A Reader.* Boston: Jones & Bartlett.

Tooley, M. (1983) *Abortion and Infanticide.* New York: Oxford University Press.

Tupa, A. (2009) Killing, letting die, and the morality of abortion. *Journal of Applied Philosophy* 26: 1–26.

Warren, M.A. (1984) On the moral and legal status of abortion. *The Monist* 57.1; with "Postscript on infanticide" from Joel Feinburg, (ed.), *The Problem of Abortion*, 2nd edn. Belmont, CA: Wadsworth.

Chapter 5 Genetic Enhancement

Anderson, W.F. (1992) Human gene therapy. *Science* 256: 808–13.

Anderson, W.F. (1998) Human gene therapy. *Nature* 392(Suppl.): 25–30.

Areen, J. (1992) The greatest rewards and the heaviest penalties. *Human Gene Therapy* 3: 277–8.

Boylan, M. and Brown, K.E. (2013) *Genetic Engineering: Ethics and Science on the New Frontier*, 2nd edn. Malden, MA, and Oxford: Wiley-Blackwell.

Brassington, I. (2010) Enhancing evolution and *Enhancing Evolution. Bioethics* 24: 395–402.

Cosset, F-L. and Russell, S.J. (1996) Targeting retrovirus entry. *Human Gene Therapy* 3: 946–56.

Delaney, J.J. (2011) Possible people, complaints, and the distinction between genetic planning and genetic engineering. *Journal of Medical Ethics* 37: 410–14.

Epstein, S.L. (1991) Regulatory concerns in human gene therapy. *Human Gene Therapy* 2: 243–9.

Fisher, K.J., Jooss, K., Alston, J., *et al.* (1997) Recombinant adeno-associated virus for muscle directed gene therapy. *Nature Medicine* 3: 306–12.

Fletcher, J.C. and Anderson, W.F. (1992) Germ-line gene therapy: a new stage of debate. *Law, Medicine & Health Care* 20(Spring/Summer): 26–39.

Fletcher, J.C. and Richter, G. (1996) Human fetal gene therapy: moral and ethical questions. *Human Gene Therapy* 7: 1605–14.

Gunderson, M. (2007) Seeking perfection: a Kantian look at human genetic engineering. *Theoretical Medicine and Bioethics: Philosophy of Medical Research and Practice* 28: 87–102.

Juengst, E.T. (ed.) (1991) Human germ-line engineering—special issue. *Journal of Medicine and Philosophy* 16: 587–694.

Ledley, F.D. (1993) Are contemporary methods for somatic gene therapy suitable for clinical applications? *Clinical and Investigative Medicine* 16: 78–88.

Murphy, T.F. (2012) The ethics of impossible and possible changes to human nature. *Bioethics* 26: 191–7.

Palmer, J.G. (1991) Liability considerations presented by human gene therapy. *Human Gene Therapy* 2: 235–42.

Sandel, M.J. (2010) The case against perfection: ethics in the age of genetic engineering. *The Linacre Quarterly: Journal of the Catholic Medical Association* 77: 115–16.

Tauer, C.A. (1990) Does human gene therapy raise new ethical questions? *Human Gene Therapy* 1: 411–18.

Von Tongeren, P.J.M. (1991) Ethical manipulations: an ethical evaluation of the debate surrounding genetic engineering. *Human Gene Therapy* 2: 71–5.

Walters, L. (1991) Ethical issues in human gene therapy. *Journal of Clinical Ethics* 2: 267–74.

Zohar, N.J. (1991) Prospects for 'genetic therapy'—can a person benefit from being altered? *Bioethics* 5: 275–8.

Chapter 6 Healthcare Policy

A. The right to healthcare

Bayer, R., Caplan, A.L. and Daniels, N. (eds) (1983) *In Search of Equity Health Needs and the Health Care System. The Hastings Center Series in Ethics.* New York: Plenum Press.

Beauchamp, T.L. and Faden, R.R. (1979) The right to health and the right to health care. *Journal of Medicine and Philosophy* 4: 118–31.

Bole, T.J. and Bondeson, W.B. (eds) (1991) *Rights to Health Care.* Philosophy and Medicine Series, vol. 38. Dordrecht, The Netherlands: Kluwer Academic.

Bradley, A. (2010) Positive rights, negative rights and health care. *Journal of Medical Ethics* 36: 838–41.

Brody, B. (1989) The President's Commission: the need to be more philosophical. *Journal of Medicine and Philosophy* 14: 369–83.

Callahan, D. (1990) *What Kind of Life: The Limits of Medical Progress.* New York: Simon & Schuster.

Daniels, N. (1985) *Just Health Care. Studies in Philosophy and Health Policy.* Cambridge: Cambridge University Press.

Dula, A. and Goering, S. (1994) *It Just Ain't Fair: The Ethics of Health Care for African Americans.* Westport, CT: Praeger Publishers.

Engelhardt, H.T. (ed.) (1979) Rights to health care. *Journal of Medicine and Philosophy* 4: 113–215.

Fried, C. (1976) Equality and rights in medical care. *Hastings Center Report* 6: 29–34.

Gruenewald, D.A. (2012) Can health care rationing ever be rational? *Journal of Law, Medicine & Ethics* 40: 17–25.

Jecker, N.S. and Berg, A. (1992) Allocating medical resources in rural America: alternative perceptions of justice. *Social Science and Medicine* 34: 467–74.

Kirby, N. (2010) Access to healthcare services as a human right. *Medicine Law* 294: 487–96.

MacNaughton, G. (2009) Untangling equality and non-discrimination to promote the right to health care for all. *Health & Human Rights: An International Journal* 11: 47–63.

Menzel, P.T. (1990) *Strong Medicine: The Ethical Rationing of Health Care.* New York: Oxford University Press.

Menzel, P.T. (2011) The cultural moral right to a basic minimum of accessible health care. *Kennedy Institute of Ethics Journal* 21: 79–119.

Pan American Health Organization (1990) A human right to health under international law. *Bulletin of the Pan American Health Organization* 24: 624–8.

Porter, S. (1987) Does everyone merit health care? *Ohio Medical Journal* 83: 16–18.

Roemer, R. (1988) The right to health care—gains and gaps. *American Journal of Public Health* 78: 241–7.

Sterba, J.P. (1995) Justice. In: W.T. Reich (ed.), *Encyclopedia of Bioethics*, rev. edn. New York: Simon & Schuster Macmillan; pp. 1308–15.

B. The organ allocation problem

Aaron, H.J. and Schwartz, W.B. (1984) *The Painful Prescription: Rationing Hospital Care.* Washington, DC: Brookings Institution.

Benjamin, M., Cohen, C., and Growchowski, E. (1994) What transplantation can teach us about health care reform. *New England Journal of Medicine* 330: 858–60.

Caplan, A.L. (1992) If I were a rich man could I buy a pancreas? Problems in the policies and criteria used to allocate organs for transplantation in the United States. In: A.L. Caplan (ed.), *If I Were a Rich Man Could I buy a Pancreas? and Other Essays on the Ethics of Health Care*. Bloomington, IN: Indiana University Press; pp. 158–77.

Cherkassky, L. (2011) Does the United States do it better? A comparative analysis of liver allocation protocols in the United Kingdom and the United States. *Cambridge Quarterly of Healthcare Ethics* 20: 418–33.

Childress, J.F. (1995) Policies for allocating organs for transplantation: some reflections. *Biolaw* 11: 29–39.

Daniels, N. (1988) *Am I My Parent's Keeper? An Essay on Justice Between the Young and Old*. Oxford: Oxford University Press.

Evans, R.W. (1993) Organ transplantation and the inevitable debate as to what constitutes a basic health care benefit. In: P. Teresaki and J.M. Cecka (eds), *Clinical Transplants*. Los Angeles, CA: UCLA Typing Laboratory; pp. 359–91.

Fabry, T.L. and Klion, F.M. (1992) *Guide to Liver Transplantation*. New York: Igaku-Shoin, 1992.

Jarvis, R. (1995) Join the club: a modest proposal to increase availability of donor organs. *Journal of Medical Ethics* 21: 199–204.

Kilner, J.F. (1990) *Who Lives? Who Dies? Ethical Criteria in Patient Selection*. New Haven, CT: Yale University Press.

Kubo, S., Ormaza, S.M., Francis, G.S., *et al.* (1993) Trends in patient selection for heart transplantation. *Journal of the American College of Cardiology* 21: 975–81.

Margolis, R.E. (1993) Are transplanted organs being allocated unfairly and illegally? *HealthSpan* 10: 14–17.

Moskowitz, E. (1995) In the courts: livers. *Hastings Center Report* 25: 48.

O'Connell, D.A. (1991) Ethical implications of organ transplantation. *Critical Care Nursing Quarterly* 13(February): 1–7.

Pope, T.M. (2010) Legal briefing: organ donation and allocation. *Journal of Clinical Ethics* 21: 243–63.

Ravelingien, A. and Krom, A. (2005) Earning points for moral behavior: organ allocation based on reciprocity. *International Journal of Applied Philosophy* 19: 75–83.

Rescher, N. (1969) The allocation of exotic medical lifesaving therapy. *Ethics*. 79: 173–86.

Scarantino, A. (2010) Inductive risk and justice in kidney allocation. *Bioethics* 24: 421–30.

Schmidt, V.H. (1998) Selection of recipients for donor organs in transplant medicine. *Journal of Medicine and Philosophy* 23: 50–74.

Swazey, J.P. and Fox, R. (1993) Allocating scarce gifts of life. *Trends in Health Care, Law & Ethics* 8(4): 29–34.

Wilkinson, T.M. (2007) Racist organ donors and saving lives. *Bioethics* 21: 63–74.

C. International public health policy and ethics

Gostin, L.O. (2007) Why rich countries should care about the world's least healthy people. *Journal of the American Medical Association* 298: 89–92.

Mackenbach, J.P. (2007) Public health ethics in times of global environmental change: time to look beyond human interests. *Scandinavian Journal of Public Health* 35: 1–3.

Schuftan, C. (2009) The role of ethics and ideology in our contribution to global health. *Global Health Action* 2: 1–7.

Stewart, K.A., Keusch, G.T., and Kleinman, A. (2010) Values and moral experience in global health: bridging the local and the global. *Global Public Health* 5: 115–21.

Swazo, N.K. (2007) The right to health, international law, and economic justice. *Internet Journal of Law, Healthcare & Ethics* 5; DOI: 10.5580/1c1d.